Diabetes Digital Health

Diabetes Digital Health

Edited by

David C. Klonoff
Mills-Peninsula Medical Center, San Mateo, CA, United States

David Kerr
Sansum Diabetes Research Institute, Santa Barbara, CA, United States

Shelagh A. Mulvaney
Vanderbilt University, Nashville, TN, United States

ELSEVIER

Elsevier
Radarweg 29, PO Box 211, 1000 AE Amsterdam, Netherlands
The Boulevard, Langford Lane, Kidlington, Oxford OX5 1GB, United Kingdom
50 Hampshire Street, 5th Floor, Cambridge, MA 02139, United States

British Library Cataloguing-in-Publication Data
A catalogue record for this book is available from the British Library

Library of Congress Cataloging-in-Publication Data
A catalog record for this book is available from the Library of Congress

ISBN: 978-0-12-817485-2

For Information on all Elsevier publications
visit our website at https://www.elsevier.com/books-and-journals

Publisher: Stacy Masucci
Acquisitions Editor: Stacy Masucci
Editorial Project Manager: Pat Gonzalez
Production Project Manager:
    Sreejith Viswanathan
Cover Designer: Mark Rogers

Typeset by MPS Limited, Chennai, India

Working together
to grow libraries in
developing countries

www.elsevier.com • www.bookaid.org

Contents

List of contributors

Michael D. Abràmoff The Robert C Watzke Professor of Ophthalmology and Visual Sciences at the University of Iowa, Retina Service, UI Hospital Clinics, Iowa City, IA, United States; Founder and Executive Chairman, IDx, Coralville, IA, United States

S. Will Acuff Department of Medicine, Vanderbilt University Medical Center, Nashville, TN, United States

Nancy A. Allen University of Utah College of Nursing, Salt Lake City, UT, United States

David G. Armstrong Department of Surgery, Southwestern Academic Limb Salvage Alliance (SALSA), Keck School of Medicine of University of Southern California, Los Angeles, CA, United States

Eirik Årsand Norwegian Centre for E-health Research, University Hospital of North Norway, Tromsø, Norway; Faculty of Science and Technology, Department of Computer Science, UiT The Arctic University of Norway, Tromsø, Norway

Mariam Askari Netspective Media LLC, Silver Spring, MD, United States

Arielle G. Asman Ferkauf Graduate School of Psychology, Yeshiva University, Bronx, NY, United States

Syed Umer Abdul Aziz Netspective Media LLC, Silver Spring, MD, United States

Samantha A. Barry-Menkhaus University of California, San Francisco, San Francisco, CA, United States

Meghan Bradway Norwegian Centre for E-health Research, University Hospital of North Norway, Tromsø, Norway; Faculty of Health Sciences, Department of Clinical Medicine, UiT The Arctic University of Norway, Tromsø, Norway

Gladys Crespo-Ramos Ferkauf Graduate School of Psychology, Yeshiva University, Bronx, NY, United States

Mohan Deepa Madras Diabetes Research Foundation & Dr. Mohan's Diabetes Specialities Centre, WHO Collaborating Centre for Non-Communicable Diseases Prevention and Control & ICMR Center for Advanced Research on Diabetes, Chennai, India

Daniel J. DeSalvo Department of Pediatrics, Baylor College of Medicine, Texas Children's Hospital, Houston, TX, United States

Cyrus Desouza Division of Diabetes, Endocrinology & Metabolism, Department of Internal Medicine, University of Nebraska Medical Center, Omaha, NE, United States

Andjela Drincic Division of Diabetes, Endocrinology & Metabolism, Department of Internal Medicine, University of Nebraska Medical Center, Omaha, NE, United States

Dominic Ehrmann Research Institute Diabetes Academy Mergentheim (FIDAM), Diabetes Center Mergentheim, Bad Mergentheim, Germany; Department of Clinical Psychology and Psychotherapy, University of Bamberg, Bamberg, Germany

Kathryn L. Fantasia Section of Endocrinology, Diabetes, and Nutrition, Boston University School of Medicine and Boston Medical Center, Boston, MA, United States

Sherecce Fields Department of Psychological and Brain Sciences, Texas A&M University, College Station, TX, United States

Elia Gabarron Norwegian Centre for E-health Research, University Hospital of North Norway, Tromsø, Norway

Jeffrey S. Gonzalez Ferkauf Graduate School of Psychology, Yeshiva University, Bronx, NY, United States; Departments of Medicine (Endocrinology) and Epidemiology and Population Health, Albert Einstein College of Medicine, Bronx, NY, United States; The Fleischer Institute for Diabetes and Metabolism, Albert Einstein College of Medicine, Bronx, NY, United States; The New York Regional Center for Diabetes Translation Research (NY-CDTR), Albert Einstein College of Medicine, Bronx, NY, United States

Michael A. Harris Oregon Health & Science University, Portland, OR, United States; Harold Schnitzer Diabetes Health Center, Portland, OR, United States

Ben Healy IDEO, Chicago, IL, United States; Michener Center for Writers at the University of Texas at Austin, Austin, TX, United States; American Studies, Brown University, Providence, RI, United States

Erin Henkel Industrial Design, California College of the Arts, San Francisco, CA, United States; IDEO, Chicago, IL, United States

Marisa E. Hilliard Department of Pediatrics, Baylor College of Medicine, Texas Children's Hospital, Houston, TX, United States

Claire J. Hoogendoorn Ferkauf Graduate School of Psychology, Yeshiva University, Bronx, NY, United States

Victoria Hsiao University of California, San Francisco, CA, United States

David Kerr Sansum Diabetes Research Institute, Santa Barbara, CA, United States

David C. Klonoff Diabetes Research Institute, Mills-Peninsula Medical Center, San Mateo, CA, United States

Michelle L. Litchman University of Utah College of Nursing, Salt Lake City, UT, United States

Janice MacLeod Clinical Advocacy, Companion Medical, San Diego, CA, United States

William "Brad" Marsh U.S. Army, Washington, DC, United States

William Martinez Department of Medicine, Vanderbilt University Medical Center, Nashville, TN, United States; Center for Health Behavior and Health Education, Vanderbilt University Medical Center, Nashville, TN, United States

Lindsay S. Mayberry Department of Medicine, Vanderbilt University Medical Center, Nashville, TN, United States; Center for Health Behavior and Health Education, Vanderbilt University Medical Center, Nashville, TN, United States; Center for Diabetes Translation Research, Vanderbilt University Medical Center, Nashville, TN, United States; Department of Biomedical Informatics, Vanderbilt University Medical Center, Nashville, TN, United States

Jennifer Merickel Mind & Brain Health Labs, Department of Neurological Sciences, University of Nebraska Medical Center, Omaha, NE, United States

Katherine L. Modzelewski Section of Endocrinology, Diabetes, and Nutrition, Boston University School of Medicine and Boston Medical Center, Boston, MA, United States

Viswanathan Mohan Madras Diabetes Research Foundation & Dr. Mohan's Diabetes Specialities Centre, WHO Collaborating Centre for Non-Communicable Diseases Prevention and Control & ICMR Center for Advanced Research on Diabetes, Chennai, India

Maureen Monaghan Children's National Hospital, Washington, DC, United States

Grant A. Murphy Department of Surgery, Southwestern Academic Limb Salvage Alliance (SALSA), Keck School of Medicine of University of Southern California, Los Angeles, CA, United States

Bijan Najafi Division of Vascular Surgery and Endovascular Therapy, Michael E. DeBakey Department of Surgery, Interdisciplinary Consortium for Advanced Motion Performance (iCAMP), Baylor College of Medicine, Houston, TX, United States

Lyndsay A. Nelson Department of Medicine, Vanderbilt University Medical Center, Nashville, TN, United States; Center for Health Behavior and Health Education, Vanderbilt University Medical Center, Nashville, TN, United States

Yarmela Pavlovic Manatt, Phelps & Phillips, LLP, San Francisco, CA, United States

Jessica Randazza-Pade IDEO, Chicago, IL, United States; Communications Studies, University of Alabama at Birmingham, Birmingham, AL, United States

Matthew Rizzo Mind & Brain Health Labs, Department of Neurological Sciences, University of Nebraska Medical Center, Omaha, NE, United States

Ashutosh Sabharwal Department of Electrical and Computer Engineering, Rice University, Houston, TX, United States

Pablo Salazar McKinsey & Company, New York, NY, United States

Shahid N. Shah Netspective Media LLC, Silver Spring, MD, United States

Muralidharan Shruti Madras Diabetes Research Foundation & Dr. Mohan's Diabetes Specialities Centre, WHO Collaborating Centre for Non-Communicable Diseases Prevention and Control & ICMR Center for Advanced Research on Diabetes, Chennai, India

Adam Somauroo McKinsey & Company, New York, NY, United States

Mary-Catherine Stockman Section of Endocrinology, Diabetes, and Nutrition, Boston University School of Medicine and Boston Medical Center, Boston, MA, United States

Maggie Stoeckel The Children's Program, Portland, OR, United States

Christine Sublett Sublett Consulting, San Mateo, CA, United States

Mark Swerdlow Department of Surgery, Southwestern Academic Limb Salvage Alliance (SALSA), Keck School of Medicine of University of Southern California, Los Angeles, CA, United States

Anthony L. Threatt Health Information Technology, Vanderbilt University Medical Center, Nashville, TN, United States

Sacha Uelmen Diabetes Education and Prevention Programs, Association of Diabetes Care & Education Specialists (ADCES), Arlington County, VA, United States

David V. Wagner Oregon Health & Science University, Portland, OR, United States

Hope Warshaw Hope Warshaw Associates, LLC, Asheville, NC, United States

Elissa R. Weitzman Division of Adolescent/Young Adult Medicine, Boston Children's Hospital (BCH), Boston, MA, United States; Computational Health Informatics Program, Boston Children's Hospital (BCH), Boston, MA, United States; Department of Pediatrics, Harvard Medical School (HMS), Boston, MA, United States

Lauren E. Wisk Division of Adolescent/Young Adult Medicine, Boston Children's Hospital (BCH), Boston, MA, United States; Department of Pediatrics, Harvard Medical School (HMS), Boston, MA, United States; Division of General Internal Medicine & Health Services Research, David Geffen School of Medicine, University of California, Los Angeles (UCLA), Los Angeles, CA, United States

Connie Wong Children's National Hospital, Washington, DC, United States

Preface

Digital health represents the convergence of health care with devices and software such that wearable devices, information technology and electronic communication tools, such as smartphones, come together to support people with diabetes and the practice of medicine. An increasing number of wearable sensors are able to transmit accurate physiologic data to progressively more sophisticated smartphones, which in turn contain increasingly intelligent embedded software to transmit information to the cloud to support diabetes care. Digital health utilizes software applications (apps) to process and deliver information, provide decision support advice, and automatically control systems such as insulin delivery.

Our world is increasingly utilizing data from sensors. Medical sensors are also becoming ubiquitous and their connections with each other, as well as with actuators, smartphones, and the cloud together are known as the Internet of Medical Things (IoMT). The field of digital health and diabetes, as part of the IoMT, has the potential to provide real-time information and advice. This decision support function can assist people with diabetes by promoting healthy behaviors between traditional clinic visits and maximizing personal benefits from prescribed treatments.

Digital health is a rapidly developing area. We believe that the subject has matured sufficiently that the time has come to create a book that explores the current status and future potential for digital health for diabetes in particular. To achieve this goal, we have assembled an international team of expert authors based in the United States, Europe, and India who are at the forefront of digital health for diabetes. We believe that the design, evaluation, and evolution of a thriving ecosystem of digital tools depend on input from a wide variety of stakeholders across industry, academia, clinical care, and law, including patients, families, prescribers, developers, informaticians, investors, and regulators.

Overall best practices in digital health will safely and effectively link wearable physiologic sensors, mobile apps, and wireless mobile communication platforms to achieve meaningful and improved outcomes for people with diabetes. We hope this book will provide useful information for a variety of audiences about current best practices and future trends in digital health for diabetes.

Section 1

Building digital health tools for diabetes

Chapter 1

Reducing the global burden of diabetes using mobile health

Mohan Deepa, Muralidharan Shruti and Viswanathan Mohan
Madras Diabetes Research Foundation & Dr. Mohan's Diabetes Specialities Centre, WHO Collaborating Centre for Non-Communicable Diseases Prevention and Control & ICMR Center for Advanced Research on Diabetes, Chennai, India

Abbreviations

ADA	American Diabetes Association
BCW	Behavior Change Wheel
BMI	body mass index
CVD	cardiovascular disease
D-CLIP	Diabetes Community Lifestyle Improvement Program
DQDPS	Da Qing Diabetes Prevention Study
DPP	Diabetes Prevention Program
DPS	Diabetes Prevention Study
eHealth	electronic health
GSMA	Groupe Spécial Mobile—Global System for Mobile Communications
HbA1c	glycated hemoglobin
HPFS	Health Professionals Follow-Up Study
IDEAS	Integrate, Design, Assess, and Share
IDF	International Diabetes Federation
IDPP	Indian Diabetes Prevention Program
IGT	impaired glucose tolerance
IMB	information−motivation−behavioral skills model
LSM	lifestyle management
mHealth	mobile health
MVPA	moderate and vigorous physical activity
SMS	short message services
T2D	type 2 diabetes
WAT	wearable activity trackers

Diabetes Digital Health. DOI: https://doi.org/10.1016/B978-0-12-817485-2.00001-8

Key points

- Digital health can play an important role in improving the lifestyle behaviors and thereby helps in the prevention and management of type 2 diabetes.
- Current evidence supports the role of mobile health devices as a complementary tool in diabetes-intervention studies.
- Though digital health applications seem promising, there is a need for long-term studies to evaluate their efficacy, sustainability, patient satisfaction, and cost-effectiveness.

Introduction

The marked increase in prevalence rates of type 2 diabetes (T2D) that is now reaching epidemic proportions is one of the major global health challenges today. Once considered a disease of affluence, diabetes is now more prevalent in emerging economies than in the industrialized nations of the world. The rapid rise in diabetes prevalence is due to greater access to unhealthy and high-calorie foods and decreased physical activity coupled with population growth and improved longevity [1]. There are several randomized clinical trials showing that the prevention of diabetes is possible. The challenge is to scale these up at a population level, to reach millions of people. With recent advances in information technology and mobile health (mHealth) or the use of mobile communications for health information and services, prevention of diabetes should become possible even at a population level. This chapter will provide an overview of the prevalence and risk factors of T2D and the role of mHealth in reducing the burden of T2D.

Global prevalence of type 2 diabetes

The number of people with diabetes is increasing due to population growth, improved longevity, urbanization, physical inactivity, unhealthy diets, and the consequent increase in prevalence of obesity. Wild et al. [2] estimated that in 2004, the global prevalence of T2D across all age groups was 2.8%. More recently, these figures have risen sharply and the projection is that it will rise still higher, in the next decade [3]. According to the International Diabetes Federation (IDF) Diabetes Atlas (2017), now 425 million adults aged 20−79 years have diabetes and the number projected for the year 2045 is 629 million people with diabetes [4].

Epidemiology of type 2 diabetes—ethnic and regional differences in the prevalence

China and India have the largest numbers of people with T2D [3]. The highest prevalence rates are in the Pacific Islands and the Middle East. South and

Central America and Africa, although currently having relatively lower numbers, are expected to experience a very rapid increase in prevalence rates [4]. Individuals of certain ethnicities are more prone to develop T2D, for example, South Asians, Pima Indians, Pacific Islanders, and Hispanics [2,5]. Studies have shown that Asian-Indian immigrants have a higher prevalence of T2D compared to the white US population and Europeans [6,7]. There can also be variation between immigrants within a region. In Canada the risk for diabetes was higher among immigrants from South Asia, Latin America, the Caribbean, and sub-Saharan Africa than immigrants from Western Europe and North America [8]. The "South Indian phenotype" suggests that South Asians develop diabetes at younger ages, progressing faster from pre-diabetes to diabetes, when compared to white Caucasians of similar body mass index [9].

Type 2 diabetes—a modifiable pandemic

Economic development in many countries has led to environmental factors that promote obesity and diabetes. These include a marked decrease in physical activity levels along with unhealthy diets rich in carbohydrates (sugars), fat, and excess calories. Additional risk factors include depression, smoking, inadequate sleep, lack of adequate built environment and green areas, and increasing exposure to environmental pollutants, all of which are associated with an increase in T2D. Many of the factors are modifiable, and thus addressing them can lead to prevention of diabetes. Three major modifiable risk factors—physical inactivity, diet, and built environment—are discussed here.

1. *Physical inactivity*: Physical inactivity has been shown to increase the risk of T2D across all ethnicities [10]. The absence of recreational physical activity has not yet become a major risk factor in some developing nations, where the level of occupational physical activity remains high. Recreational physical activity, for instance, is reported to be less than 10% in India [11]. Nevertheless, even in these countries, mechanization and industrialization have resulted in a major decline in physical activity. Studies have shown that sedentary individuals are at a higher risk for T2D compared to individuals leading an active lifestyle [12]. A systematic review reported that achieving the recommended physical activity levels of 150 minutes of moderate aerobic physical activity led to 26% decrease in T2D incidence after adjusting for body weight [13]. A global economic analysis of physical inactivity showed that it costs the world economy, US$67.5 billion per year in health-care costs, in addition to lost productivity [14]. Thus, the need for increasing physical activity is very clear.

2. *Dietary factors*: Nutrition transition has been linked to rapid economic development leading to increased consumption of fast foods, sweetened

beverages, and foods high in calories, and this disproportionately affects people living in urban areas and younger individuals. Traditionally, the staple diet in several parts of the world was unpolished whole grains that were rich in fiber and thus had a low glycemic index and glycemic load. Unfortunately, there has been a shift to the use of refined polished grains owing to the availability of food-processing technologies. This led to a decrease in intake of fiber, fruits, and vegetables and an increase in the intake of polished rice, wheat, and other unhealthy carbohydrates (carbs) in addition to sweetened beverages and unhealthy fats [15].

An increased intake of plant-based diets, low glycemic load, fruits and vegetables, whole grains, and low-fat dairy products has been associated with a lower risk of T2D. The Health Professionals Follow-up Study (HPFS) that looked at the relationship between intakes of dairy products concluded that the risk for T2D was lower with increased dairy intake [16]. Another study showed that replacing soft drinks and sweetened milk beverages with unsweetened tea or coffee can result in a decrease in T2D [17].

3. *Built environment*: The term "built environment" refers to the human-made surroundings that provide the setting for human activity, ranging in scale from buildings and parks or green space to neighborhoods. The built environment influences physical activity of the population and thus their health [18]. A study conducted in Toronto, Canada assessed the impact of neighborhood walkability on diabetes incidence and concluded that, independent of age and income, built environment was a strong predictor of diabetes and people living in low-walkability areas had higher rates of diabetes than those who lived in high-walkability areas [19]. A 10-year follow-up of an urban South Indian study, where individuals in one community were given standard lifestyle advice on increasing physical activity and improving their diet, while the other community increased their physical activity by building a park, showed that this leads to a 277% increase in exercise levels of the residents in the intervention group [20] with a modest 24% increase in diabetes prevalence 10 years later compared to the "Control" community, where there was a 135% increase in diabetes prevalence [21]. Recent recommendations [22–24] emphasize the need to make active transport safe, attractive, affordable, and desirable giving priority to pedestrian paths and nonmotorized transport (e.g., cycle lanes) over motorized transport and ensuring urban design that makes neighborhoods safe and attractive to walk, and with adequate green spaces and parks.

Prevention of type 2 diabetes

Reduction in modifiable risk factors in those with prediabetes can lead to primary prevention of T2D. The Chennai Urban Rural Epidemiology

Study [25] evaluated the contribution of various modifiable risk factors to the partial population attributable risk for T2D in an Asian-Indian population and concluded that physical inactivity and unhealthy diet could explain 51.7% of "preventable" diabetes. Several randomized control trials [26–30] across different population have demonstrated that diabetes prevention is possible (Table 1.1). After 6 years of follow-up in a nonrandomized trial conducted in 260 men with impaired glucose tolerance (IGT) (the Malmo study), the cumulative diabetes prevalence was 10% lower in the intervention group when compared to the control group [30]. The Da Qing IGT and Diabetes study, one of the first few randomized control trials, showed that the risk for diabetes was reduced by 46% in individuals who exercised, over a 6-year period [26]. Further, after 20 years of follow-up in the Da Qing Diabetes Prevention Study (DQDPS) [26], a 43% risk reduction was reported in the intervention group. The Finnish Diabetes Prevention Study (DPS) [29] and the US Diabetes Prevention Program (DPP) [28] both showed that weight loss by diet and exercise reduced incidence of diabetes by 58%. The Indian Diabetes Prevention Program (IDPP) showed that the reduction in risk for diabetes was greater with lifestyle management (28.5%) than with metformin (26.4%) [27]. The Diabetes Community Lifestyle Improvement Program (D-CLIP), a randomized control trial that used a culturally tailored DPP curriculum alongside stepwise addition of metformin (500 mg twice daily), resulted in a relative risk reduction in the incidence of diabetes of 32% [31]. These findings underscore the feasibility of prevention of diabetes by adopting simple lifestyle changes. The next big challenge is how to scale up these activities in order to reach millions of people.

Role of mobile health technology in diabetes prevention

mHealth is an area of electronic health (eHealth) and it is the provision of health services and information via mobile technologies such as mobile phones and personal digital assistants [32]. According to the second global survey on eHealth, the most frequently reported types of mHealth initiatives globally were health call centers/health-care telephone help lines (59%), emergency toll-free telephone services (55%), emergencies (54%), and mobile telemedicine (49%) [32].

According to the Global System for Mobile Communications (GSMA—Groupe Spécial Mobile) intelligence data, there are now over 8.98 billion mobile connections worldwide, which surpasses the current (2019) world population of 7.69 billion as shown by the UN digital analyst estimates [33]. Notably, 66.7% of the world's population is mobile subscribers, making mobile technology the fastest growing man-made technology. Mobile phone technologies include text messaging, video messaging, voice calling, and internet connectivity. Of these, text messaging is the most widely used. In a systematic review of published articles on text messaging, eight out of nine

TABLE 1.1 Summary of "face-to-face" diabetes prevention trials.

Study	Published year	Number of people	Type of intervention	Medications	Targets	Effect of intervention
Da Qing, China [26]	2008	577	Diet, exercise, or both	—	BMI <23 kg/m², healthier diet	Reduction in diabetes incidence per group: 31%
IDPP [27]	2006	531	Diet and exercise metformin; diet, exercise, and metformin	—	Unspecified weight loss, reduced calorie and fat intake, and moderate physical activity	Reduction in diabetes incidence in LSM—28.5%; Metformin Group—26.4%; and LSM + Metformin—28.2%
DPP, United States [28]	2002	3234	Diet, exercise	Metformin	7% of weight loss, low-fat diet, and 150 min exercise/week	Decreased progression to diabetes per group; 58% diet and exercise (71% in people aged >70) >metformin. 3.8 kg weight loss diet + exercise. 1.8 kg weight loss metformin
DPS, Finland [29]	2001	522	Diet, exercise	—	5% of weight loss, decrease fat intake, and increase fiber intake >150 min exercise/week	Reduction in diabetes incidence in intervention group—58% (63% in men and 54% in women) 3.5 kg weight loss after 2 years
Malmo, Sweden [30]	1991	181 (men only)	Diet, exercise	—	Unspecified weight loss	Reduction in diabetes incidence in intervention group 37% 2.0–3.3 kg weight loss

BMI, Body mass index; DPP, Indian Diabetes Prevention Programme; LSM, lifestyle management.

sufficiently powered studies were found to support evidence of the widely accessible, relatively inexpensive tool of text messaging as a tool for health behavior change and these effects exist across age, minority status, and nationality [34]. The use of short message services (SMS) has made an effective contribution to advance behavior change in many prevention programs, including obesity prevention, smoking cessation, and physical activity programs.

Table 1.2 summarizes the studies [35−48] using SMS technology in the prevention or management of T2D. The major advantages of SMS are its relatively low cost, widespread usage, and applicability to every model of mobile phone.

Mobile technologies have narrowed the gap of access to health care in many resource-constrained sectors. mHealth technology is thus cost-effective and enables easy access to millions of individuals [49]. However, different technological barriers have been reported, including user experience and user interface difficulties, suggesting that interventions need to be tailor made. There is also a need for standardized protocols to be adapted to deliver mHealth interventions.

Recent mHealth interventions targeting diabetes include insulin-management applications, automated text messages, health diaries, and virtual health coaching [50]. mHealth offers new channels for delivering and complementing existing interventions that target lifestyle-related risk factors for diabetes and chronic diseases such as physical activity, dietary habits, sedentary time, and sleep. The most commonly used technology in T2D prevention includes wearable activity trackers (WATs) and mobile applications.

Smartphone application and wearable activity tracker

Monitoring physical activity has been made easier with advancements in technology. Initially, pedometers (simple step-counting devices) were used. Later, accelerometers came into the market. They measure physical activity under free-living conditions. With the growing numbers of smartphone users, physical activity trackers and interventions are increasingly being used to promote physical activity. Recent advancements in mHealth include the wearable activity monitors owing to their ability to incorporate effective, behavior change techniques [51]. These devices provide periodic (daily/weekly) feedback via a monitor display, with e-mail or text messages.

A recent systematic review by Shin et al. [52] has combined the prevailing research on WATs, and it provides an excellent summary based on common themes and approaches, by analyzing 463 articles. The six key themes (topics) of WAT research identified by the topic modeling methods were (1) technology focus, (2) patient treatment and medical settings, (3) behavior change, (4) acceptance and adoption (abandonment), (5) self-monitoring data centered, and (6) privacy. The studies on "technology focus" theme mainly

TABLE 1.2 Summary of studies using mHealth and short message service (SMS) technology.

Study	Published year	Country/ region	Study design	Sample size	Age group	Follow-up period	Subject description	Outcomes
Haider et al. [35]	2019	Global	Systematic review and metaanalysis	1710	Mean age: 52.2 ± 3.6 years	Studies with at least 4 weeks follow-up (11 RCTs)	Trials involving participants with Type 1 diabetes mellitus, prediabetes or gestational diabetes, or other forms of telemedicine were excluded. Studies employing bidirectional messaging were excluded	Five studies showed a significant improvement in HbA1c with the intervention. The remaining studies demonstrated a trend to improvement in HbA1c. Metaanalysis on 9 of the 11 randomized controlled trials found an overall reduction in HbA1c of 0.38% (−0.53; −0.23, $P < .001$). Overall result—lifestyle-focused text messaging is effective, with a significant improvement in HbA1c
Lari et al. [36]	2018	Iran	Quasi-experimental study	73	Adults	3 months	SMS group consists of 37 T2D subjects and control group consists of 36 T2D subjects. Eligibility	Improved perceptions of self-efficacy and family support and reduced barriers to physical activity

Study	Year	Country	Design	N	Age	Duration	Inclusion/Exclusion criteria	Findings
Fang and Deng [37]	2018	China	Convenience sample study with randomized group assignment	189	≥ 18 years	12 months	included having no diabetic foot ulcers and duration of diabetes ≥ 1 year; T2D accompanied by renal failure, infection, serious heart failure, respiratory failure, or cerebral infarction that had occurred in the month prior were excluded	among diabetic patients, subsequently increasing their level of physical activity. However, SMS were not effective in improving perceived benefits of physical activity or support of friends for physical activity; Regular smartphone communication had a favorable impact on cardiovascular risk factors in patients with T2D
Pfammatter et al. [38]	2016	India	A prospective, parallel cohort design	1925	≥ 18 years	6 months	Subjects opted to receive text messages as motivation to improve diabetes risk behaviors and increase awareness	Intervention group reported an improvement in diabetes risk behaviors, specifically in fruit, vegetable, and fat consumption

(Continued)

TABLE 1.2 (Continued)

Study	Published year	Country/region	Study design	Sample size	Age group	Follow-up period	Subject description	Outcomes
							about the causes and complications of diabetes	
Peimani et al. [39]	2016	Iran	Three-arm randomized controlled trial	150	Adults	12 weeks	T2D subjects randomized into three groups—tailored SMS, nontailored SMS, and the control group. Exclusion criteria—subjects with renal insufficiency with a creatinine level >1.5 mg/dL, hepatic insufficiency, severe visual impairment due to diabetes complication, or psychiatric diseases	Sending short text messages as a method of education in conjunction with conventional diabetes treatment can improve glycemic control and positively influence other aspects of diabetes self-care

Study	Year	Country	Study design	n	Population	Duration	Inclusion criteria	Findings
Bin Abbas et al. [40]	2015	Saudi Arabia	Nonrandomized experimental trial	100	Adults with a mean age of 41 ± 9.5 years	4 months	Adults with T2D diagnosed for over a year with no complications	HbA1c decreased from 9.9% to 9.5%, a significant increase in patient knowledge
Haddad et al. [41]	2014	Iraq	Feasibility study	42	Adults	29 weeks	Participants were recruited from an outpatient clinic and were in the first year following diagnosis (mean—6 months), regardless of microvascular complications and were treated with diet and antidiabetic drugs	Mean knowledge increased from 8.6 to 9.9, and the mean HbA1c deceased from 9.3% to 8.6%
Arora et al. [42]	2014	United States	Randomized control trial	128	Adults	6 months	Participants with T2D with HbA1c ≥ 8% speak and read English or Spanish and uses text messages on their mobile phones	Intervention (TExT-MED) group showed decrease of 1.05% in HbA1c when compared to the control group (0.60%). Among secondary outcomes the TExT-MED group showed increased medication adherence

(Continued)

TABLE 1.2 (Continued)

Study	Published year	Country/ region	Study design	Sample size	Age group	Follow-up period	Subject description	Outcomes
Wong et al. [43]	2013	China	Pilot single blinded randomized control trial	104	Adults	12 and 24 months	Chinese professional drivers identified with prediabetes within the previous 3 months and if accessible by a mobile phone that could receive Chinese text messages	6% developed T2D in the intervention group compared to 16% in the control group. Number needed to treat was 9.1
Ramachandran et al. [44]	2013	India	Prospective, parallel-group, and randomized controlled trial	537	35–55 years	—	Working men with ownership/ability to read and understand mobile phone messages in English, a positive family history of T2D and BMI ≥ 23 kg/m^2	18% developed T2D in the intervention group compared to 27% in the controls ($P = .015$). Significant changes in HDL level and total energy intake in the intervention group were also observed

Study	Year	Country	Study design	N	Age	Duration	Inclusion criteria	Outcome
Goodarzi et al. [45]	2012	Iran	Randomized control trial	81	>30 years	12 weeks	Self-reported subjects with T2D, glycated hemoglobin (HbA1c) >7% with no complications for more than a year, and owning a mobile phone with ability to handle SMS feature	Significant changes in HbA1c, LDL-C, blood urea nitrogen, microalbumin, knowledge, practice, and self-efficacy when compared to control group
Hussein et al. [46]	2011	Middle East	Feasibility study	34	≥18 years	3 months	Newly diagnosed T2D, HbA1c ≥7.5%, and/or insulin	Significant difference in HbA1c between the groups resulting in a 1.16% decrease in HbA1c compared to the controls
Faridi et al. [47]	2008	United States	Randomized control trial	30	≥18 years	—	Controlled diabetes, BMI >25, HbA1c <8%, no insulin use, and serum creatinine <1.5 mg/dL	Improvement in HbA1c and self-efficacy was reported in comparison to controls

(Continued)

TABLE 1.2 (Continued)

Study	Published year	Country/ region	Study design	Sample size	Age group	Follow- up period	Subject description	Outcomes
Kim and Kim [48]	2008	Korea	Quasi- experimental study	40	Adults	1 year	Individuals with diabetes according to the ADA criteria, BMI >23 kg/m², participants were required to be able to self-monitor blood glucose, self-inject in the case of insulin, and should have owned mobile phone	Mean decrease in HbA1c at all testing points in the intervention group, however, not significantly different from the control group

ADA, American Diabetes Association; HbA1c, glycated hemoglobin; RCT, randomized controlled trial; T2D, type 2 diabetes.

assessed the technological operation of WAT and the quality of data generated in terms of accuracy, validity, and essential features associated with data collection. The authors state that although there is rapid improvement in the development of WAT, studies on the precision of the various devices are still not fully established. The studies under the theme "patient treatment and medical settings" suggest that the use of WAT overcomes barriers of conventional health measurements and allows collection of new types of patient monitoring information. It was also suggested that these data would create new prospects for clinicians, as they need not rely on the information based on patient questionnaires. This offers new promise of incorporating WAT into medical applications in the future. The studies reviewed under the topic theme "behavior change" suggest that WAT enables users to track their health patterns and brings a behavioral change toward self-improvement. It was also discussed that as an interventional tool, WAT may not induce sustainable change without researcher training and technology access. The "acceptance and adoption (abandonment)" research theme suggests that effective design of an all-purpose, worldwide WAT is presently an unreasonable expectation. Instead, variability in design patterns and information models should emerge with preferences of various user groups. The "self-monitoring data centered" theme focused more on WAT for the collection and analysis of personal data than on their technological feature. The studies addressed under the "privacy" theme received least attention and the article emphasizes the need to balance privacy and security issues with the potential benefits to customers, the health-care system, and the health and wellness of society as a whole. This review, however, included only commercially available activity-tracking devices and not all types of digital technologies, applications, and platforms that may provide similar functionalities.

A recent systematic review by Brickwood et al. [53] elucidated the effects of interventions that utilize consumer-based WAT compared with a nonactivity tracker–based control group on physical activity participation in adults. This review defined the consumer-based WAT as an electronic device that monitors physical activity and provides automated real-time feedback and may also include interactive behavior change tools via a smartphone or Web-based platform. Studies that included the use of a consumer-based WAT as either the basis of the intervention or as a component of a multifaceted intervention were included. Studies that included the use of established behavioral change techniques such as group or individual counseling or information sessions, financial incentives, or telephone counseling were classified as multifaceted interventions. Interventions that included tools such as regular emails, text messages, online algorithms, or smartphone apps were classified as wearable-based interventions. Twenty-eight randomized controlled trials were reviewed with respect to daily step count, moderate and vigorous physical activity (MVPA), energy expenditure, and sedentary behavior. Of these 28 studies, 12 reported on step counts, 10 measured

MVPA objectively, 5 on energy expenditure using either Paffenbarger Physical Activity Questionnaire or the International Physical Activity Questionnaire to obtain self-reported physical activity levels, and 8 reported on the changes in sedentary behavior. The metaanalysis concluded that participants who received an intervention, including a consumer-based WAT, demonstrated a significant improvement in daily steps, MVPA, and energy expenditure when compared with control groups. The results hold good both when the consumer-based WAT was utilized as the primary component of an intervention and a part of a broader physical activity intervention in increasing physical activity participation. The results show a significant improvement in all measures of physical activity participation when compared with control groups, even when interventions were separated into wearable-based and multifaceted. However, intervention groups that were multifaceted in nature appeared to have a greater effect on physical activity participation when compared with control groups than those that included just the use of a consumer-based WAT. The review suggests that consumer-based WAT may be complementary to traditional intervention modalities such as group-based education and telephone counseling. They thus have the potential to be included as an effective tool to assist health professionals provide monitoring and support to patients.

There are many reports discussing the efficiency of the recent technologies that have largely focused on healthy populations. The systematic review by Kirk et al. [54] evaluated the efficacy of wearable device interventions in improving physical activity in individuals diagnosed with cardiometabolic chronic disease. The authors reviewed 35 studies and specifically, 9 studies with relevance to cardiovascular disease (CVD), 10 studies pertaining to obesity/metabolic syndrome, and 16 studies related to T2D. Four categories of devices were determined—pedometer, uniaxial accelerometer, triaxial accelerometer, and other (e.g., heart rate monitor). It has been reported that Fitbit wristband was the most commonly used commercial device, and a total of 12 studies have reported the use of updated mobile technology along with the wearable device. Sensitivity analysis revealed that (1) the length of the intervention had no significant impact on steps/day or weight, (2) health coaching (motivational support) did not have any further impact on MVPA or steps/day, and (3) patients with CVD showed a higher increase in steps/day than the participants with T2D or obesity. Overall, this review indicates that wearable technology holds promise in contributing to the increase of physical activity in chronic disease management. It also suggested the use of wearable technology as a means to stimulate the physical activity behavior changes among adults, particularly with CVD and T2D.

Behavioral theory in designing mHealth solutions

Digital health plays a vital role in changing the behavior and increasing adherence to recommended treatments. However, many digital health products provide lack of emphasis on behavioral theory. Klonoff [55] reported on the four theories that were capable of enhancing the performance of digital health tools for diabetes. These include (1) Integrate, Design, Assess, and Share (IDEAS); (2) the Behavior Change Wheel (BCW); (3) the informa-tion—motivation—behavioral skills (IMB) model; and (4) gamification. The IDEAS, a framework and toolkit of strategies to change health behavior, was based on five concepts, including (1) behavioral theory, (2) design thinking, (3) user-centered design, (4) rigorous evaluation, and (5) dissemination. BCW, a method for characterizing and linking behavior frameworks and behavioral change interventions, was based on a wheel-shaped figure with three layers: (1) sources of behavior, (2) intervention functions, and (3) policy categories. In the IMB model the performance of health-promotion behavior is supported by being (1) well informed about the behavior, (2) highly motivated to per-form the behavior, and (3) sufficiently skillful to perform the behavior. Gamification is a process that uses elements of game design, such as competi-tion, rules, points, and rewards, to achieve a goal. Incorporating these theories and greater appreciation of its importance could help achieve the required behavioral changes and increase adherence to therapy.

The way forward

With advances in mHealth technology the use of mHealth tools could play an important role in the prevention and management of T2D in the future. More work is needed to determine the factors that could improve the efficacy of the mHealth-intervention tools. Current evidence supports the role of mHealth devices as a complementary tool in planning diabetes-intervention studies. However, more studies are needed to consider mHealth as a stand-alone intervention tool for diabetes prevention and management. Also, these studies should have robust study designs like randomized controlled trials, with prospective cohort studies, long follow-up period, large sample size, and wider range of age groups. There are several factors that need to be stud-ied while designing the mHealth applications, such as behavioral factors (probably, the most important factor), general and health literacy, racial/eth-nic groups, culture, and socioeconomic status. In addition to personalized or tailor-made content, social support and application of game design elements to motivate participation and engagement of patients are also important fac-tors. Thus mHealth tools need to be tailored to the specific needs of the tar-get population, through the application of behavior theory. Their usage can be improved with more attention provided on maintaining privacy, regula-tion, and security issues.

Conclusion

There is an urgent need to institute T2D prevention, especially in high risk groups. However, currently, there are several challenges to the implementation of prevention programs. These challenges include identifying individuals at risk for T2D and adopting culturally specific and acceptable methods. Although several interventions have proven to be effective, the main challenges are sustainability and scalability of these interventions. The need of the hour, therefore, is to implement cost-effective strategies such as the use of mHealth technology both to identify high risk groups and to provide diabetes prevention strategies.

References

[1] Herman WH. The global agenda for the prevention of type 2 diabetes. Nutr Rev 2017;75 (Suppl. 1):13−18.

[2] Wild S, Roglic G, Green A, Sicree R, King H. Global prevalence of diabetes: estimates for the year 2000 and projections for 2030. Diabetes Care 2004;27(5):1047−53.

[3] Kaiser AB, Zhang N, Der Pluijm WV. Global prevalence of type 2 diabetes over the next ten years (2018−2028). Diabetes 2018;67(Suppl. 1). Available from: https://doi.org/ 10.2337/db18-202-LB.

[4] International Diabetes Federation. IDF diabetes atlas. 8th ed. Brussels, Belgium: International Diabetes Federation; 2017. <https://diabetesatlas.org/resources/2017-atlas.html>.

[5] Bennett PH. Type 2 diabetes among the Pima Indians of Arizona: an epidemic attributable to environmental change. Nutr Rev 1999;57:S51−4.

[6] Shah AD, Vittinghoff E, Kandula NR, Srivastava S, Kanaya AM. Correlates of prediabetes and type II diabetes in US South Asians: findings from the Mediators of Atherosclerosis in South Asians Living in America (MASALA) study. Ann Epidemiol 2015;25(2):77−83.

[7] Unnikrishnan R, Anjana RM, Mohan V. Diabetes in South Asians: is the phenotype different? Diabetes 2014;63(1):53.

[8] Laberge M, Leclerc M. Immigration factors and potentially avoidable hospitalizations in Canada. SSM Popul Health 2018;7:100336.

[9] Sattar N, Gill JM. Type 2 diabetes in migrant south Asians: mechanisms, mitigation, and management. Lancet Diabetes Endocrinol 2015;3(12):1004−16.

[10] Shi L, Shu XO, Li H, Cai H, Liu Q, Zheng W, et al. Physical activity, smoking, and alcohol consumption in association with incidence of type 2 diabetes among middle-aged and elderly Chinese men. PLoS One 2013;8(11):e77919.

[11] Anjana RM, Pradeepa R, Das AK, Deepa M, Bhansali A, Joshi SR, et al. Physical activity and inactivity patterns in India—results from the ICMR-INDIAB study (Phase-1) [ICMR-INDIAB-5]. Int J Behav Nutr Phys Act 2014;11(1):26.

[12] Joseph JJ, Echouffo-Tcheugui JB, Golden SH, Chen H, Jenny NS, Carnethon MR, et al. Physical activity, sedentary behaviors and the incidence of type 2 diabetes mellitus: the Multi-Ethnic Study of Atherosclerosis (MESA). BMJ Open Diabetes Res Care 2016;4(1): e000185.

[13] Wahid A, Manek N, Nichols M, Kelly P, Foster C, Webster P, et al. Quantifying the association between physical activity and cardiovascular disease and diabetes: a systematic review and meta-analysis. J Am Heart Assoc 2016;5(9):e002495.

[14] Ding D, Lawson KD, Kolbe-Alexander TL, Finkelstein EA, Katzmarzyk PT, van Mechelen W, et al. The economic burden of physical inactivity: a global analysis of major non-communicable diseases. Lancet 2016;388(10051):1311−24.

[15] Popkin BM. Nutrition transition and the global diabetes epidemic. Curr Diabetes Rep 2015;15(9):64.

[16] Choi HK, Willett WC, Stampfer MJ, Rimm E, Hu FB. Dairy consumption and risk of type 2 diabetes mellitus in men: a prospective study. Arch Intern Med 2005;165 (9):997−1003.

[17] O'Connor L, Imamura F, Lentjes MA, Khaw KT, Wareham NJ, Forouhi NG. Prospective associations and population impact of sweet beverage intake and type 2 diabetes, and effects of substitutions with alternative beverages. Diabetologia 2015;58(7):1474−83.

[18] Creatore MI, Glazier RH, Moineddin R, Fazli GS, Johns A, Gozdyra P, et al. Association of neighborhood walkability with change in overweight, obesity, and diabetes. JAMA 2016;315:2211−20.

[19] Auchincloss AH, Roux AVD, Mujahid MS, Shen M, Bertoni AG, Carnethon MR. Neighborhood resources for physical activity and healthy foods and incidence of type 2 diabetes mellitus: the Multi-Ethnic study of Atherosclerosis. Arch Intern Med 2009;169 (18):1698−704.

[20] Mohan V, Shanthirani C, Deepa M, Datta M, Williams O, Deepa R. Community empowerment-a successful model for prevention of non-communicable diseases in India—the Chennai Urban Population Study (CUPS-17). J Assoc Physicians India 2006;54:858−62.

[21] Deepa M, Anjana RM, Manjula D, Narayan KV, Mohan V. Convergence of prevalence rates of diabetes and cardiometabolic risk factors in middle and low income groups in urban India: 10-year follow-up of the Chennai Urban Population Study. J Diabetes Sci Technol 2011;5(4):918−27.

[22] Giles-Corti B, Vernez-Moudon A, Reis R, Turrell G, Dannenberg AL, Badland H, et al. City planning and population health: a global challenge. Lancet 2016;388 (10062):2912−24.

[23] Stevenson M, Thompson J, de Sá TH, Ewing R, Mohan D, McClure R, et al. Land use, transport, and population health: estimating the health benefits of compact cities. Lancet 2016;388(10062):2925−35.

[24] Sallis JF, Bull F, Burdett R, Frank LD, Griffiths P, Giles-Corti B, et al. Use of science to guide city planning policy and practice: how to achieve healthy and sustainable future cities. Lancet 2016;388(10062):2936−47.

[25] Anjana RM, Sudha V, Nair DH, Lakshmipriya N, Deepa M, Pradeepa R, et al. Diabetes in Asian Indians—how much is preventable? Ten-year follow-up of the Chennai Urban Rural Epidemiology Study (CURES-142). Diabetes Res Clin Pract 2015;109:253−61.

[26] Li G, Zhang P, Wang J, Gregg EW, Yang W, Gong Q, et al. The long-term effect of lifestyle interventions to prevent diabetes in the China Da Qing Diabetes Prevention Study: a 20-year follow-up study. Lancet 2008;371(9626):1783−9.

[27] Ramachandran A, Snehalatha C, Mary S, Mukesh B, Bhaskar AD, Vijay V, et al. The Indian Diabetes Prevention Programme shows that lifestyle modification and metformin prevent type 2 diabetes in Asian Indian subjects with impaired glucose tolerance (IDPP-1). Diabetologia 2006;49(2):289−97.

[28] Knowler WC, Barrett-Connor E, Fowler SE, Hamman RF, Lachin JM, Walker EA, et al. Reduction in the incidence of type 2 diabetes with lifestyle intervention or metformin. N Engl J Med 2002;346(6):393−403.

[29] Tuomilehto J, Lindström J, Eriksson JG, Valle TT, Hämäläinen H, Ilanne-Parikka P, et al. Prevention of type 2 diabetes mellitus by changes in lifestyle among subjects with impaired glucose tolerance. N Engl J Med 2001;344(18):1343−50.

[30] Eriksson K-F, Lindgärde F. Prevention of type 2 (non-insulin-dependent) diabetes mellitus by diet and physical exercise: the 6-year Malmö feasibility study. Diabetologia 1991;34 (12):891−8.

[31] Weber MB, Ranjani H, Staimez LR, Anjana RM, Ali MK, Narayan KV, et al. The step-wise approach to diabetes prevention: results from the D-CLIP randomized controlled trial. Diabetes Care 2016;39(10):1760−7.

[32] World Health Organization. mHealth: new horizons for health through mobile technolo-gies: second global survey on eHealth. Available from: <http://www.who.int/goe/publica-tions/goe_mHealth_web.pdf>; 2011.

[33] WorldoMeters. U.N. data, GSMA intelligence. <https://www.bankmycell.com/blog/how-many-phones-are-in-the-world>; 2019 [accessed 17.04.19].

[34] Cole-Lewis H, Kershaw T. Text messaging as a tool for behavior change in disease pre-vention and management. Epidemiol Rev 2010;32(1):56−69.

[35] Haider R, Sudini L, Chow CK, Cheung NW. Mobile phone text messaging in improving glycaemic control for patients with type 2 diabetes mellitus: a systematic review and meta-analysis. Diabetes Res Clin Pract 2019;150:27−37.

[36] Lari H, Noroozi A, Tahmasebi R. Impact of short message service (SMS) education based on a health promotion model on the physical activity of patients with type II diabetes. Malays J Med Sci 2018;25(3):67−77.

[37] Fang R, Deng X. Electronic messaging intervention for management of cardiovascular risk factors in type 2 diabetes mellitus: a randomised controlled trial. J Clin Nurs 2018;27 (3−4):612−20.

[38] Pfammatter A, Spring B, Saligram N, Davé R, Gowda A, Blais L, et al. mHealth interven-tion to improve diabetes risk behaviors in India: a prospective, parallel group cohort study. J Med Internet Res 2016;18:e207.

[39] Peimani M, Rambod C, Omidvar M, Larijani B, Ghodssi-Ghassemabadi R, Tootee A, et al. Effectiveness of short message service-based intervention (SMS) on self-care in type 2 diabetes: a feasibility study. Prim Care Diabetes 2016;10(4):251−8.

[40] Bin Abbas B, Al Fares A, Jabbari M, El Dali A, Al Orifi F. Effect of mobile phone short text messages on glycemic control in type 2 diabetes. Int J Endocrinol Metab 2015;13: e18791.

[41] Haddad NS, Istepanian R, Philip N, Khazaal FA, Hamdan TA, Pickles T, et al. A feasibil-ity study of mobile phone text messaging to support education and management of type 2 diabetes in Iraq. Diabetes Technol Ther 2014;16:454−9.

[42] Arora S, Peters AL, Burner E, Lam CN, Menchine M. Trial to examine text message-based mHealth in emergency department patients with diabetes (TexT-MED): a random-ized controlled trial. Ann Emerg Med 2014;63:745−754.e6.

[43] Wong CK, Fung CS, Siu SC, Lo YY, Wong KW, Fong DY, et al. A short message service (SMS) intervention to prevent diabetes in Chinese professional drivers with pre-diabetes: a pilot single-blinded randomized controlled trial. Diabetes Res Clin Pract 2013;102:158−66.

[44] Ramachandran A, Snehalatha C, Ram J, Selvam S, Simon M, Nanditha A, et al. Effectiveness of mobile phone messaging in prevention of type 2 diabetes by lifestyle modification in men in India: a prospective, parallel-group, randomised controlled trial. Lancet Diabetes Endocrinol 2013;1:191−8.

[45] Goodarzi M, Ebrahimzadeh I, Rabi A, Saedipoor B, Jafarabadi MA. Impact of distance education via mobile phone text messaging on knowledge, attitude, practice and self

efficacy of patients with type 2 diabetes mellitus in Iran. J Diabetes Metab Disord 2012;11:10.

[46] Hussein WI, Hasan K, Jaradat AA. Effectiveness of mobile phone short message service on diabetes mellitus management; the SMS-DM study. Diabetes Res Clin Pract 2011;94: e24−6.

[47] Faridi Z, Liberti L, Shuval K, Northrup V, Ali A, Katz DL. Evaluating the impact of mobile telephone technology on type 2 diabetic patients' self-management: the NICHE pilot study. J Eval Clin Pract 2008;14(3):465−9.

[48] Kim SI, Kim HS. Effectiveness of mobile and internet intervention in patients with obese type 2 diabetes. Int J Med Inf 2008;77(6):399−404.

[49] Muralidharan S, Ranjani H, Anjana R, Allender S, Mohan V. Mobile health technology in the prevention and management of type 2 diabetes. Indian J Endocrinol Metab 2017;21 (2):334−40.

[50] Shan R, Sarkar S, Martin SS. Digital health technology and mobile devices for the management of diabetes mellitus: state of the art. Diabetologia 2019;62:877−87.

[51] Lyons EJ, Lewis ZH, Mayrsohn BG, Rowland JL. Behavior change techniques implemented in electronic lifestyle activity monitors: a systematic content analysis. J Med Internet Res 2014;16(8):e192.

[52] Shin G, Jarrahi MH, Fei Y, Karami A, Gafinowitz N, Byun A, et al. Wearable activity trackers, accuracy, adoption, acceptance and health impact: a systematic literature review. J Biomed Inf 2019;93:103153.

[53] Brickwood KJ, Watson G, O'Brien J, Williams AD. Consumer-based wearable activity trackers increase physical activity participation: systematic review and meta-analysis. JMIR Mhealth Uhealth 2019;7:e11819.

[54] Kirk MA, Amiri M, Pirbaglou M, Ritvo P. Wearable technology and physical activity behavior change in adults with chronic cardiometabolic disease: a systematic review and meta-analysis. Am J Health Promot 2019;33:778−91.

[55] Klonoff DC. Behavioral theory: the missing ingredient for digital health tools to change behavior and increase adherence. J Diabetes Sci Technol 2019;13(2):276−81.

Chapter 2

Diabetes education reimagined: educator-led, technology-enabled diabetes population health management services

Sacha Uelmen[1] and Janice MacLeod[2]

[1]*Diabetes Education and Prevention Programs, Association of Diabetes Care & Education Specialists (ADCES), Arlington County, VA, United States,* [2]*Clinical Advocacy, Companion Medical, San Diego, CA, United States*

Abbreviations

ADA	American Diabetes Association
ADCES	Association of Diabetes Care & Education Specialists
CDCES	Certified Diabetes Care & Education Specialist
CPT	current procedures terminology
DSMES	diabetes self-management education and support
FDA	Food and Drug Administration
PGHD	patient-generated health data
RPM	remote patient monitoring
TES	technology enabled self-management

Key points

- Digital health highlights a leadership opportunity for enterprising diabetes care and education specialists to redesign their traditional diabetes education services to incorporate technology-enabled population health management options that can lead the health-care team to efficiently provide better care at lower cost to a growing diabetes population.
- To be of value, evidence-based digital health tools and the resulting patient-generated health data (PGHD) must be integrated into clinical practice, becoming the standard of care and the vehicle for how care is delivered.

Diabetes Digital Health. DOI: https://doi.org/10.1016/B978-0-12-817485-2.00002-X

- Educator-led, technology-enabled diabetes population health management services are diabetes education reimagined.

Overview of digital health in diabetes education—addressing unmet needs

Complex chronic conditions, such as diabetes, require regular follow-up and ongoing therapy adjustments along with extensive self-management. The ubiquitous nature of smartphone technology supporting the delivery of automated, tailored coaching at the right time and place enables individuals to share their data and connect with their care team when needed between scheduled touch points, whether remotely or face-to-face. To be useful, the data must be summarized into actionable information in an interface that allows patients and providers to easily share and act on the insights collaboratively. Ultimately, technology has the potential to enable care teams to deliver individualized, evidence-based care to entire populations cost-effectively.

As the transition to value-based care and payment accelerates, there is an increased demand for diabetes care and education services outside of traditional, "brick-and-mortar" hospital-based diabetes self-management education and support (DSMES) programs. These programs have long been underutilized. Only 5% of Medicare beneficiaries with newly diagnosed diabetes receive DSMES services, and only 6.8% of individuals with type 2 diabetes and private health insurance receive DSMES services within the first year of diagnosis [1]. Low participation is due to multiple factors, including low levels of referrals from physicians to education services, inconvenience in terms of timing and location, and cost concerns, among others.

Health plan case managers, health system population health managers, patient-centered medical home care coordinators, and occupational health coaches, although not specifically trained or experienced in diabetes care, are increasingly expected to deliver diabetes education at the point of care. The increasing complexity of diabetes therapy and the extensive ongoing self-management support necessary for individuals living with diabetes to thrive has led to a growing interest in the potential for digital health to assist health-care teams. Digital health has the potential to support these evolving care models to more effectively manage diabetes populations with the goal of achieving the quadruple aim. This means to improve population health, reduce costs, and enhance the patients' experience with providers [2].

The new role of technology

The Association of Diabetes Care & Education Specialists (ADCES) (formerly known as The American Association of Diabetes Educators [AADE]) has defined the diabetes eHealth ecosystem, illustrated in Fig. 2.1, as the use

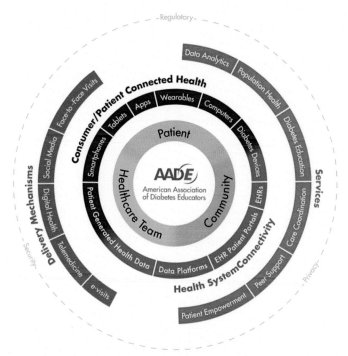

FIGURE 2.1 Diabetes eHealth ecosystem graphic. *American Association of Diabetes Educators (AADE) 2016 Technology Workgroup. Based on Architecture for Integrated Mobility Framework (AIM). Reprinted by permission of the AADE.*

of information and communication technologies for health [3]. Extending well beyond diabetes devices, the eHealth ecosystem includes personal health devices such as physical activity and sleep trackers, smart implantables, smart home assistants, cloud-connected monitoring systems, data management platforms, telehealth services, digital education, mobile apps, digital therapeutics, and social media platforms.

According to the 2019 American Diabetes Association's (ADA) Standards of Medical Care in Diabetes, diabetes technology refers to the hardware, devices, and software that when used appropriately can help people with diabetes "manage blood glucose levels, stave off diabetes complications, reduce the burden of living with diabetes, and improve quality of life" [4]. Recognizing the complexity and rapid change of the diabetes technology landscape, the 2019 Standards of Medical Care in Diabetes devoted a new section to diabetes technology initially with a focus on insulin delivery and glucose monitoring but with plans to expand to include software as a medical device, technology-enabled diabetes education and support, telemedicine, and other issues regarding technology use in diabetes care (Table 2.1).

TABLE 2.1 Multiple technology-enabled solutions for diabetes and prediabetes education and care have been made available in recent years.

Delivery methods	Audience/offerings	Third-party attributes	Accessibility	Metabolic data
• Self-paced • Group based (set or chosen schedule) • Individualized coaching • Automated coaching based on PGHD • Clinical guidance from licensed professional (RN, RDN, CDCES) • Videos • Articles • Interactive tools • Phone/app • Internet	• Prediabetes • Type 1 diabetes • Type 2 diabetes • Peer support community • Analyzed data by report or cloud accessible to the health-care team • Ability for two-way communication between the patient and health-care team	• FDA cleared • Digital therapeutic • ADA recognized DSMES • CDC recognized DPP • ADCES licensed curriculum • DTSec certified	• Open to public • Referral required • Prescription required • Membership required • Integration with individual's local health-care team	• Glucose • Smart insulin pen doses • Insulin pump data • Heart rate • Blood pressure • Labs *Food and fitness trackers* • Food • Sleep • Stress • Notes (ability to track factors affecting daily diabetes care) • Social determinants • Other

Key considerations are described in the table. *ADA*, American Diabetes Association; *ADCES*, Association of Diabetes Care & Education Specialists; *CDCES*, Certified Diabetes Care & Education Specialist; *DSMES*, diabetes self-management education and support; *FDA*, Food and Drug Administration; *PGHD*, patient-generated health data.

While digital health will become a major part of the solution for transforming diabetes care, it is currently a rapidly growing space that is constantly changing. Many diabetes digital health applications provide the ability to track and monitor data of day-to-day cardiometabolic care, including blood glucose, blood pressure, heart rate, weight, food, physical activity, medication usage, dosage, and timing, sleep, symptoms, and mood. However, most offer minimal data analysis, interpretation, or guidance to patients and as such, most are categorized by the Food and Drug Administration (FDA) as general health and wellness apps not requiring regulation [5].

New category of therapy: digital therapeutics

A new category of therapy called "digital therapeutics" has emerged in recent years. Digital therapeutics are defined by the Digital Therapeutics Alliance as solutions that "deliver evidence-based therapeutic interventions to patients that are driven by high-quality software programs to prevent, manage, or treat a medical disorder or disease. They are used independently or in concert with medications, devices, or other therapies to optimize patient care and health outcomes". Five criteria are required to meet the definition of a digital therapeutic. Such an intervention must [6].

1. provide data analysis and feedback that are evidence- and theory-based and tailored to the individual's clinical needs, goals, and lifestyle;
2. connect the individual with their own health-care team;
3. demonstrate safety and efficacy in randomized clinical trials appearing in peer-reviewed publications;
4. ensure the safety and security of the patient-generated health data (PGHD);
5. obtain FDA clearance when used as a medical device and be developed in accordance with appropriate quality standards; and
6. embody user-friendly and engaging design.

The evidence for digital health in diabetes education

According to the evidence from a 2017 systematic review of 25 review studies published since 2013 evaluating technology-enabled DSMES, there were significant reductions in A1C, by as much as -0.8% [7]. This review identified four key elements that were incorporated into the most effective interventions. They included: (1) two-way communication in a continuous feedback loop, (2) analyses of PGHD, (3) tailored education, and (4) individualized feedback. The authors referred to this as a technology-enabled self-management feedback loop (Fig. 2.2). This loop connects people with their health-care providers. The authors also suggested that these factors be

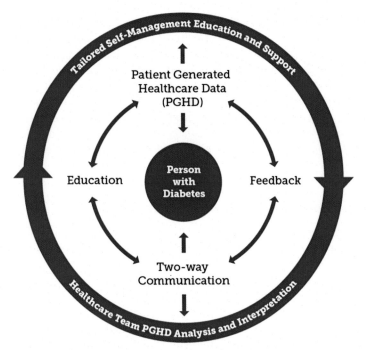

FIGURE 2.2   TES feedback loop. *TES*, Technology-enabled self-management. *Adapted from Greenwood DA, Gee PM, Fatkin KJ, Peeples M. A systematic review of reviews evaluating technology-enabled diabetes self-management education and support. J Diabetes Sci Technol 2017;11(5):1015—27 [7].*

considered when designing studies investigating the effectiveness of technology-enabled diabetes education initiatives.

A 2018 randomized clinical study of 359 African American participants with type 2 diabetes included a telemedicine intervention specifically designed to address clinical inertia in chronic disease management. In spite of nurse-led efforts leveraging technology to minimize barriers to treatment intensification and to provide self-management education, at least 67% of encounters resulted in inappropriate nonintensification of treatments when treatment changes were indicated. Researchers speculate that health system design lacking decision support, visit planning, and outreach systems contributed to these results. The authors also speculated that a lack of practice-based planning, care coordination, and integration of analyzed, actionable PGHD into the workflow contributed to the study findings [8].

An earlier systematic review showed that randomized clinical trials with telehealth remote patient monitoring (RPM) interventions incorporating structured blood glucose monitoring and access to actionable, real-time PGHD for patients with diabetes, compared to basic care that did not incorporate PGHD in the interactions, resulted in greater A1C improvements [9].

In a telehealth RPM intervention compared to usual care in adults with type 2 diabetes, a statistically significant improvement in A1C was found [10]. This trial provided subjects with an intervention consisting of remote monitoring and instructions on a structured self-monitoring of blood glucose approach. The structured approach included "checking in pairs" that empowered participants to perform daily experiments to learn how their blood glucose responded to changes in eating and activity. Nurses in the study had access to the blood glucose data and were able to reach out to participants using a shared decision-making approach to discuss medication changes with patients in response to their data. Thirty percent of participants required medication changes. In a 1-year randomized controlled trial providing a behavioral mobile coach application for metabolic and lifestyle self-management combined with analyzed PGHD integrated with evidence-based guidelines for the care team for subjects with type 2 diabetes, there was an overall reduction in A1C of 1.9% compared to 0.7% in the control group. The initial A1C concentrations in the two groups were control group 9.1% and intervention group 9.9% [11].

Focus on the patient

With technology-enabled diabetes solutions, the new focal point becomes the person as the collector of data. Instead of traditional, episodic, and time-bound care, the PGHD drives tailored ongoing guidance, education, and support. This timely "nudge" reaches the individual at a teachable moment, at the point of decision in their daily lives—helping them build problem-solving skills [12]. Traditionally, the educator facilitates a scheduled session with patients, often in a data vacuum, but digital health offers the opportunity to reimagine diabetes education. Digital tools can prompt the patient to reach out to the health-care team when data patterns needing attention are identified, and the educator or other members of the care team are able to engage the individual with a focused conversation that supports problem-solving skills for that event. The learning and care plan adjustments are individualized to that person and presented contextually. This approach builds self-management skills and fosters collaboration between the patient and their care team.

> As the research indicates, to be of value, evidence-based digital health tools and the resulting PGHD must be integrated into clinical practice, becoming the standard of care and the vehicle for how care is delivered.

Because of the growing evidence that digital health interventions can improve A1C and other diabetes-related outcomes, both the 2017 National

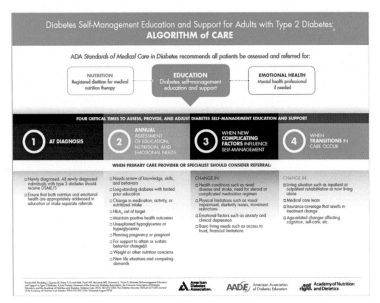

FIGURE 2.3   Critical times to refer to DSMES [15]. *DSMES*, Diabetes self-management education and support.

Standards for DSMES [13] and the 2019 ADA Standards of Medical Care in Diabetes [14] encourage inclusion of technology-enabled solutions to deliver diabetes care and education. Technology-enabled solutions may help to assure timely access to DSMES [15] (Fig. 2.3).

The power and potential of patient-generated health data/remote patient monitoring

Traditional care requires in-person visits with patients bringing their data to their care team in logbooks or stored in meters. In contrast, however, apps or digital solutions can collect and transmit manually tracked PGHD or data from connected devices such as insulin pumps, smart insulin pens, blood pressure cuffs, heart rate monitors, continuous glucose monitors, activity trackers, sleep monitors, and weight scales.

PGHD has been key in diabetes self-management and the optimization of diabetes treatment plans since the introduction of the blood glucose meter in the early 1970s. Diabetes care and education specialist have led the efforts to inform self-management decisions based on this data and are well positioned to bring this expertise to bear with the broader array of PGHD, which is now available to facilitate more effective self-management in multiple chronic conditions [16]. The full potential of PGHD is realized only when (1) the data is analyzed, (2) actionable insights are gleaned from the data, and (3) these insights are presented to both patients and their care teams. These insights can and should be used in shared decision-making with the patient to inform collaborative treatment decisions that strengthen the patient-provider relationship and increase the likelihood of patient buy-in. Timely, better informed, mutually agreed-upon optimization of the care plan has the potential to lead to improved outcomes with patients more likely to have the ability and willingness to manage their health and act on their care teams' recommendations. The new domain of PGHD can be integrated into clinical data for continuous health monitoring and personalized treatment decisions to support a person-centered, rather than a disease-centered approach.

As the use of technology in health care grows, payment models for virtually delivered diabetes health services will evolve. Medicare now incentivizes remote patient care within its merit-based incentive payment. This program recognizes the use of digital tools to monitor PGHD with clinically validated tools that include an active feedback loop providing actionable information to patients and their care teams [17].

Starting in 2018, Medicare "unbundled" an existing Part B current procedures terminology (CPT) code, 99091 into three new CPT codes: 99453, 99454, and 99457. These pay separately for RPM done by qualified providers including physicians, nurse practitioners, physician assistants, and clinical nurse specialists. Providers can be paid for a cumulative time of 30 min/month (12 months/year) to 1) review biometric data that the patient and/or caregiver digitally transmits and 2) communicate the findings and care plan recommendations to the patient and/or caregiver. Additional new care coordination and remote monitoring codes introduced in 2019 and 2020 further expand payment to support staff to allow reimbursement for initial set up and ongoing coordination of data collection each month. These new codes reflect the growing potential of using connected health tools to better support health-care teams in population health services, including using technology to connect with patients at home and gather data for care management and coordination [18].

Social media

Social media platforms provide an avenue for people to share information about their health with family and friends in a nonregulated, unmonitored way. Collectively, this data has the potential to provide new sources of understanding about an individual's health outside of the traditional health-care environment [19]. In contrast to data collected only during in-person clinic visits, PGHD presents a more accurate and holistic view into a person's health and quality of life. PGHD also provides an opportunity to gain deeper insights enabling quicker responses to identified health issues.

Research reports that nonmedical factors, including social, behavioral and environmental determinants of health, consistently play a substantially larger role than medical factors in health outcomes. Collecting and analyzing PGHD from patients with burdensome, high-cost conditions such as diabetes can provide insight into these nonmedical factors [20].

Transforming role of diabetes care and education specialists

Diabetes Care & Education Specialists are well positioned to lead in leveraging evidence-based digital health solutions to increase access and effectiveness of diabetes care and education services. The diabetes care and education specialist can provide expert consultation to lead health-care transformation in evolving care payment models such as integrated delivery systems, population health programs, patient-centered medical homes, and accountable care organizations. The enterprising diabetes care and education specialists can mentor and lead other members of the health-care team in the use of the ever-expanding PGHD with the goal to connect individuals with their care teams to optimize diabetes self-management and treatment. Diabetes educators are already trained to provide person-centered care, including empowering individuals in building diabetes self-management and problem-solving skills [21].

While the diabetes care & education specialist has been the distribution channel for placing evidence-based technology tools into the hand of their patients to ensure optimal use, preparing diabetes care and education specialists to navigate and lead within the continuously evolving digital health and payment landscape will be critical. Training is needed on how to integrate evidence-based technology tools into practice, including how to use expanded PGHD to optimize individual care plans. It will be necessary to leverage aggregated population-level data to assess the overall health status of a population, supporting quality improvement and population health initiatives. Technology-enabled care enables the shift to data-driven versus time-bound episodic encounters. Educators will need to expand and develop new skills to provide remote (virtual) care and learn how to effectively leverage RPM codes in their practice setting [22]. ADCES's multiyear Project Vision initiative seeks to optimize outcomes through the integration of diabetes technology, clinical management, education, prevention, and support. As technology continues to become the vehicle of care, the ADCES is working to expand the skillset of its membership to meet the needs of people with diabetes and prepare diabetes care and education specialists to be the technology experts, data interpreters, trainers, and consultants for all areas of diabetes-related technology.

Recognizing the needs of its membership, in 2018 the ADCES launched DANA [23]. Danatech is a hub for diabetes care and education specialists and other health-care providers, as well as industry to come together to learn about the latest devices, medications, mobile apps, and technology-focused research so they can serve patients and caregivers more effectively.

DANA includes resources in four functional areas targeted at a professional health-care audience: device training, resource library, education, and evolving and emerging technology.

Conclusion

Technology is rapidly transforming health care. Opportunities are here for health-care teams to leverage these tools to improve diabetes outcomes for their diabetes population. Diabetes care and education specialists, with their extensive experience in the practical use of PGHD, person-centered diabetes care, and self-management training, are uniquely positioned to lead in integrating their services enabled by evidence-based technology tools into clinical practice. Technology-enabled diabetes population health management services led by a diabetes care and education specialist are diabetes education reimagined.

References

[1] Chrvala CA, Sherr D, Lipman RD. Diabetes self-management education for adults with type 2 diabetes mellitus: A systematic review of the effect on glycemic control. Patient Educ Counseling 2016;99(6):926–43.

[2] Kavookjian J. New vision for the specialty focuses on achieving the quadruple aim. American Association of Diabetes Educators; 2019 [updated March 12, 2019. Available from: <https://www.diabeteseducator.org/news/aade-blog/aade-blog-details/aade/2019/03/12/new-vision-for-the-specialty-focuses-on-achieving-the-quadruple-aim>.

[3] Peeples M, Greenwood D, Gee PM. Technology-enabled diabetes self-management education & support. p. 1.

[4] American Diabetes Association. 7. Diabetes technology: standards of medical care in diabetes—2019. Diabetes Care 2019;42(Suppl. 1):S71–80.

[5] Health C for D and R. Guidances with digital health content. FDA [Internet]. 2019 [cited 2019 Jun 28]. Available from: <http://www.fda.gov/medical-devices/digital-health/guidances-digital-health-content>.

[6] McKinsey. Digital therapeutics: preparing for takeoff. McKinsey [Internet] [cited 2018 Oct 20]. Available from: <https://www.mckinsey.com/industries/pharmaceuticals-and-medical-products/our-insights/digital-therapeutics-preparing-for-takeoff>.

[7] Greenwood DA, Gee PM, Fatkin KJ, Peeples M. A systematic review of reviews evaluating technology-enabled diabetes self-management education and support. J Diabetes Sci Technol 2017;11(5):1015–27.

[8] Barton AB, Okorodudu DE, Bosworth HB, Crowley MJ. Clinical inertia in a randomized trial of telemedicine-based chronic disease management: lessons learned. Telemed J E Health 2018;24(10):742–8.

[9] Greenwood DA, Young HM, Quinn CC. Telehealth remote monitoring systematic review: structured self-monitoring of blood glucose and impact on A1C. J Diabetes Sci Technol 2014;8(2):378–89.

[10] Greenwood DA, Blozis SA, Young HM, Nesbitt TS, Quinn CC. Overcoming clinical inertia: a randomized clinical trial of a telehealth remote monitoring intervention using paired glucose testing in adults with type 2 diabetes. J Med Internet Res 2015;17(7):e178.

[11] Quinn CC, Shardell MD, Terrin ML, Barr EA, Ballew SH, Gruber-Baldini AL. Cluster-randomized trial of a mobile phone personalized behavioral intervention for blood glucose control. Diabetes Care 2011;34(9):1934−42.

[12] The growing value of digital health [Internet] [cited 2018 Oct 20]. Available from: <https://www.iqvia.com/institute/reports/the-growing-value-of-digital-health>.

[13] Beck J, Greenwood DA, Blanton L, Bollinger ST, Butcher MK, Condon JE, et al. National standards for diabetes self-management education and support. Diabetes Care 2017; 2017 Jul 27;dci170025.

[14] American Diabetes Association. 5. Lifestyle management: standards of medical care in diabetes-2019. Diabetes Care 2019;42(Suppl. 1):S46−60.

[15] Powers MA, Bardsley J, Cypress M, Duker P, Funnell MM, Fischl AH, et al. Diabetes self-management education and support in type 2 diabetes: a joint position statement of the American Diabetes Association, the American Association of Diabetes Educators, and the Academy of Nutrition and Dietetics. Diabetes Care 2015;38(7):1372−82.

[16] Peeples M. Patient-generated health data: an overview and the opportunity for diabetes educators. Cut Edge Newsl Am Dietetic Association's Diabetes Care Educ Pract Group 2016;37(6):13−17.

[17] Improvement activities requirements − QPP [Internet] [cited 2019 May 9]. Available from: <https://qpp.cms.gov/mips/improvement-activities>.

[18] American Medical Association. AMA releases 2019 CPT code set [Internet]. American Medical Association [cited 2019 May 9]. Available from: <https://www.ama-assn.org/press-center/press-releases/ama-releases-2019-cpt-code-set>.

[19] Iyengar V, Wolf A, Brown A, Close K. Challenges in diabetes care: can digital health help address them? Clin Diabetes 2016;34(3):133−41.

[20] Taylor LA, Tan AX, Coyle CE, Ndumele C, Rogan E, Canavan M, et al. Leveraging the social determinants of health: what works? PLoS One 2016;11(8):e0160217.

[21] MacLeod J, Peeples M. Are you ready to be an eEducator? AADE Pract 2017;5(5):30−5.

[22] Nochomovitz M, Sharma R. Is it time for a new medical specialty?: The medical virtualist. JAMA 2018;319(5):437−8.

[23] AADE Technologies. DANA [Internet] [cited 2018 Oct 20]. Available from: <https://www.danatech.org/>.

Chapter 3

Digital technologies to support behavior change: challenges and opportunities

Ashutosh Sabharwal[1], Sherecce Fields[2], Marisa E. Hilliard[3] and Daniel J. DeSalvo[3]

[1]Department of Electrical and Computer Engineering, Rice University, Houston, TX, United States, [2]Department of Psychological and Brain Sciences, Texas A&M University, College Station, TX, United States, [3]Department of Pediatrics, Baylor College of Medicine, Texas Children's Hospital, Houston, TX, United States

Abbreviations

AID automated insulin delivery
BFST-D behavioral family systems therapy for diabetes
CDM continuous diet monitor
CGM continuous glucose monitor
CoYoT1 Colorado young adults with type 1 diabetes
CST coping skills training
HbA1c hemoglobin A1C
HBM health belief model
IDEAS integrate, design, assess, and share framework
SCT social cognitive theory
SDT self-determination theory
T1D type 1 diabetes
T2D type 2 diabetes
TPB theory of planned behavior
TTM transtheoretical model

Key points

- Behavior plays a key role in the optimal self-management of diabetes, but continues to remain a very challenging aspect on a day-to-day basis.
- Quantification of important behaviors and understanding of context for those behaviors are crucial for the development of effective interventions.

Diabetes Digital Health. DOI: https://doi.org/10.1016/B978-0-12-817485-2.00003-1

● From a digital health perspective, findings from recent research have the potential to be the foundation for significant breakthroughs for personalized interventions that could be scaled in a cost-effective manner.

Introduction

Engagement in health behaviors has a significant impact on both short and long-term health outcomes in diabetes. Daily self-management behaviors, for example, choosing healthy foods and undertaking physical activity, require careful planning, because each decision can have a significant impact on daily health outcomes. Everyday challenges accumulate and can impact long-term glycemic outcomes. Therefore, in the presence of a high hemoglobin A1C (HbA1c) value, an important task is to determine which self-management behaviors might be changed to achieve lower values. Furthermore, given the many factors contributing to glycemic outcomes—including but not limited to engagement in complex health behaviors—this can be extremely difficult and can contribute to diabetes distress.

Successful diabetes management is a significant challenge, and approximately two out of three people with diabetes have suboptimal glycemic control. In search of methods to ease the burden of diabetes management and improve glycemic outcomes, researchers continue to explore the potential value of technology.

When considering health behavior change efforts, an important first step is to identify factors that influence one's ability to engage in health behaviors that are amenable to change. A large body of research has focused on behavior change strategies to increase adherence to diabetes management requirements, including blood glucose monitoring, insulin administration, and physical activity. The pediatric self-management model [1] provides a framework for considering the degree to which different influences on self-management behaviors have the potential to be modified through behavioral or clinical interventions. For example, individual influences on engagement in health behaviors can include a person's cognitive abilities (nonmodifiable) and one's knowledge or beliefs about their condition (modifiable). Family/personal network influences on engagement in health behaviors can include household income (nonmodifiable) and involvement/support of family members around one's disease management (modifiable). While this model focuses on pediatric health behaviors, the concepts clearly apply across the lifespan.

Technology-based approaches to behavior change intervention may have particular promise for some of these modifiable influences. For example, technology tools, that track physical activity, share the data with one's friend network, and provide encouraging feedback can target modifiable individual and interpersonal influences, including motivation, confidence, and social support. Electronic medication containers can date-stamp and time-stamp openings. These types of containers can provide the foundation for behavioral interventions to support medication adherence by providing data that can increase individual awareness of behavior patterns or guide goal-setting and problem-solving to target barriers to taking medications.

In this chapter, we focus on the design of technologies for behavior change, through both the lens of behavioral theory and practice as well as the lens of technology. We find ourselves in a territory where there are more gaps than effective solutions for technology-based behavior change. Given the state of the field, major advances in diabetes care will require close collaborations between behavioral scientists, practitioners and clinical, and engineering researchers. This chapter will review and discuss research on technology-based strategies and tools to target the modifiable influences on health behavior in order to support behavior change and promote optimal diabetes outcomes, as well as potential avenues for joint research.

Behavioral theories

Human behavior refers to physical and emotional activities. A behavior can be described as *what* happened *when* and *why*. For example, a person can make a dietary choice (*what*) at 8:30 p.m. (*when*) because they are at a restaurant with their friends (*why*). In the context of diabetes, many daily behaviors are of importance, and thus, like any chronic health problem, we also need to understand *how* the behaviors impact health.

To reach a large population in a cost-effective way, electronic health (eHealth; health-care services provided electronically via the Internet) and mobile health (mHealth; a general term for the use of mobile phones and other wireless technology in medical care) will play an important role; however, research about the effectiveness of eHealth/mHealth interventions is mixed [2]. Although theoretically informed interventions and programs tend to be more effective in changing health behavior, most web- and app-based programs are not grounded in behavioral theory [3]. To solve this problem the IDEAS (integrate, design, assess, and share) framework was proposed to guide the development and evaluation of mobile health behavior change interventions [4]. Of its 10 phases, grounding mobile interventions in behavioral theory is a primary focus [3].

Behavioral theories aim to understand why individuals engage (or do not engage) in health behaviors, such as screenings and medication adherence. There are five common theories that have potential implications for technology-based behavior change: *self-determination theory* (SDT) [5], *social cognitive theory* (SCT) [6], the *health belief model* (HBM) [7], the *theory of planned behavior* [8], and the *transtheoretical model* (also referred to as the stages of change model) [9].

A taxonomy of behavior-change techniques argues that there are similarities in many theories, and multiple theories can ground many techniques.

TABLE 3.1 Behavior change techniques as related to health behavior theories.

Behavior change technique	Technology examples	SDT	SCT	HBM	TPB	TTM
Reward and threat (includes providing incentives, identification of future negative outcomes, identification of positive outcomes, and identification of discrepancies between current behaviors and goals)	• Notifications when in "danger zones" (aka just-in-time interventions)			X		X
Feedback and monitoring (includes observings or recording behaviors, feedback on behavior and outcomes of behavior, self-monitoring of behavior and behavioral outcomes, and receiving biofeedback)	• App and text message reminders • Sensor-based tracking • App-based diaries			X		X
Scheduled consequences (includes rewarding completion of a task, rewarding alternative behaviors, and removing punishment)	• Gamification/points for engaging in health behaviors			X		X
Goals and planning (includes setting target goals, action planning, and problem solving)	• Goal trackers	X	X		X	
Social support (includes encouraging target behaviors, receiving practical help from friends, relatives, or staff, and receiving emotional support)	• Social networking via online forums or apps	X			X	
Comparison of behavior (includes providing examples of the performance of behavior, allowing comparison between individual performance and the example, and providing information about what others think about the behavior)	• Sharing health behavior tracking with friends via apps		X		X	
Self-belief (includes providing evidence that the person is capable of performing the behavior, practicing imagining	• Summaries of health behavior with encouraging messages via tracking apps	X	X		X	

BCT category and definition	Technique example		
performance of the behavior, focusing on past success, and promoting positive self-talk)			
Shaping knowledge (includes providing advice or agreement on how to perform a behavior, information about situations or events that lead to the behavior, and providing alternative explanations for behavior)	• App-based accessible information and tips	X	
Regulation (includes advising on ways of reducing negative emotions, minimizing demands on mental resources, and managing stress)	• Text message—based stress management strategies • Guided meditation apps	X	X	X

HBM, Health belief model; SCT, social cognitive theory; SDT, self-determination theory; TPB, theory of planned behavior; TTM, transtheoretical model.
Source: Adapted from Michie S, Richardson M, Johnston M, Abraham C, Francis J, Hardeman W, et al. The behavior change technique taxonomy (v1) of 93 hierarchically clustered techniques: building an international consensus for the reporting of behavior change interventions. Ann Behav Med 2013;46(1):81—95.

We adapted Table 3.1 from Michie et al. [10] to illustrate this point and offer examples of how each theory could be applied to technologies for behaviors that could be modifiable through digital behavioral health interventions. Note that many techniques have not been explored with technology tools (to our knowledge) and hence offer a potential for future research (see the "Research directions" section).

Digital technology–based behavior change interventions

This section reviews examples of behavior change interventions delivered to people with diabetes via digital health technologies. When applicable, we highlight the theories that underpin the behavioral interventions. Digital health technologies have the potential to promote and support diabetes-related behavior change by (1) decreasing barriers to accessing behavior change support, (2) providing individualized and tailored interventions around health behaviors, and (3) delivering these interventions in a timely manner. Digital health technologies are commonly used by people with diabetes to support self-management. Research on adolescents with type 1 diabetes (T1D) and their parents shows that most use some form of technology for diabetes management, most frequently they use text messaging. Those who reported more frequent use of diabetes-related social networking, websites, or device-integrated software (e.g., insulin pumps and blood glucose meters) reported more engagement in diabetes self-management behaviors (also sometimes referred to as treatment adherence). This study assessed 15 behaviors related to diabetes self-management but did not report associations between technology use and any specific health behaviors. In a survey of nearly 2000 people with diabetes, over half of people with T1D and one-third of people with type 2 diabetes (T2D) reported using diabetes apps for self-management. Diabetes self-management behaviors were significantly higher among app-users than nonusers, especially following healthy eating guidelines, engaging in regular physical activity, and frequent blood glucose monitoring [11]. The majority of work in this area has been with youth who have T1D. Currently, research shows high feasibility and acceptability of these approaches, and the following sections summarize the existing evidence regarding improvements in diabetes self-management behaviors or glycemic outcomes.

Technology-enabled diabetes management

Use of diabetes management devices, including insulin pumps, continuous glucose monitors (CGMs), and smart pens has increased in recent years. While CGM technology is not a behavior change technology, it has become a key component of behavioral interventions, because the continuous glucose information allows users to adapt their diabetes management behaviors in real-time to achieve better outcomes. Multiple studies have reported improved medical outcomes, such as lower HbA1c and less hypoglycemia with CGM use, and there may also be psychosocial benefits, such as reduced diabetes distress [12].

Telemedicine, which uses web-based video conferencing for health-care delivery, is a strategy to deliver patient-centered clinical care with less travel time and missed school or work. The Colorado Young Adults with T1D (CoYoT1) Clinic provides a unique telemedicine clinic model incorporating individual appointments with a diabetes professional and shared virtual visits with a certified diabetes educator. In a pilot study, young adults participating in the CoYoT1 Clinic reported high satisfaction, reduced travel time, and reduced time away from work and school; however, there was no control group, so efficacy was not assessed [13]. One online specialty medical clinic for adults with T2D recommends carbohydrate restriction for diabetes management and provides patients with (1) access to a health coach and physician, (2) online peer support, and (3) ongoing information and feedback on their health. In an observational study of participants in this program's remote care model at the 1-year mark, HbA1c was reduced (7.6% to 6.3%), weight declined by an average of 13.8 kg, insulin therapy was reduced or eliminated in 94% of users, and T2D medication prescriptions other than metformin declined from 56.9% to 29.7% [14]. Telemedicine may also be deployed for the delivery of behavioral interventions.

Behavioral interventions delivered via the Internet

Several empirically supported behavioral interventions for youth with T1D have been adapted for delivery via the Internet. Behavioral family systems therapy for diabetes (BFST-D) is a 6-month program that teaches families of adolescents' communication and problem-solving skills to manage diabetes-related challenges. Coping skills training (CST) is a six-session group intervention for youth with T1D that teaches skills for managing diabetes-related stressors in social situations, including social problem-solving, cognitive and behavioral strategies, and conflict resolution. When adapted for web-based delivery, feasibility and acceptability were high for teens, but at 6 months there were no differences in HbA1c or quality of life compared to web-based diabetes education [15]. BFST-D and CST use aspects of SCT, including learning and applying skills, setting goals, and accessing support. Their adaptations to web-based delivery use the same theoretical foundations.

There are also behavioral interventions designed specifically for the Internet. For example, Mulvaney et al. developed an interactive web-based program based in SCT and SDT, in which teens with T1D learned problem-solving skills, were prompted to use those skills to manage diabetes-related scenarios, and were connected with other teens with diabetes for social support [16]. Compared to usual care, in a per-protocol analysis (but not in an intent-to-treat analyses) participants receiving the intervention significantly improved their self-management behaviors compared to the control group. Mean glycemia in the intervention group remained constant, while that of the control group significantly worsened.

Together, these examples suggest the high appropriateness of remote/web-based behavioral intervention delivery for youth and potential for impact on health behaviors and outcomes. However, the optimal content (e.g., educational vs behavioral skills or youth- vs family-focused) for this format is not yet evident.

Mobile technologies for behavior change support

Diabetes behavior change support can also be delivered using individualized diabetes-related feedback (similar to what HBM recommends) via mobile apps. Mulvaney et al. developed an app that collects psychosocial data via ecological momentary assessment from teens with T1D and provides personalized feedback on glucose trends and psychosocial assessments [17]. The engagement was high, and more improvements were related to greater participation, but overall there was no change in self-management behaviors or HbA1c concentrations.

Mobile technologies including smartphones and wearable devices provide highly scalable new approaches to diabetes management. Several mobile apps provide blood glucose monitoring strips that link to a mobile phone application and provide remote health coaching by a diabetes educator. One system provides real-time, in-app educational and behavioral messaging to people with T2D via automated decision support from an artificial intelligence algorithm, in response to individually analyzed blood glucose values and lifestyle behaviors [18].

Diabetes-specific mobile apps and text messaging may also provide support for behavior change. For example, MyT1Dhero, developed at Michigan State University, aims to encourage adolescents with T1D to self-manage their diabetes and improve communication with parents [19]. Texting-based interventions to promote self-management in youth with T1D have mixed results: high feasibility and participant satisfaction, but less evidence for impact on behavioral and outcome metrics, such as self-management and HbA1c concentrations. Most research has been on pilot studies of reminder-oriented text messaging interventions or multicomponent interventions that include text-messaging for reminders, support, or education [20]. When teens engage more with text reminders for blood glucose checks, there may be benefits for HbA1c. Thus this approach may be useful for some youth who are amenable to receiving reminders. There is a need to tailor the frequency, timing, and content of text messages to the intervention recipient. As with all technologies, software issues can interfere with text message delivery and effectiveness. Using personalized text messages to enhance/boost impact of other behavior change/supportive interventions may be helpful; for example, in the Novel Interventions in Children's Healthcare program for high-risk youth with social and medical vulnerabilities, interventionists send personal text−based communication to their patients to solidify skills learned in other contacts, provide support, and act as a reminder/accountability for engaging in self-management behaviors [21].

The American Diabetes Association (ADA) psychosocial position statement [22] recommends routine psychosocial screening in diabetes clinic for depressive symptoms, anxiety/worry about diabetes-specific concerns, disordered eating behaviors, and diabetes distress. Using tablet computers or web-based systems integrated with the electronic medical record can facilitate efficient conduct of psychosocial screening in clinic settings.

Research directions

The most common use of technology falls in three major categories: (1) *measurement*, for example, of *what* and *when* of a behavior, like using activity trackers for physical activity measurement or *how* of health, like using CGMs to assess how a variable such as stress impacts glucose level; (2) *prediction and insights*, for example, data analytics for detecting dangerous glycemic events; and (3) *delivering interventions*, for example, activating an insulin pump to adjust insulin delivery or sending a message to warn the user, see Fig. 3.1. However, technology cannot yet understand the *why* behind a behavior. Behavioral theories posit that the *why* often relates to user decisions, attitudes, or capacities, or to environmental constraints, and thus in many cases, the only way to learn the *why*, is to ask the individual (self-reports).

The above discussion points us to an important question: if automation does not allow us to collect all needed pieces of the information (*what* and

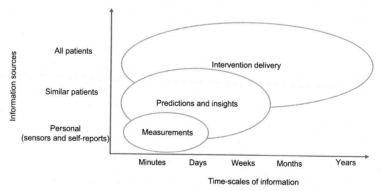

FIGURE 3.1   Technology often serves three roles: (1) *measurement*, (2) *prediction and insights*, and (3) *intervention delivery*. In the context of diabetes the above figure provides an organization of time-scales and types of data for each of the roles.

when, but not *why),* is there a possibility of positive behavior change? The history of glucose meters provides an encouraging answer, since each advance in size, cost, accuracy, number of readings per unit time and comfort provided new avenues for better clinical interventions. For example, self-management of diabetes became possible in the 1980s only because technology advances allowed patients to operate the glucose meters themselves. Thus technology innovations can expand what we can measure and predict when to deliver interventions, all with the aim of reducing human workload and, if done well, can lead to improved health outcomes for more people.

Measurement: For many people with diabetes a significant source of stress stems from daily decisions regarding diet and exercise. For many dietary choices, there is no easy and accurate method to estimate their carbohydrate content. Furthermore, the glucose response is modulated by the fat and fiber in the food and rate of glucose consumption. These measures are further complicated because the same food item can cause different glycemic responses for each individual. Thus both the "input" (diet composition) and "output" (expected glucose response) are difficult to estimate accurately. This motivates two complementary research directions. The first direction is to develop methods to estimate food composition based on either descriptions or photographs. This could be accomplished by pointing a smartphone camera at a food item. A machine learning—based system would then estimate its ingredients. Components of such systems have already been proposed, and their accuracy may improve as research in this area accelerates. The second direction is to develop a wearable sensor for dietary intake that could leverage biochemical measurements to *automatically* estimate the composition (carbohydrates, fat, and protein) of food consumed by an individual, which we label as a continuous diet monitor (CDM). This approach could become a reality by adding methods to measure fat and protein intake, such as measuring triglycerides and certain amino acids, in addition to blood glucose. This idea is still in its infancy because of the complexity of human metabolism, and much remains to be done.

Prediction and insights: One of main values of quantitative measurement is that it permits quantitative predictions and thereby becomes the foundation for data-driven insights. We envision at least three major directions for digital health predictive systems. First, if the person with diabetes is provided a CGM or CDM, then an exciting avenue for research is to develop methods to estimate the expected glucose response to a food item *before* consuming it. This prediction could be performed based on past data of the device user (using both sensor and self-report data) and potentially shared data from other users who may be most phenotypically similar. Such ability to predict expected glucose response could become the basis for many behavioral interventions, where the individual can evaluate their options before consuming them. Alternately, if only one food option was available, then the predictive methods could help estimate the recommended quantity of food, appropriate medicine, and/or exercise to maintain desired glycemic control. Second, the past information about the diet−glucose relationship could be converted into personalized insights for the individual, who can in turn leverage these insights to adapt their future behaviors. For example, if an algorithm detects frequent out-of-range glucose values on Mondays, then this historical information could allow the individual to reflect on their Monday routines and make changes for better glycemic control, in their living context.

Finally, with more data of diverse forms, for example, exercise, diet, and physiology, a key challenge is how to present the data or derived insights such that the data consumer (person with diabetes, caregiver, or physician) can extract the maximum value. The value of the data to the consumer is not a fixed construct and depends on the individual. For example, data presentation to children and infirm elderly has to match their cognitive abilities. Despite years of attention, products continue to have poor designs, often with little attention to human factors. Thus it is important to have increased emphasis on the design of human−computer interfaces to extract maximum value from data. User-centered research incorporates the expectations, desired features, potential benefits, perceived burdens, and lived experiences of digital health technologies. This type of research has begun to inform automated insulin delivery (AID) systems development, which may lead to optimal user−system interactions and ultimately help users achieve improved glycemic outcomes [23].

Intervention delivery: The primary goal for technology-development discussion in this chapter is behavioral interventions. We discuss three research directions, loosely classified based on the time-scale of intervention and types of data used in the development of intervention. First, a much researched and anticipated next step in diabetes-specific device technology involves closing the loop between the CGM and insulin pump via an AID system. In the ideal case the system will become personalized by learning from the past data of the user. In addition to improving medical outcomes, such AID systems may also improve health-related quality of life by reducing the mental and psychosocial burden of managing diabetes [24]. The AID system research has gained impetus from the Do-It-Yourself community, where people with diabetes are "hacking" their devices to develop systems that work for them. A potential research and development *methodology* question has thus appeared, on how community-developed ideas can provide input to commercial product development and accelerate the process of creating fully automated AID systems.

Second, potential behavioral interventions based in theory, some of which are already delivered via technology-based tools, must be developed. A number of the techniques presented in Table 3.1 still lack sufficient empirical evidence. Some could be expanded on for future interventions. In addition, Michie et al.'s taxonomy of behavior-change methods suggest techniques not listed in our table that could be amenable to technology development [10]. A major research challenge is not only developing new forms of interventions, but also triggering the right intervention for the right person at the right time, based on the context. For example, CGM use may be enhanced by the development of contextually aware methods to mitigate alert fatigue, sleep interruptions, and unnecessary alarms during work or school. Furthermore, the right intervention often requires learning the *why* behind specific gaps in care, and this is where individual's input is often required. Users are often asked to document their choices, especially *why* behind the *when* and *what*. This information is needed to guide the next steps for individualized intervention delivery. Another key research challenge is how to reduce the documentation burden for all stakeholders and still obtain sufficient information for effective implementation of interventions.

Finally, as health-care systems collect more data using a combination of Internet-connected diabetes technology and mobile devices, there is an opportunity to develop methodologies to convert health-care systems into *learning* systems, which can learn from all patients. Specifically, as we deploy ideas from randomized controlled trials into larger populations, there is a potential to use recent advances in statistical methods to make causal inferences using observed data. These inferences could inform (1) optimization of clinical workflows, for example, when should a patient visit their doctor and using which method; (2) adaptive messaging, for example, what type of messages (automated or health-care system initiated) may be useful for a patient based on their recent data; and (3) generation of new hypotheses to be rigorously tested.

Conclusion

Any clinician will attest that optimal care requires personalization to an individual's needs and living context, but development of personalized therapy requires significant time and financial resources. Thus technology has a clear role to play in addressing the growing chronic disease epidemic. The key challenge lies in the development of technologies that can both scale to millions of people who need them, and still do it effectively for each of them. We noted that an important opportunity for technology development lies in achieving personalization, specifically by understanding the context in which patients live, and then leveraging the context to develop effective technology for improved health outcomes.

References

[1] Modi AC, Pai AL, Hommel KA, Hood KK, Cortina S, Hilliard ME, et al. Pediatric self-management: a framework for research, practice, and policy. Pediatrics 2012;129(2): e473–85.

[2]   Pal K, Eastwood SV, Michie S, Farmer AJ, Barnard ML, Peacock R, et al. Computer-based diabetes self-management interventions for adults with type 2 diabetes mellitus. Cochrane Database Syst Rev 2013;(3):CD008776.

[3]   Klonoff DC, King F, Kerr D. New opportunities for digital health to thrive. J Diabetes Sci Technol 2019;13(2):159–63.

[4]   Mummah SA, Robinson TN, King AC, Gardner CD, Sutton S. IDEAS (integrate, design, assess, and share): a framework and toolkit of strategies for the development of more effective digital interventions to change health behavior. J Med Internet Res 2016;18(12): e317.

[5]   Deci EL, Ryan RM. Self-determination theory: a macrotheory of human motivation, development, and health. Can Psychol 2008;49(3):182–5.

[6]   Bandura A. The explanatory and predictive scope of self-efficacy theory. J Soc Clin Psychol 1986;4(3):359–73.

[7]   Becker MH. The health belief model and sick role behavior. Health Educ Monogr 1974;2 (4):409–19.

[8]   Ajzen I. The theory of planned behavior. Organ Behav Hum Decis Process 1991;50 (2):179–211.

[9]   Prochaska JO, DiClemente CC. Stages and processes of self-change of smoking: toward an integrative model of change. J Consult Clin Psychol 1983;51(3):390–5.

[10] Michie S, Richardson M, Johnston M, Abraham C, Francis J, Hardeman W, et al. The behavior change technique taxonomy (v1) of 93 hierarchically clustered techniques: building an international consensus for the reporting of behavior change interventions. Ann Behav Med 2013;46(1):81–95.

[11] Kebede MM, Pischke CR. Popular diabetes apps and the impact of diabetes app use on self-care behaviour: a survey among the digital community of persons with diabetes on social media. Front Endocrinol (Lausanne) 2019;10:135.

[12] Polonsky WH, Hessler D, Ruedy KJ, Beck RW, Group DS. The impact of continuous glucose monitoring on markers of quality of life in adults with type 1 diabetes: further findings from the DIAMOND randomized clinical trial. Diabetes Care 2017;40 (6):736–41.

[13] Reid MW, Krishnan S, Berget C, Cain C, Thomas JF, Klingensmith GJ, et al. CoYoT1 Clinic: home telemedicine increases young adult engagement in diabetes care. Diabetes Technol Ther 2018;20(5):370–9.

[14] Hallberg SJ, McKenzie AL, Williams PT, Bhanpuri NH, Peters AL, Campbell WW, et al. Effectiveness and safety of a novel care model for the management of type 2 diabetes at 1 year: an open-label, non-randomized, controlled study. Diabetes Ther 2018;9(2):583–612.

[15] Whittemore R, Jaser SS, Jeon S, Liberti L, Delamater A, Murphy K, et al. An Internet coping skills training program for youth with type 1 diabetes: six-month outcomes. Nurs Res 2012;61(6):395–404.

[16] Mulvaney SA, Rothman RL, Wallston KA, Lybarger C, Dietrich MS. An Internet-based program to improve self-management in adolescents with type 1 diabetes. Diabetes Care 2010;33(3):602–4.

[17] Mulvaney SA, Vaala S, Hood KK, Lybarger C, Carroll R, Williams L, et al. Mobile momentary assessment and biobehavioral feedback for adolescents with type 1 diabetes: feasibility and engagement patterns. Diabetes Technol Ther 2018;20(7):465–74.

[18] Quinn CC, Shardell MD, Terrin ML, Barr EA, Ballew SH, Gruber-Baldini AL. Cluster-randomized trial of a mobile phone personalized behavioral intervention for blood glucose control. Diabetes Care 2011;34(9):1934–42.

[19] Holtz BE, Murray KM, Hershey DD, Dunneback JK, Cotten SR, Holmstrom AJ, et al. Developing a patient-centered mHealth app: a tool for adolescents with type 1 diabetes and their parents. JMIR Mhealth Uhealth 2017;5(4):e53.

[20] Herbert LJ, Mehta P, Monaghan M, Cogen F, Streisand R. Feasibility of the SMART project: a text message program for adolescents with type 1 diabetes. Diabetes Spectr 2014;27 (4):265–9.

[21] Wagner DV, Barry SA, Stoeckel M, Teplitsky L, Harris MA. NICH at its best for diabetes at its worst: texting teens and their caregivers for better outcomes. J Diabetes Sci Technol 2017;11(3):468–75.

[22] Young-Hyman D, de Groot M, Hill-Briggs F, Gonzalez JS, Hood K, Peyrot M. Psychosocial care for people with diabetes: a position statement of the American Diabetes Association. Diabetes Care 2016;39(12):2126–40.

[23] Naranjo D, Suttiratana SC, Iturralde E, Barnard KD, Weissberg-Benchell J, Laffel L, et al. What end users and stakeholders want from automated insulin delivery systems. Diabetes Care 2017;40(11):1453–61.

[24] Tanenbaum ML, Hanes SJ, Miller KM, Naranjo D, Bensen R, Hood KK. Diabetes device use in adults with type 1 diabetes: barriers to uptake and potential intervention targets. Diabetes Care 2017;40(2):181–7.

Further reading

Vaala SE, Hood KK, Laffel L, Kumah-Crystal YA, Lybarger CK, Mulvaney SA. Use of commonly available technologies for diabetes information and self-management among adolescents with type 1 diabetes and their parents: a web-based survey study. Interact J Med Res 2015;4(4):e24.

Chapter 4

Agile science: what and how in digital diabetes research

Lyndsay A. Nelson[1,2], Anthony L. Threatt[3], William Martinez[1,2],
S. Will Acuff[1] and Lindsay S. Mayberry[1,2,4,5]

*[1]Department of Medicine, Vanderbilt University Medical Center, Nashville, TN, United States,
[2]Center for Health Behavior and Health Education, Vanderbilt University Medical Center,
Nashville, TN, United States, [3]Health Information Technology, Vanderbilt University Medical
Center, Nashville, TN, United States, [4]Center for Diabetes Translation Research, Vanderbilt
University Medical Center, Nashville, TN, United States, [5]Department of Biomedical
Informatics, Vanderbilt University Medical Center, Nashville, TN, United States*

Abbreviations

HbA1c hemoglobin A1c
MOST multiphase optimization strategy
PI principal investigator
RCT randomized controlled trial
SMART sequential, multiple assignment, randomized trial
SUS System Usability Scale
UX user experience

Key points

- Integrating agile methods into digital diabetes research can allow for more rapid intervention development that accounts for users' needs and expectations.
- An agile mindset and agile processes can be applied at any phase of the research, including study design, usability testing, evaluation, and team management.
- When evaluating a digital health intervention, anticipate problems with the technology and prepare to iterate continuously. We recommend performing regular, reproducible, and evolving checks of the data inputs and outputs to ensure that the intervention is delivered as intended.

Diabetes Digital Health. DOI: https://doi.org/10.1016/B978-0-12-817485-2.00004-3

What is agile?

Imagine your research team received a grant to develop and evaluate a digital intervention to support diabetes self-care. Your team spends a few months designing an intervention based on your previous studies and a literature review. Next, you work with a development team to build exactly what you designed; however, it takes 3 months longer than originally anticipated. When the intervention is ready, you conduct a feasibility study to ensure that the intervention is acceptable and can be successfully delivered before beginning your randomized controlled trial (RCT). Your goal was to recruit 50 participants over 2 months and ask them to use the intervention for 3 months, but it takes an additional 2 months to acquire the full sample. Results from your feasibility study indicate that participants were generally satisfied with the intervention and it seemed to work as intended, so you hurriedly begin the recruitment for the RCT to get back on track. When evaluating the results of your RCT, you learn that 20% of participants never used the intervention; another 50% used it for only a few months of the 12-month intervention experience. In addition, content intended to be tailored to participant characteristics was incorrectly sent to at least half of the participants. The intervention was not effective at improving self-care, but you do not know whether this finding was due to limited use, poor usability, incorrect content, and/or something else entirely.

This imaginary scenario illustrates many of the problems encountered by research teams. In the product and software development industry, this approach is called the "waterfall" methodology, describing a linear process in which steps are completed sequentially without returning to previously completed steps to make changes. This way of working can lead to frustration because work efforts are often siloed, communication is poor, and it requires a great deal of upfront analysis, design, and specification documentation. In these scenarios, product teams dutifully deliver a product after working for months only to find out that their product did not fully meet user or business needs. In contrast, agile is a methodology used to design and deliver products rapidly and iteratively. The agile methodology was developed at a time when "waterfall" or more traditional design process methodologies were presenting problems for both developers and customers. To change the status quo, in February 2001, the writers of the Agile Manifesto developed a new working philosophy, in which they emphasize individuals and interactions over processes and tools, functioning software over comprehensive documentation, customer collaboration over contract negotiation, and responding to change over following a plan [1].

Agile is defined as a very iterative, incremental, and collaborative approach to delivering projects, often used by small, cross functional teams. Specific processes and tools are often used to help facilitate this approach (Table 4.1). For example, these teams will often "timebox" (i.e., designate a

TABLE 4.1 Common agile processes and methods.

Type	Purpose/description
Meetings	
Planning meetings	To discuss problems, desired outcomes, what will be worked on, and committed timeline
Daily stand-ups	To discuss work completed, blockers, and next work
Work review meetings	After a set timebox, review the work completed to determine next steps
Retrospective meetings	Review meeting to discuss team dynamics or how everyone communicated and worked together on the last timeboxed effort
Tools	
Timebox	Verb: to designate a defined period to complete a task
	Noun: amount of time designated for a task or between planning and retrospective meetings
Story cards	Delineate specific tasks, help to visualize the work, and serve as a communication device
Backlog	A list of ideas or requirements that might be worked on in the future; often broken into story cards when they become a priority
Work lanes	Communicate the status of the story cards among team members (e.g., to do, doing, and done)
The Sprint	The planning meeting and retrospective meeting bookend the timebox; collectively this is referred to as The Sprint (as in "what are we going to focus on for our next Sprint?")
Mindset and method	
Iteration	Each revision of an idea or solution with input from team members, end users, and/or data
Continual end-user evaluation and feedback	Collecting quantitative and qualitative data about the solutions that are developed and applying information learned to inform next steps
Value	Intentionally increased at each step of the development process; value can be customer-, technical-, or revenue-focused

defined period to complete a task), so that they can iteratively create and deliver customer value quickly. Teams using an agile approach are often made up of people from different disciplines with different skills, each representing an aspect of the product or process. Collaboration among team members is key and includes end users who provide input on the most valuable work to be completed next. Ultimately, the end product, whether a capability, technology, or intervention, is developed with the goal of increasing functionality, usability, and/or value [2,3].

Since the Agile Manifesto was written, other methodologies have been developed to increase the speed with which teams are able to deliver validated ideas and value. These methods include Scrum (*Agile Software Development with Scrum* written by Ken Schwaber) [2], Kanban (*Kanban* written by David J. Anderson) [3], Lean start-up (*The Lean Start-Up* written by Eric Ries) [4], and Design Sprints (*Sprint* written by Jake Knapp) [5].

Why bring agile to research?

In a traditional research study the study design is cemented prior to evaluation and the knowledge to be gained focuses on efficacy and acceptability of the intervention as designed. The agile approach assumes that we do not know all the right questions to ask at the start of any project. Therefore agile design processes continually collect data in the form of user feedback with iterative rounds of revisions, leading to more data generation, more questions answered, and more discovery of questions that were not initially asked (i.e., hypothesis generation). It has been our team's experience that real-world pragmatic studies, essential for testing of digital health interventions, face an ever-changing human landscape compounded by the fast-paced changes of technology development and availability. Agile brings a malleable framework for getting things done efficiently when there is a moderate-to-high level of uncertainty that is (should be) the case with digital interventions in diabetes.

Applications of agile methods in digital diabetes research

Agile science principles can be applied to all phases of the research process to facilitate more iterative and efficient work. In the following sections, we present examples from our own work conducting trials with text message−delivered and web−delivered interventions for diabetes.

Agile intervention design

The five-phase design sprint methodology (Fig. 4.1) [5] is an excellent application of the agile approach to design digital health interventions. Design sprints allow 6- to 8-member teams composed of researchers, collaborators, and stakeholders [e.g., user experience (UX) designers, programmers, project managers, relevant organizational leaders, and end users] to quickly test ideas with user feedback as a fundamental piece of the design process. Originally developed by a team from Google Ventures, design sprints are intended to take place over the course of 5 days (1 day for each of the five

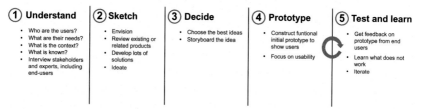

FIGURE 4.1 The five phases in a design sprint. *Adapted from Knapp J, Zeratsky J, Kowitz B. Sprint: how to solve big problems and test new ideas in just five days. Simon and Schuster; 2016 [5].*

phases) [5]. The design sprint methodology overcomes significant limitations of alternative design approaches, namely, design sprints help mitigate time and cost in relation to the rapidly evolving pace of technology and results in products that better reflect users' needs and expectations.

In phase 1 a preappointed facilitator (e.g., UX designer or project manager) organizes team discussions and interviews with expert stakeholders, including end users, to generate a deep understanding of target users' needs and the challenges they face. The facilitator then assists the team to *understand* how the intervention might overcome those challenges. In phase 2 the team reviews existing solutions, architecture, and designs from healthcare and other industries that might inform their own design. For example, when creating the My Diabetes Dashboard within a patient portal [6], our study team reviewed existing technology-based solutions for displaying actionable data and providing alerts and reminders from healthcare and other industries (e.g., finance and education). The study team then applies what they learn from their review, and from expert stakeholders in phase 1, to individually *sketch* potential intervention designs. In phase 3 the team reviews the proposed designs and a preappointed decider [usually the principal investigator (PI)] *decides* which design(s) have the greatest potential to successfully meet users' needs and overcome challenges in the long term. Then, the team adapts the chosen design to create a storyboard or systematic plan for their prototype. In phase 4 the UX designer collects assets (e.g., stock imagery or icons) and, using a presentation- or design-based software program (e.g., PowerPoint, keynote, and Sketch), stitches all the components together into an initial *prototype* that is ready for usability testing in phase 5.

Agile usability testing

Usability testing is critical to ensure the intervention works as intended and a null effect in subsequent evaluations is not due to usability challenges [7]. Iterative usability testing achieves goals similar to traditional feasibility studies by ensuring that recruitment and data collection methods are feasible but goes further with improving and learning more about the intervention itself

[8,9]. Although there are many approaches to usability testing, we highlight two specific methods: task-based usability testing and longitudinal, real-world usability testing. We also share examples using either method from our own research.

In task-based usability testing, users are asked to accomplish real tasks using a prototyped intervention under controlled conditions. In usability testing for the diabetes dashboard, we asked users to perform standardized tasks in the prototype that a real patient might do when visiting their dashboard [e.g., log in, retrieve hemoglobin A1c (HbA1c) data, and message their doctor] [6]. We recorded the interactions and later, two coders reviewed and coded each user's task performance using a basic rating scale (i.e., from "successful/straightforward" to "gives up"). We repeated this process with a new group of users for three rounds of testing which included collecting and analyzing interview data and used the findings to revise the prototype between each round. We then compared performance among the users in the first round who tested the initial prototype and the users in the third round who tested the final prototype (Fig. 4.2) [6]. Because usability testing typically involves a small sample of participants, it is not possible to test for statistical significance; however, this is one approach for assessing change in performance. Notably, the prototypes are not fully programmed digital interventions but rather emulate a UX with a digital product; thus time spent by developers between rounds of testing is minimized.

Longitudinal "real-world" usability testing is well-suited to assess usability of a fully programmed digital health intervention and uncover any concerns not evident in the prototyped version prior to a more formal evaluation. This form of usability testing simulates how users will engage with the intervention in the real world and over time and allows for a comprehensive assessment of users' experience, barriers to use, and reasons for nonuse. For usability testing of a text message—delivered diabetes self-care intervention, we recruited patients to participate in one of three rounds of testing

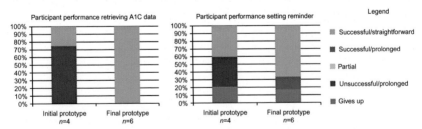

FIGURE 4.2   Task-based usability ratings for initial and final prototype iterations for the diabetes dashboard. *Data from Martinez W, Threatt AL, Rosenbloom ST, Wallston KA, Hickson GB, Elasy TA. A patient-facing diabetes dashboard embedded in a patient web portal: design sprint and usability testing. JMIR Hum Factors 2018;5(3):e26. doi: 10.2196/humanfactors.9569 [6]. https://humanfactors.jmir.org/2018/3/e26/. Licensed under Creative Commons Attribution cc-by 4.0.*

[10]. During each round a group of patients experienced the intervention for 2 weeks (i.e., received and responded to tailored and targeted text message content and accessed HbA1c results via a study website or helpline). We collected user feedback and response data, which we then used to improve the intervention and UX between each round of testing [10]. For example, we revised our text message content to be more comprehensive and consistent with participants' preferences. We also modified our informed consent to help ensure participants understood how to use intervention components and that a computer, not a person, sends all the text messages.

Using a mixed-methods approach that includes quantitative and qualitative measures, researchers can assess users' experience and satisfaction with the intervention [11]. Quantitative data can inform the extent to which there were usability issues and help contextualize results relative to similar interventions, while qualitative data can provide a richer understanding of why there were issues and how to resolve them. A variety of validated usability metrics are available to help quantify the usability of an intervention, including the Computer System Usability Questionnaire [12] and the system usability scale (SUS) [13]. The SUS offers a useful quantitative metric with both high reliability and validity and a threshold score indicative of "above average" usability that can be used to benchmark an intervention or intervention aspects. The SUS is also brief (10 items) and items can be easily adapted to the specific intervention. Recently, the Health Information Technology Usability Evaluation Scale (Health-ITUES) was developed and validated for assessing the usability of mobile health technologies, specifically [14]. The Health-ITUES also contains items that are customizable and includes four subscales (impact, perceived usefulness, perceived ease of use, and user control). Finally, at the conclusion of the UX, researchers often benefit from administering semistructured interviews to qualitatively assess users' experience and suggestions for improvement. Thematic analysis of qualitative interview data can be used to reveal patterns of experiences among users [15].

Agile study designs

Several research designs and frameworks for intervention evaluation apply agile methods. Specifically, there is growing interest in using the multiphase optimization strategy (MOST) for optimizing and evaluating multicomponent behavioral intervention designs [16]. MOST is intended to produce behavioral interventions that are effective, economical, efficient, and scalable [17]. The first phase in this three-phase framework is a preparation phase in which a theoretical model is formed and a criterion for optimization is established (e.g., cost, effectiveness, or efficiency). The second phase is a refining or optimization phase that involves selecting the components and component levels that meet the optimization criterion. Often, this requires estimating the effects of the individual and combined components (e.g., an app, texts, or both). Any type of experimental design can be used in the optimization phase, but one common and efficient randomized experiment is a factorial or fractional−factorial experiment. This type of experiment requires fewer subjects than a standard RCT and reveals which components are the least/most effective and whether the presence or absence of a component impacts the effectiveness of the other components [18]. Another popular design choice for refining/testing optimization is the sequential, multiple assignment, randomized trial (SMART) (elaborated later) [19]. Finally, in the third phase of MOST, the refined/optimized intervention is evaluated in an RCT.

SMART can be used in the context of the MOST framework or on its own to evaluate adaptive interventions [19]. Unlike a traditional RCT that tests individual fully formed interventions, a SMART allows systematic comparisons of different doses, timing, and types of intervention components in the same trial. Using a sequence of decision rules, this design tailors the intervention for each individual based on certain inputs or levels of responsiveness, often at multiple times throughout the trial [20]. For instance, patients could be randomized to receive text messages or use an app, and nonresponsive patients in both groups (e.g., those not using the intervention or those without improvement on target outcomes) could be rerandomized to receive phone coaching or not after a certain amount of time. Randomizing individuals at each decision point means several adaptive interventions are embedded in a single SMART. This supports identification of treatments not producing benefit to eliminate those treatments quickly; participants can be randomized to remaining treatment options without the waste of continuing ineffective treatments for the duration of the trial.

These agile study designs are particularly useful for digital health interventions, in which inputs collected from patients can be used to adapt and optimize an intervention rapidly and cost-effectively. In addition to the previously mentioned designs, researchers are using just-in-time adaptive interventions, ecological momentary assessment, and intensive adaptive interventions to capitalize on digital health for improving chronic disease and health outcomes [21,22].

Cycles of evaluation and iterative improvement often require researchers to decide at each phase (e.g., each round of testing, shifting from usability to evaluation) whether to include the same or new participants. Both are useful for different purposes. For instance, one project may benefit from an advisory board of users who partner across phases of the research process while also bringing in naïve users for certain phases. Other projects may benefit from naïve users at each phase. There are no hard and fast rules, but researchers should be cognizant of the prior experiences of trial participants, so their experiences are not contaminated by participation in an earlier usability testing experience.

Agile study management

Regardless of selected study design, the evaluation phase will be best served by application of agile methods throughout. Agile methods can be used to address common challenges in intervention evaluation, including recruitment and retention deficits, low intervention engagement, and technological advances.

Team meetings and recruitment goals

In a 15-month pragmatic trial evaluating mobile phone—delivered interventions [23], we originally planned to recruit from two community clinics. We had a long history of successful diabetes research in these clinics; however, markedly slow recruitment for this RCT forced us to reassess and strategize how to move forward. We applied an agile methodology to our recruitment approach, incorporating the following three key strategies:

1. *Consistently evaluate and view data as a team.* Each team member was responsible for preparing and presenting a PowerPoint slide reporting data on an aspect of our recruitment progress for weekly team meetings. Viewing the data allowed us to determine as a team which recruitment methods were working in which clinic and what the total potential yield was. For instance, weekly we identified the clinic(s) we should devote our efforts to, tracked progress, and revised accordingly the subsequent week. Using this data-driven iterative approach, we learned early that 15% was roughly our ceiling for enrollment within each clinic; this led us to pursue expanding our potential participant pool to reach our target sample before falling further behind.

2. *Agile meetings.* The goals of agile meetings are that everybody knows the necessary information required for quick decisions and participates actively in identifying and trouble-shooting challenges. During the recruitment phase, our meetings included research staff who brought "on the ground" knowledge of idiosyncrasies of clinics (e.g., staffing, space, and staff and patient attitudes) as well as the PI who could inform recruitment strategies and protocol changes. This approach contrasts with common models where staff meet with the project coordinator and the coordinator alone meets with the PI.

3. *Team reflections and culling the backlog to focus collective efforts.* We embedded project milestones in the weekly data slides. Comparing progress against projected milestones generated a natural rhythm for team reflection on blockers and successes, increasing our capacity to adjust and meet goals moving forward. We also intentionally discussed the team's work priorities, revising iteratively and shifting the entire team's focus for the next Sprint as needed. We could anticipate busy recruitment/retention weeks through the use of data and shift priorities accordingly.

Alternatively, we could anticipate weeks with less recruitment/retention demands and identify new goals/work packages to develop.

At the time we implemented the agile methodology, we had enrolled roughly 10% of our target RCT sample at a rate of 1−2 participants per week. After implementing these changes, our average weekly enrollment rate increased to 7−8 participants; we overcame our deficit by the 75% recruitment milestone, ultimately surpassing our recruitment goal.

Communication

It may be evident at this point that communication plays a key role in the agile process. For agile to work well, everyone should know what others are working on during any given sprint or iteration. In our experience, regular team meetings (Table 4.1) achieve this and also generate a new culture around communication and problem identification. Bringing research assistants into the decision-making and trouble-shooting processes exposes them to higher level thoughts about the research process. This, in turn, improves their ability to identify and foresee important problems while also—in our experience—improving work satisfaction and employee retention.

A critical element of this communication approach is that transparency is highly valued, which means it is key to develop a culture of honesty when challenges occur. This may be in contrast/not keeping with the hierarchical structures of many academic settings and it is incumbent upon the leader (often the PI) to establish a meeting structure for check-ins and to set the tone by welcoming transparency around mistakes and avoiding punitive responses. One of the merits leaders should support and recognize is employees' willingness to bring forth and collaborate to address problems—particularly when they themselves created or missed a problem. This is an opportunity to iterate and to "level up" the skill/knowledge of the team member, and thereby advance the entire team.

Applying the agile philosophy to your digital diabetes intervention

Throughout this chapter, we have described various approaches and examples for integrating agile methods into the research process. Next, we highlight specific lessons learned from our own experiences to strengthen future applications of agile science and avoid pitfalls.

Lessons learned from the technical builds of digital interventions

- Intervention design and usability testing are critical places to start applying agile methodology. These phases allow the most flexibility with iteration. For usability testing, marry the approach with the type of digital health intervention you plan to evaluate. In addition, a mixed-methods approach is usually necessary to assess diversity of perspectives and opinions alongside objective evidence of improvement or decline.

- The agile approach assumes that something will go awry and systematically, iteratively checks to catch and address it as quickly as possible. Do not conclude that once the technology is working well, it will continue to do so for the duration of your study. Anticipate technology problems and look for them systematically, in a reproducible way (e.g., monthly reports generated by team members) to identify problems.
- Meet with your technology partner annually or when there is turnover to ensure they understand: what is this intervention, what is integral, and what needs to be checked to ensure it is working. As things inevitably break, the fixes need to rely on an accurate understanding of the goals/core elements of the product, otherwise additional problems will be introduced.
- If pursuing a digital intervention, then we highly recommend including persons with a relevant technology background on your team. Consider reaching out to colleagues in other disciples or departments at your institution who have experience in user-interface design or other technology domains (e.g., biomedical informatics). If writing a grant for such an intervention, then these individuals' effort should be included in the initial budget.

Challenges

Although an agile approach to research has many benefits, it does come with certain challenges that should be acknowledged.

- This methodology requires a type of rhythmic consistency that can be difficult to adjust to at first. Team members need to be on the same page and open to being overly communicative, especially when first finding that rhythm. This often requires mature team dynamics and communication skills (i.e., high social and emotional intelligence). We have found that agile works best with teams that have a high degree of both flexibility and curiosity.
- An agile approach can be difficult to include in a grant application because it can contrast with standard approaches to research. If wanting to use the five-phase design sprint, you should consider balancing descriptions of the fast-paced methods with an integration of assessment measures to still demonstrate rigor in your process.
- Iterating during a clinical trial (e.g., modifying a recruitment strategy) typically means writing IRB amendments, which can considerably slow down progress. Teams need to learn to expect this and may require experience to do this well.

To learn more

In the software and product world, there are many examples of how the agile method leads to better products that meet real-world needs quickly (e.g., https://www.ideo.com). This is the result of obtaining active user feedback at every iteration, to make the product a better "market fit." However, to date, there are few examples of this approach in research. Notable exceptions include an initiative at Arizona State University, funded by the Robert Wood Johnson Foundation, focused on using agile science to design and optimize behavior change interventions [24], and The Design Lab at University of California San Diego that applies agile principles to research addressing complex societal problems [25]. We hope these initiatives and this chapter will encourage more published applications of the agile philosophy in research, so teams can operate more efficiently and interventions will meet users' needs and meaningfully impact outcomes.

References

[1] Fowler M, Highsmith J. The agile manifesto. Software development [Internet]. Available from: <http://users.jyu.fi/~mieijala/kandimateriaali/Agile-Manifesto.pdf>; 2001.
[2] Schwaber K, Beedle M. Agile software development with scrum. Saddle River, NJ: Prentice Hall Upper; 2002.
[3] Anderson DJ. Kanban: successful evolutionary change for your technology business. Blue Hole Press; 2010.
[4] Ries E. The lean startup: how today's entrepreneurs use continuous innovation to create radically successful businesses. Crown Books; 2011.
[5] Knapp J, Zeratsky J, Kowitz B. Sprint: how to solve big problems and test new ideas in just five days. Simon and Schuster; 2016.
[6] Martinez W, Threatt AL, Rosenbloom ST, Wallston KA, Hickson GB, Elasy TA. A patient-facing diabetes dashboard embedded in a patient web portal: design sprint and usability testing. JMIR Hum Factors 2018;5(3):e26. Available from: https://doi.org/10.2196/humanfactors.9569.
[7] Lyles CR, Sarkar U, Osborn CY. Getting a technology-based diabetes intervention ready for prime time: a review of usability testing studies. Curr Diabetes Rep 2014;14(10):1−12. Available from: https://doi.org/10.1007/s11892-014-0534-9.
[8] Atkinson NL, Saperstein SL, Desmond SM, Gold RS, Billing AS, Tian J. Rural eHealth nutrition education for limited-income families: an iterative and user-centered design approach. J Med Internet Res 2009;11(2):e21. Available from: https://doi.org/10.2196/jmir.1148 v11i2e21 [pii].
[9] Leon AC, Davis LL, Kraemer HC. The role and interpretation of pilot studies in clinical research. J Psychiatr Res 2011;45(5):626−9. Available from: https://doi.org/10.1016/j.jpsychires.2010.10.008.
[10] Nelson LA, Mayberry LS, Wallston K, Kripalani S, Bergner EM, Osborn CY. Development and usability of REACH: a tailored theory-based text messaging intervention for disadvantaged adults with type 2 diabetes. JMIR Hum Factors 2016;3(2):e23. Available from: https://doi.org/10.2196/humanfactors.6029.

[11]   Sarkar U, Gourley GI, Lyles CR, Tieu L, Clarity C, Newmark L, et al. Usability of com-
        mercially available mobile applications for diverse patients. J Gen Intern Med 2016;31
        (12):1417−26. Available from: https://doi.org/10.1007/s11606-016-3771-6.

[12]   Lewis JR. IBM computer usability satisfaction questionnaires: Psychometric evaluation
        and instructions for use. Int J Hu Comput Interact 1995;7(1):57−78. Available from:
        https://doi.org/10.1080/10447319509526110.

[13]   Brooke J. SUS-A quick and dirty usability scale. Usability Eval Ind 1996;189(194):4−7.

[14]   Schnall R, Cho H, Liu J. Health information technology usability evaluation scale
        (Health-ITUES) for usability assessment of mobile health technology: validation study. JMIR
        mHealth uHealth 2018;6(1):e4. Available from: https://doi.org/10.2196/mhealth.8851.

[15]   Francis JJ, Johnston M, Robertson C, Glidewell L, Entwistle V, Eccles MP, et al. What is
        an adequate sample size? Operationalising data saturation for theory-based interview stud-
        ies. Psychol Health 2010;25(10):1229−45. Available from: https://doi.org/10.1080/
        08870440903194015.

[16]   Collins LM, Kugler KC. Optimization of behavioral, biobehavioral, and biomedical inter-
        ventions. Cham: Springer International Publishing; 2018. Available from: http://dx.
        doi:10.1007/978-3-319-72206-1.

[17]   Collins LM, Kugler KC, Gwadz MV. Optimization of multicomponent behavioral and
        biobehavioral interventions for the prevention and treatment of HIV/AIDS. AIDS Behav
        2016;20(Suppl. 1):S197−214. Available from: https://doi.org/10.1007/s10461-015-1145-4.

[18]   Collins LM, Dziak JJ, Kugler KC, Trail JB. Factorial experiments: efficient tools for eval-
        uation of intervention components. Am J Prev Med 2014;47(4):498−504. Available from:
        https://doi.org/10.1016/j.amepre.2014.06.021.

[19]   Murphy SA. An experimental design for the development of adaptive treatment strategies.
        Stat Med 2005;24(10):1455−81. Available from: https://doi.org/10.1002/sim.2022.

[20]   Lei H, Nahum-Shani I, Lynch K, Oslin D, Murphy SAA. "SMART" design for building
        individualized treatment sequences. Annu Rev Clin Psychol 2012;8:21−48. Available
        from: https://doi.org/10.1146/annurev-clinpsy-032511-143152.

[21]   Nahum-Shani I, Smith SN, Spring BJ, Collins LM, Witkiewitz K, Tewari A, et al. Just-in-
        time adaptive interventions (JITAIs) in mobile health: key components and design princi-
        ples for ongoing health behavior support. Ann Behav Med 2017;52(6):446−62. Available
        from: https://doi.org/10.1007/s12160-016-9830-8.

[22]   Riley WT, Serrano KJ, Nilsen W, Atienza AA. Mobile and wireless technologies in health
        behavior and the potential for intensively adaptive interventions. Curr Opin Psychol
        2015;5:67−71. Available from: https://doi.org/10.1016/j.copsyc.2015.03.024.

[23]   Nelson LA, Wallston KA, Kripalani S, Greevy Jr. RA, Elasy TA, Bergner EM, et al.
        Mobile phone support for diabetes self-care among diverse adults: protocol for a three-
        arm randomized controlled trial. JMIR Res Protoc 2018;7(4):e92. Available from: https://
        doi.org/10.2196/resprot.9443.

[24]   Hekler EB, Klasnja P, Harlow J, Mishra S, Korinek E, Evans B. Agile science. Arizona
        State University. Available from: <http://www.agilescience.org/>, (accessed 05.07.19).

[25]   University of California San Diego. The design lab. Available from: <https://designlab.
        ucsd.edu/about/philosophy/>; 2019.

Chapter 5

Behavior change techniques for diabetes technologies

Connie Wong and Maureen Monaghan

Children's National Hospital, Washington, DC, United States

Abbreviations

App application
BG blood glucose
CGM continuous glucose monitor
HBM health belief model
IMB model information−motivation−behavioral skills model
SCT social cognitive theory

Key points

- Advances in diabetes technologies provide opportunities for persons with diabetes to sustain improvements in health and quality of life, but this promise relies on persons engaging with technology to change health-related behaviors.
- Attention to existing behavior change theories in the design and development of diabetes technologies is critical, yet existing research shows that behavior change theories are not consistently utilized and applied.
- Inclusion of appropriate and relevant behavior change techniques can result in improved outcomes for persons using diabetes technologies.

Advances in diabetes technologies can optimize self-management and care for persons with diabetes, offering capabilities such as alerts for glycemic excursions using continuous glucose monitors (CGMs), carbohydrate counting assistance or coaching support through mobile applications (apps), seamless tracking of physical activity through wearable devices, and communication with health-care professionals outside of traditional face-to-face medical visits via patient portals. The ability of linking many of these technologies wirelessly to share information across platforms further integrates data and technology into daily life with diabetes. Behavior change techniques

Diabetes Digital Health. DOI: https://doi.org/10.1016/B978-0-12-817485-2.00005-5

can be incorporated into diabetes technologies to increase opportunities for sustainable improvements in health. However, the promise of technology relies on persons with diabetes accessing, initiating, using, and sustaining the use of digital health devices and products. Furthermore, successful use of these technologies should lead to a measurable change in a desired behavior or clinical indicator. Without this person-level engagement and associated understanding of the behavioral mechanisms driving change, the benefits of established and emerging diabetes technologies are not truly realized. This chapter aims to provide a brief introduction to theories of behavior change, review key behavior change techniques, and address current behavior change research as related to diabetes technologies.

Behavior change theories

Behavior change theories offer unifying frameworks to identify key determinants of health behavior that may explain and predict how persons with diabetes engage with technologies and make health-related decisions. These theories provide a blueprint for the development, implementation, and evaluation of diabetes technologies [1]. However, evidence suggests that behavioral theories are infrequently applied to digital health and this lack of attention to theory may explain some of the current challenges with achieving optimal diabetes-related outcomes [2]. A review of all potential behavior change theories applicable to diabetes technologies is beyond the scope of this chapter. Rather, we introduce three overarching theories that have been applied in diabetes research and inform common elements of behavior change: social cognitive theory (SCT) [3], the health belief model (HBM) [4], and the information—motivation—behavioral skills (IMB) model [5].

Social cognitive theory

SCT addresses psychosocial factors and motivations influencing health behaviors and methods to promote sustained, translatable behavior change [3]. SCT is a commonly applied behavior change theory to diabetes technologies; a recent systematic review found the majority of mobile health interventions addressing diet, physical activity, or weight loss utilized SCT as the guiding framework [6]. SCT includes consideration of an individual's prior behavior, cognitions, social environment, and physical environment when predicting future behavior. Behavior change is initiated and maintained when persons feel that they are capable of executing the desired behavior (i.e., self-efficacy) and have a reasonable expectation that the behavior will result in a desired outcome (i.e., outcome expectations). Additional SCT considerations relevant for diabetes technology include (1) an individual's knowledge of health risks and benefits associated with target behavior, (2) identification of specific goals and strategies for tracking progress and realizing these goals, and (3) use of vicarious learning in which the observation of other people or models guides learning. Key pathways of influence include (1) tailoring content or behavioral targets to a participant's knowledge and efficacy level, (2) monitoring progress they are making, and (3) utilizing social support to enhance learning and motivation [3].

Health belief model

An alternate behavioral theory is the HBM. The HBM purports that behavior change is driven by an individual's motivation to meet a certain goal and their perception that meeting the goal will result in positive benefit (i.e., outcome expectancies) [4]. The HBM highlights four perceptions that influence behavior: (1) perceived susceptibility for a particular risk or condition, (2) perceived severity related to the seriousness of the risk or condition, (3) perceived barriers to engaging in a particular behavior, and (4) perceived benefits of engaging in a particular behavior. The HBM also includes specific cues to action that increase the likelihood of engaging in a particular behavior. For example, having a patient complete a self-assessment about health and then linking their results to a personalized risk index for complications (e.g., erectile dysfunction; neuropathy) may change perception of susceptibility and, thus, lead to behavior change. Patients with significant worry about hypoglycemia (perceived severity) may be more likely to utilize a CGM to avoid hypoglycemia and gain information about glycemic trends (perceived benefit). Patients may be less likely to utilize a CGM if there is perceived inaccuracy (reducing benefit) or if numerous barriers are perceived for use, such as discomfort, difficulty inserting the sensor, or financial cost [7].

Information–motivation–behavioral skills model

The IMB model [5] of health behavior change attends to (1) an individual's knowledge or information about the target behavior, (2) motivation to perform the target behavior, and (3) skills needed to execute the behavior at a high level across a variety of situations. Motivation to perform the behavior can be internal or external (e.g., via social support). Furthermore, skills encompass both the required skills to execute a behavior and an individual's perceived competence in his or her skills to engage in the target behavior.

The IMB model has been applied to increase the understanding of diabetes self-management behaviors such as medication adherence [8]. Klonoff provided examples of how the IMB model can be directly applied to build a diabetes-specific mobile app, including features such as personalized education based on current practice guidelines (i.e., information), use of a personal diabetes diary to track user experiences (i.e., internal motivation), integration of a social media component to share experiences (i.e., external motivation), and tracking of blood glucose (BG) trends to gain additional insight into glycemic variability across situations (i.e., skills) [2].

Overarching considerations for utilizing behavior change techniques

These established theoretical models offer several overarching behavioral constructs applicable to behavior change using diabetes technology. Each theory incorporates a clear focus on an individual's knowledge of and perceived ability to engage in a particular behavior (e.g., information, skills, and self-efficacy) and the importance of perceived benefit of engaging in that behavior (e.g., outcome expectancies and benefit). Furthermore, the theories identify key constructs that motivate or hinder behavior change for persons with diabetes (i.e., social support, modeling or observational learning, perceived severity, and perceived barriers).

Behavior change principles also can sharpen the focus of diabetes technologies through careful consideration of user experience and user implementation. Both of these domains reflect human factors (e.g., perceptions, beliefs, attitudes, expectations, and preferences) that drive uptake, use, and sustainability of diabetes technologies. To effectively support diabetes management, which is largely driven by behavior, technologies should be flexible to fit the individuality of self-management, and it is unrealistic to expect the individual to change their behavior to fit the technology [9]. As such, attention to the user experience, user implementation, and related human factors can aid designers and developers in creating technology that (1) meets an identified need of the population, (2) adapts to individual preferences, and (3) delivers a pragmatic and hedonic experience.

Given the central role of an individual's self-management behavior in improving diabetes outcomes, it is critical to consider specific behavior change techniques in the use of diabetes technologies. Michie et al. developed an extensive taxonomy of behavior change techniques for behavioral interventions [10], and this taxonomy has been adapted and applied to evaluate diabetes-related interventions [11]. The evaluation of behavior change techniques to diabetes technologies is evolving; yet there remains a significant gap in the utilization and application of behavior change theories and principles to optimize diabetes technologies [6]. The following sections illustrate how behavior change techniques can be applied to promote user engagement with and effective use of diabetes technologies and ultimately promote improvements in health outcomes.

Behavior change techniques for diabetes technologies

Education, skill development, repetition, and tailoring

Diabetes technologies offer novel and accessible platforms to deliver diabetes-specific education and resources, engage users in education, and promote the development of key diabetes skills through practice, repetition, and personalization. Education alone is often not sufficient to change behavior; however, digital health tools can promote interactive, sustained engagement in educational activities, and this information can promote skills in and related confidence for diabetes management. Furthermore, digital health tools can encourage a user to build beneficial habits or routines by explaining how to perform behaviors and providing the user with opportunities to practice and repeat behaviors. For example, a well-designed mobile app delivers diabetes education in multiple ways (e.g., written, auditory, or video) to engage the user and fit the user's learning preferences and literacy needs. This educational content is available outside of a traditional face-to-face medical visit and provides multiple opportunities for reinforcement of key information through repetition, animation, videos, and links to other resources for users who would like to learn more or practice skills. Ideally, the app is able to tailor education to meet the needs and goals of the individual user. A brief "getting to know you" activity when a user initiates an app can help one prioritize education resources and topics of the highest relevance and interest to the user. Content should be periodically reviewed and refreshed to ensure accuracy and capture advances in treatment technology, new research, or new practice guidelines or recommendations.

Educational offerings can be enhanced by informed suggestions based on a user's own data. Pairing education about insulin adjustment or dietary intake with information and feedback from a user's glucose data leverages a user's unique up-to-date glucose information to identify potential behavioral modifications that can enhance glycemic control. For example, guided review of interactive glucose charts and reports available through CGM software promotes the development of advanced problem-solving skills required to identify and interpret glucose trends and identify potential opportunities for intervention. Content also can be targeted based on user inputs to the app via user-input or by wireless connection with devices such as physical activity monitors. For example, if physical activity is logged, then a push notification could link the user with education around managing diabetes during hot-weather exercise or recommended snacks with protein. Patient portals also provide patients with education and resources specific to an individual's diagnosis and treatment plan (e.g., instructions on how to download the patient's specific brand of meter and education about target ranges for lab values completed at the most recent medical visit). Advances in technology that seamlessly integrate a user's glucose, dietary, and activity data with patient portals or electronic health records can minimize user burden and improve treatment planning for persons with diabetes.

Behavioral goal setting, monitoring, feedback, and tracking

Behavior change principles such as goal setting, monitoring, and feedback/tracking are essential to maximize the impact of diabetes technologies.

These behavioral techniques cultivate internal and external motivation for behavior change by allowing users to monitor their performance, use feedback to change or maintain behavior, track activity and accomplishments, and realize progress toward meaningful goals. For example, CGMs provide users with real-time information about glucose levels and alerts if glycemic levels are trending out of an individual user's set target range. This feedback can be a powerful behavior change tool if users are knowledgeable about how to interpret and act on trends and use these data to shape future behavior [12]. Improving the ease of monitoring glucose trends through streamlined glucose device downloading and review and linking glucose data with key contributors to glycemic control, such as physical activity or mood, can improve diabetes outcomes [13]. Research has demonstrated that persons with diabetes who regularly download devices and review data have lower hemoglobin A1c concentrations [14], likely because of increased opportunities to monitor glucose trends, identify and enact effective interventions, and experience positive benefit from these interventions.

Apps and wearable activity monitors also allow the user to set goals and receive feedback about progress toward a target goal (e.g., logging the number of glucose checks per day in relation to the user's target goal for number of glucose checks per day or tracking the number of minutes of physical activity per week). Goals that are set by the user are the most meaningful and have the highest likelihood of being achieved. Furthermore, apps can incorporate a coach function to help the user set and achieve goals by giving personalized feedback on behavior and encouragement (e.g., tells the user that they are a certain percentage closer to reaching their goal). Coaching with a personal or individualized connection with participants may be the most effective and bring a human touch to digital health [15]. Users benefit from guidance on setting appropriate goals and adjusting goals based on progress or lack thereof. Goals that align with the seven core guidelines for diabetes self-management behavior as indicated by the American Association of Diabetes Educators hold promise for behavior change [16].

Cues and rewards

Digital health technologies also provide external cues and rewards for engaging in behaviors that promote health and well-being. Reminders and cues that prompt a user to engage in an activity can encourage the user to build sustainable habits over time. For example, a common feature of apps is providing alerts or reminders for the user to adhere to a component of diabetes management (e.g., an alarm linked to medication/insulin administration or a reminder to refill a prescription). Many apps also incorporate contingency management, or the use of rewards and reinforcement, to increase external motivation and promote behavior change. Reinforcement may be tangible (e.g., points to earn badges or access to a new level or financial incentives) or intangible (e.g., praise and motivational messages for meeting goals). However, it is critical to understand what is reinforcing specific users and that appropriate behaviors are reinforced in a systematic way. For example, an adolescent with type 1 diabetes may set a goal of checking BG levels at least four times per day, and each BG check is reinforced with a digital coin immediately as soon as the level is entered or transmitted into the app. The coins can be cashed in for access to games, new badges, or other incentives. Once the specific goal is met and sustained for a set duration of time, reinforcers can be offered less frequently, eliminated, or changed to address progress toward a new goal and maintain user interest. Reinforcement may be delivered through gamification, in which mobile apps utilize gaming techniques to reward growth in knowledge through education tasks (e.g., quizzes or games to demonstrate knowledge), progress toward a goal, or achievement of an outcome. For example, apps can create competition between users by allowing users to compare progress through elements such as leaderboards; daily or weekly leaderboards offer frequent opportunities for recognizing progress and accomplishments. Character-driven games or virtual environments also improve opportunities for vicarious learning, as users can help a character enact a specific skill or make a positive choice [17]. Furthermore, the addition of contingency management via incentivizing use with cash rewards or donations to charity has been associated with modest increases in activity but it is challenging to sustain gains when the incentive is removed [18].

Social connectivity

Diabetes technologies provide opportunities for behavior change by enabling users to connect with others by sharing data, goals, or behaviors. For example, CGMs can share glucose data in real time with other users, such as parents or partners, to promote shared diabetes management, accountability, and support. Facilitation of social support via online communities also may help device users feel more comfortable with diabetes management and improve integration of diabetes into their identity [19]. Apps can facilitate this social support by allowing the user to share their behaviors with peers on social media or in forums. Peers can "like" progress toward a goal, leave supportive messages, or engage in online conversations about challenges or barriers. Apps can also facilitate connections with providers by enabling users to export and share data directly with electronic health records. Similarly, patient portals facilitate increasing support from the diabetes care team by allowing patients and their health-care professionals to easily access shared data and communicate about treatment needs. Furthermore, wearable devices that track steps or physical activity can incorporate a social aspect to learning, where individuals can engage in social competition and collaboration with others, providing effective feedback loops and improving motivation to engage in physical activity [20].

Barriers to uptake and use

While diabetes technologies hold promise, uptake of technologies such as diabetes devices and patient portals remains challenging [7,21]. Structural, psychological, and demographic barriers impact uptake and sustained use of technology [7]. For example, barriers associated with diabetes devices, such as negative attitudes about technology, disliking wearing a device, the cost of devices, and perceived hassles of use have been associated with lower uptake of diabetes technologies [7,22]. Identified barriers to portal use include challenges accessing portals, low functionality of portal platforms, perceived barriers to using messaging system, lack of integration with diabetes devices (e.g., BG monitors and activity monitors), and concerns about who can access the information (e.g., parents of adolescents) [23]. However, these barriers are potentially modifiable if identified. For example, seamlessly interfacing portals with current diabetes technologies and modifying devices to reduce burdensome tasks (e.g., redundancy of entering glucose data into an insulin pump for dosing) can increase benefits and opportunities for behavior change.

In addition, education and psychosocial interventions can play a role in addressing barriers. Education should focus on potential benefits of and barriers to use of diabetes technologies to guide realistic expectations and promote sustained engagement with technology. While physical and demographic barriers may not be modifiable through psychosocial intervention, interventions can target users' ability to cope with barriers, reducing distress associated with technology use, and increasing self-efficacy to improve attitudes toward diabetes technologies, which can improve motivation and, ultimately, adherence [22].

Considerations for accessibility

While digital health technology can be an effective platform for implementing behavior change, not all individuals have the same level of access to and comfort with use of technology. Often, the same groups who suffer from the greatest burden of diabetes and have worse health outcomes—racial minorities and individuals with limited financial resources—are the least likely to have access to the internet and technology [24]. Furthermore, few diabetes technologies (e.g., mobile apps) attend to principles of health literacy and numeracy and may not present information at a level commensurate with the user's abilities [16]. In addition, the feasibility of using technology changes among age groups (i.e., children, adolescents, young adults, and older adults), and devices need to fit the environments in which they will be used (e.g., school, workplace, or home). Technology can be an especially important tool for delivering healthcare and education, because rural communities may have limited access to specialized care. Therefore as behavior change techniques are applied to digital health, researchers should consider the adaptability of these techniques for both varying frequencies of device use and device use in different environments. These considerations are especially important for addressing the specific needs of at-risk populations who may have limited access to technology.

Conclusion

Diabetes technologies offer significant promise to improve health and well-being for persons with diabetes, but sustained improvements using technology have been elusive to date. It is critical to understand key strategies for behavior change and how these strategies can be implemented into diabetes technology design and use. As guided by human factors research, targeted assessment of potential benefits of and barriers to use of diabetes technologies is needed to ensure alignment of technology with a person's current needs and lifestyle. Features of diabetes technologies can be designed to incorporate facilitators of behavioral change, including attention to opportunities for skill development, individualized goal setting, receiving feedback, and enhancing social support. It is likely not feasible for a diabetes technology to accommodate all of the discussed strategies for behavior change; however, the use of theory to guide key elements of behavior change relevant to a particular diabetes technology or user group can elucidate mechanisms of change and inform efficacious strategies. Greater attention to behavior change techniques also can advance desired outcomes beyond glycemic control to encompass patient-reported outcomes such as quality of life, diabetes distress, and self-efficacy. Furthermore, assessment of an individual's engagement with and use of digital health technologies informs the mechanism of change in health outcomes. Health-care providers play an important role in educating patients on how to effectively and optimally use technology to improve their disease management [25]. This education includes enhancing knowledge and skills needed to tailor device features to adapt to patients' individualized lifestyle and preferences.

The landscape of diabetes technologies is rapidly evolving and the emerging Internet-of-things concept will offer expanded possibilities for connectivity across devices and platforms and increasingly personalized assessment of users' unique environments, routines, and needs. These technological advances will enhance behavior change techniques and inform precision behavioral medicine, with data-driven interventions tailored to meet the unique needs of a particular patient at a particular time. Diabetes technologies also can optimize the utilization of data to deliver just-in-time interventions to provide targeted education, motivation, and feedback for an individual based on a behavior at the present moment.

Diabetes technologies offer novel, accessible, and effective platforms for behavior change. Behavior change theories allow for personalization of these technologies for any individual to facilitate healthy behaviors. Multicomponent interventions utilizing diabetes technologies that provide education with tailored support, feedback, and development of skills coupled with a human component are likely to be the most successful to promote sustained behavior change.

References

[1] Janevic M, Connell C. Individual theories. In: Hilliard M, Riekert K, Ockene J, Pbert L, editors. The handbook of health behavior change. 5th ed. New York: Springer Publishing Company; 2018. p. 3−24.

[2] Klonoff DC. Behavioral theory: the missing ingredient for digital health tools to change behavior and increase adherence. J Diabetes Sci Technol 2019;13(2):276−81.

[3] Bandura A. Health promotion by social cognitive means. Health Educ Behav 2004;31 (2):143−64.

[4] Rosenstock IM, Strecher VJ, Becker MH. Social learning theory and the health belief model. Health Educ Q 1988;15(2):175−83.

[5] Fisher J, Fisher W. The information-motivation-behavioral skills model. In: DiClemente R, Crosby R, Kegler M, editors. Emerging theories in health promotion practice and research: strategies for improving public health. San Francisco, CA: Jossey Bass Publishers; 2002. p. 40−70.

[6] Riley WT, Rivera DE, Atienza AA, Nilsen W, Allison SM, Mermelstein R. Health behavior models in the age of mobile interventions: are our theories up to the task? Transl Behav Med 2011;1(1):53−71.

[7] Naranjo D, Tanenbaum ML, Iturralde E, Hood KK. Diabetes technology: uptake, outcomes, barriers, and the intersection with distress. J Diabetes Sci Technol 2016;10 (4):852−8.

[8] Mayberry LS, Osborn CY. Empirical validation of the information−motivation−behavioral skills model of diabetes medication adherence: a framework for intervention. Diabetes Care 2014;37(5):1246−53.

[9] Liberman A, Barnard K. Diabetes technology and the human factor. Diabetes Technol Ther 2019;21(S1):S138−47.

[10] Michie S, Richardson M, Johnston M, et al. The behavior change technique taxonomy (v1) of 93 hierarchically clustered techniques: building an international consensus for the reporting of behavior change interventions. Ann Behav Med 2013;46(1):81−95.

[11] Yang CH, Maher JP, Conroy DE. Implementation of behavior change techniques in mobile applications for physical activity. Am J Prev Med 2015;48(4):452−5.

[12] American Diabetes Association. Diabetes technology: standards of medical care in diabetes—2019. Diabetes Care 2019;42(Suppl. 1):S71−80.

[13] Clements MA, Staggs VS. A mobile app for synchronizing glucometer data: impact on adherence and glycemic control among youths with type 1 diabetes in routine care. J Diabetes Sci Technol 2017;11(3):461−7.

[14] Wong JC, Neinstein AB, Spindler M, Adi S. A minority of patients with type 1 diabetes routinely downloads and retrospectively reviews device data. Diabetes Technol Ther 2015;17(8):555−62.

[15] Veazie S, Winchell K, Gilbert J, et al. Rapid evidence review of mobile applications for self-management of diabetes. J Gen Intern Med 2018;33(7):1167−76.

[16] Ye Q, Khan U, Boren SA, Simoes EJ, Kim MS. An analysis of diabetes mobile applications features compared to AADE7: addressing self-management behaviors in people with diabetes. J Diabetes Sci Technol 2018;12(4):808–16.

[17] Swartwout E, El-Zein A, Deyo P, Sweenie R, Streisand R. Use of gaming in self-management of diabetes in teens. Curr Diab Rep 2016;16(7):59.

[18] Finkelstein EA, Haaland BA, Bilger M, et al. Effectiveness of activity trackers with and without incentives to increase physical activity (TRIPPA): a randomised controlled trial. Lancet Diabetes Endocrinol 2016;4(12):983–95.

[19] Litchman ML, Walker HR, Ng AH, et al. State of the science: a scoping review and gap analysis of diabetes online communities. J Diabetes Sci Technol 2019;13(3):466–92.

[20] Patel MS, Asch DA, Volpp KG. Wearable devices as facilitators, not drivers, of health behavior change. JAMA 2015;313(5):459–60.

[21] Jones JB, Weiner JP, Shah NR, Stewart WF. The wired patient: patterns of electronic patient portal use among patients with cardiac disease or diabetes. J Med Internet Res 2015;17(2):e42.

[22] Tanenbaum ML, Hanes SJ, Miller KM, Naranjo D, Bensen R, Hood KK. Diabetes device use in adults with type 1 diabetes: barriers to uptake and potential intervention targets. Diabetes Care 2017;40(2):181.

[23] Sun R, Korytkowski M, Sereika S, Saul M, Li D, Burke L. Patient portal use in diabetes management: literature review. JMIR Diabetes 2018;3(4):e11199.

[24] Cotter AP, Durant N, Agne AA, Cherrington AL. Internet interventions to support lifestyle modification for diabetes management: a systematic review of the evidence. J Diabetes Complications 2014;28(2):243–51.

[25] Beck J, Greenwood DA, Blanton L, et al. 2017 National standards for diabetes self-management education and support. Diabetes Educ 2018;44(1):35–50.

Chapter 6

Integrating behavior and context with glucose data to advance behavioral science and clinical care in diabetes

Claire J. Hoogendoorn[1], Dominic Ehrmann[2,3], Gladys Crespo-Ramos[1], Arielle G. Asman[1] and Jeffrey S. Gonzalez[1,4,5,6]

[1]*Ferkauf Graduate School of Psychology, Yeshiva University, Bronx, NY, United States,* [2]*Research Institute Diabetes Academy Mergentheim (FIDAM), Diabetes Center Mergentheim, Bad Mergentheim, Germany,* [3]*Department of Clinical Psychology and Psychotherapy, University of Bamberg, Bamberg, Germany,* [4]*Departments of Medicine (Endocrinology) and Epidemiology and Population Health, Albert Einstein College of Medicine, Bronx, NY, United States,* [5]*The Fleischer Institute for Diabetes and Metabolism, Albert Einstein College of Medicine, Bronx, NY, United States,* [6]*The New York Regional Center for Diabetes Translation Research (NY-CDTR), Albert Einstein College of Medicine, Bronx, NY, United States*

Abbreviations

AGP	ambulatory glucose profile
CGM	continuous glucose monitoring
EMA	ecological momentary assessment
FDA	US Food and Drug Administration
HbA1c	hemoglobin A1c
JITAIs	just-in-time adaptive interventions
NA	negative affect
PA	positive affect
PRO	patient-reported outcome
SMBG	self-monitoring of blood glucose
SMS	short message service
SR	self-report
T1D	type 1 diabetes
T2D	type 2 diabetes

Diabetes Digital Health. DOI: https://doi.org/10.1016/B978-0-12-817485-2.00006-7

Key points

- The examination and layering of fluctuations in experiences, behavior, and glucose concentrations that occur in an individual over time (i.e., individual differences from day-to-day) may advance the understanding of dynamic temporal associations (e.g., glycemic variability and variability in experience across a day) and possible causal patterns (e.g., glucose affecting mood vs mood affecting glucose) to improve diabetes therapy and outcomes.
- While technological advances have made it easier to collect complex psychological, contextual, behavioral, and glycemic data over time, more standardization is needed in terms of (1) methodological best practices; (2) the selection of variables and their validity and reliability; and (3) the aggregation of data, when it comes to modeling dynamic relationships.
- As the clinical value of assessing experiences, behavior, and context in daily life in relation to glycemic variability is not yet established, researchers and clinicians should focus on identifying meaningful and detailed individual trajectories that can facilitate patient-centered clinical care and the development of individualized interventions.

Introduction

Diabetes has long been recognized for providing an important paradigm for behavioral science research exploring the effects of behavior and psychological states on glucose regulation and control [1]. Mechanisms underlying these associations are believed to be bidirectional, and both physiological and behavioral in nature. A central aspect of diabetes management is psychological, as individuals with diabetes must cope with having a chronic condition that requires constant treatment and attention. Psychological states, such as feeling distressed, can directly affect glucose concentrations via physiological pathways and can also indirectly influence glucose through their negative effects on diabetes self-care behaviors (e.g., adherence to diet, physical activity, and medication). Today, with new technologies developing rapidly, the examination of dynamic influences between experience, behavior, and glucose concentrations is more possible than ever before.

The development of continuous glucose monitoring (CGM) systems has allowed individuals with diabetes more immediate and complete knowledge of their glucose levels. These systems provide feedback about trends that can inform compensatory actions to avoid hyper- and hypoglycemic states. In this way, technology directly contributes to the dynamic relationship between experience and behavior. CGM also provides clinicians the opportunity to assess a variety of glucose metrics beyond hemoglobin A1c (HbA1c), which reflects mean glucose levels over the prior 3 months, including CGM-derived glycemic variability, % time in range (70−180 mg/dL), % time in hypoglycemia (<70 mg/dL), and % time in hyperglycemia (>180 mg/dL). Measures capturing fluctuations and variability in glucose are important to consider, because glycemic variability has been postulated to be an HbA1c-independent risk factor for diabetic complications [2] and is associated with quality of life and treatment satisfaction [3]. Further, these metrics allow clinicians, researchers, and individuals with diabetes to better understand how glucose levels and variability relate to daily experience and behavior.

A person's experiences and expectations are central to the successful adoption of new diabetes therapy regimens and technologies, which in turn influence diabetes outcomes. For example, negative perceptions, experiences, or expectations toward insulin therapy among individuals with type 2 diabetes (T2D) affect willingness to accept insulin treatment, which was coined "psychological insulin resistance" [4]. In type 1 diabetes (T1D), research shows that the successful adoption of new technologies such as CGM and continuous subcutaneous insulin injection therapy is closely associated with expectations and early experiences with these technologies [5]. For these reasons, patient-reported outcomes (PROs) that capture individual experiences are important. The US Food and Drug Administration (FDA) emphasizes that systematic inclusion of PROs can provide valuable information to inform evaluations of treatments and technologies in ways that are important to individuals with diabetes [6]. Current influential treatment recommendations from the American Diabetes Association emphasize that glycemic targets and treatment selection should be based on a person's "preferences, needs, and values" [7]. This increased focus on PROs is in line with patient-centered care and the goal of developing individualized treatment. While PROs are often examined in relation to distal diabetes health outcomes (e.g., HbA1c concentrations, complications, and mortality), less research has been conducted on moment-to-moment relationships between experience and behavior, the role of situational and social context (e.g., time of day or the presence of others), and their real-time associations with parameters of glycemic control.

In this chapter, we first review why it is important to assess variability in experience, self-care behavior, and glucose concentrations that occur for individuals over time and in different situations, and we review technology options for measurement. Next, we discuss the role of contextual factors like time of day that can be related to variation in peoples' experiences, mood, behavior, and glycemic control. We also discuss the clinical value of assessing experiences, behavior, and context in daily life in relation to glycemic variability to facilitate patient-centered clinical care and the development of individualized interventions. Finally, future directions are identified. In our review of the literature, we have integrated studies of T1D and T2D given limited research conducted and the equivalence of methods for data collection. However, generalizing findings of this research from one condition to the other is premature, based on the available evidence.

Variability in experience, behavior, and glucose in diabetes

Clinicians and researchers are interested in people's daily real-world experiences and behaviors surrounding their diabetes, yet traditional research methods often involve asking individuals to report global, retrospective self-reports (SRs) of experience and behavior in a laboratory room or doctor's office (e.g., level of depression over the past 2 weeks). This traditional emphasis on global assessments limits our ability to accurately characterize dynamic day-to-day and hour-to-hour changes in experience, self-care behavior, and glucose concentrations as life is lived [8]. One's mood and experiences, self-care behaviors, and glucose values are known to fluctuate throughout the day and week, and these fluctuations are influenced by context. Self-care behaviors to maintain glycemic control need to be carried out in a variety of contexts, including places such as work/school/home and often around meals. In addition, to maintain good glycemic control, self-care behaviors need to be carried out independent from mood or feeling motivated or not. For these reasons, it is important that dynamic relationships between experience and behavior are measured close to (in time and context) when they naturally occur [8]. This approach requires novel methodology facilitated by technology that repeatedly (1) assesses experience, behavior, glucose concentrations, and context and (2) documents temporal sequences to identify individual trajectories, rather than the traditional focus on differences between persons and groups based on one or two assessments.

The omnipresence of smartphones has allowed researchers to more easily implement and fine-tune novel methodological approaches to data collection that repeatedly measure experiences, behavior, and context in real-time as part of the patient's daily routine. This process is referred to as ecological momentary assessment (EMA) or experience sampling. EMA variables are often based on a person's SRs, and thus many EMA variables could be considered momentary PROs. In fact, EMA has been referred to as the gold standard for the assessment of PROs because data is collected in the individual's daily environment, leading to increased ecological validity. Furthermore, assessment of in-the-moment experiences limits recalls biases and error inherent in most SR and interview methods [8]. EMA can also capture contextual factors, such as whether a person is alone or with others, or if they are at work/school/home, or another location. While self-reported contextual variables may not fit the FDA definition of a PRO [6], such questions can identify individually based modifiable conditions that are associated with both optimal and suboptimal self-care. In this way, EMA methodology advances our capability to more proximally and specifically evaluate and address contextual barriers and facilitators of diabetes self-care.

EMA approaches examining moment-to-moment associations between different parameters of glycemic control and experience, behavior, and context allow for a more detailed and dynamic understanding of established cross-sectional relationships. Cross-sectional relationships based on traditional questionnaire methods are well-documented between glycemic control and PROs such as depressive symptoms, diabetes distress, and poor adherence to self-care. A methodological approach, such as EMA that captures granular data for individual persons over time in various contexts, can help further elucidate these established associations in ways that are more applicable to the daily life of people with diabetes. Initial findings from studies repeatedly assessing experience, behavior, and glucose concentrations within one person suggest that measures of variability are important. For example, previous EMA work suggests that mental health disorders like depression are associated with greater daily variability in negative affect (NA) [9], and this may influence the established relationships between depression, poor adherence to self-care, and poor glycemic control. Further, a study involving a small sample of 50 Latinos with T2D using blinded CGM for 7 days showed that higher variability in self-care was associated with a higher percentage of glucose values out of range (either <70 or >180 mg/dL) [10].

However, only a handful of studies have been conducted that assess variability in experience, behavior, and glucose concentrations among individuals with diabetes. Many of these studies have small sample sizes and are focused on dynamic relationships between affect or mood and changes in glucose concentrations. One study of 45 insulin-treated adults with T2D showed that the rate of change in glucose concentration after breakfast and dinner was associated with momentary NA but not with positive affect (PA) 1 hour later over a 4-week period [11]. A blinded CGM study of 36 adults with T1D showed that current glucose values and area under the curve during the prior hour were associated with momentary PA and NA, while glycemic variability was not associated with PA or NA [12]. This matches a more recent finding where glycemic variability assessed by blinded CGM over 7 days showed no associations with momentary PA or NA among 50 Latino adults with T2D [10]. Overall, the authors only found associations between NA variability and higher mean glucose concentrations and lower % time in range, as well as an association between PA variability and lower % time in hypoglycemia [10]. Jointly, findings indicate that NA may show a stronger association with glucose concentrations than PA, and associations between mood and glycemic variability have not been convincingly shown in blinded CGM studies in which information about variability is not accessible to participants. Additional studies are needed using larger samples of people with diabetes that integrate variability in affect and glucose concentrations with self-care behavior and context.

Various forms of technology can be used to assess a person's experiences, context, behavior, and glycemic variability in daily life. Continuously tracking glucose concentrations is important for the accurate assessment of glycemic variability, and CGM data can be used to further calculate a variety of glycemic parameters that are related to glycemic variability including mean glucose concentrations and % time in range [13]. The use of a smartphone app is particularly common for collecting participant experiences and context, because participants can answer the questions directly on their smartphone, and passive contextual data can be easily integrated. Behaviors associated with glycemic control such as physical activity, medication-taking, and sleep can be tracked daily using smart devices, wearables, and apps, with commonly used technologies listed in Table 6.1.

Contextual factors

Daily life involves many contextual factors that may affect patient experience, behavior, and glucose values. Collection of real-time data using technology provides a unique opportunity to assess potential contextual influences. As technology makes it possible to track individuals continuously, specific barriers and facilitators of adherence to self-care behaviors can be identified [14]. Such information could then inform the development of interventions that can be tailored to times of the day that are individually relevant and can provide situational prompts or skills (e.g., planning) that could assist the individual in overcoming barriers to adherence behaviors [15]. Yet, studies are limited that examine contextual influences on adherence to self-care among individuals with diabetes in a granular manner and in real-time.

The roles of time of day or week, current activities, location, and presence of others may be important for studies examining psychosocial factors and glycemic variability. For example, diurnal physiological fluctuations may influence affect and behavior throughout the day, while affect, symptoms, and behaviors may also fluctuate based on time of day or week for reasons related to context, such as increased fatigue in the evening or increased happiness on Saturday versus Monday. While some work has examined daily fluctuations in affect among working women [16], studies that examine diurnal patterns in affect among individuals with diabetes could not be located. Similarly, no consistent diurnal glucose concentration pattern has emerged among those with diabetes [17]. However, big data collected from 2.2 million glucose monitors worldwide showed that the highest glucose values occurred during the weekend (Friday−Sunday), with hyperglycemia being most likely to occur at 11:00 p.m. on Saturday and hypoglycemia most likely to occur at 02:00 a.m. on Thursday [18]. The same report showed a peak frequency of glucose testing between 05:00 and 09:00 a.m. and its lowest point between 01:00 and 03:00 a.m. Among adolescents with T1D, one study [15] found that mornings were a time that many adolescents forgot to administer insulin or perform self-monitoring of blood glucose (SMBG), while evening time was associated with the highest adherence to these behaviors. In addition, bedtime was associated with lower adherence to app questions

TABLE 6.1 Commonly used technologies to assess daily glucose parameters, experiences, self-care behaviors and context.

Construct	Measures of interest	Technologies used	Considerations
Glycemic parameters	<ul><li>Glycemic variability</li><li>Time in range</li><li>Time in hypo- and hyperglycemia</li></ul>	<ul><li>Blinded or open continuous glucose monitors</li></ul>	<ul><li>Can assess variation continuously</li><li>Large amount of data</li><li>Ideal assessment intervals</li></ul>
Patient-reported outcomes	<ul><li>Presence of clinical disorders (e.g., depression)</li><li>Affect and mood</li><li>Motivation and coping</li><li>Self-rated health</li><li>Quality of life</li></ul>	<ul><li>Smartphone applications</li><li>SMS-delivered online surveys</li><li>Computer-based surveys</li><li>Audio recording devices, including voice recognition technology</li><li>Phone-based interviews</li></ul>	<ul><li>Reduces bias, more ecologically valid</li><li>Measures are often unvalidated</li><li>Burden and ease of use for participants</li></ul>
Context	<ul><li>Time of day</li><li>Presence of others</li><li>Current activities</li><li>Location</li></ul>	<ul><li>Smartphone applications (SR, passive)</li><li>SMS-delivered online surveys (SR)</li><li>Wearable wristbands (activity)</li><li>Geolocation (location)</li><li>Audio recording devices</li></ul>	<ul><li>Contextual data can often be collected passively</li><li>Data can be sensitive to error (e.g., timestamps)</li></ul>
Medication adherence	<ul><li>Oral medications</li><li>Injectable medications (e.g., insulin and glucagon like peptide-1 receptor agonists)</li><li>Inhaled insulin</li></ul>	<ul><li>Smartphone applications (SR)</li><li>SMS-delivered online surveys (SR)</li><li>Electronic medication caps</li><li>Smart insulin pens</li><li>Insulin pump data</li><li>Blood glucose monitors with wireless data transmission</li></ul>	<ul><li>No "gold standard" (e.g., SR vs objective) for assessing medication adherence</li><li>Smart devices can send a bluetooth signal alerting nonadherence and facilitate just-in-time adaptive interventions</li></ul>

(Continued)

TABLE 6.1 (Continued)

Construct	Measures of interest	Technologies used	Considerations
Physical activity	<ul><li>Steps taken</li><li>Heart rate</li><li>Heart rate variability</li><li>Sedentary behavior</li></ul>	<ul><li>Smartphone applications (SR)</li><li>SMS-delivered online surveys (SR)</li><li>Wearable wristbands</li></ul>	<ul><li>Many technology options</li><li>Accuracy of measures unclear</li><li>Large amount of data (e.g., every minute)</li></ul>
Diet and food choices	<ul><li>Calories consumed</li><li>Carbohydrates consumed</li><li>Protein and fat consumed</li><li>Food choices (e.g., soda and vegetables)</li></ul>	<ul><li>Smartphone applications (SR)</li><li>SMS-delivered online surveys (SR)</li><li>Cameras</li><li>CGM monitors (excursions)</li></ul>	<ul><li>Large amount of data</li><li>Often requires additional coding (e.g., images)</li><li>Selective or incomplete use of monitoring technology can often be a problem</li></ul>
Sleep	<ul><li>Hours slept</li><li>Time in REM</li><li>Number of awakenings</li><li>Sleep quality</li></ul>	<ul><li>Smartphone applications (SR)</li><li>SMS-delivered online surveys (SR)</li><li>Wearable wristbands</li></ul>	<ul><li>Wearables allow for objectively quantifying sleep, though sleep is assessed indirectly, high noise</li></ul>

REM, Rapid eye movement; SR, self-report; SMS, short message service.

compared to mealtimes [19]. Current activities and social context can also influence patient experience, self-care behaviors, and glucose concentrations [20]. Examination of potential barriers to self-care behaviors associated with a time of day, activity, or social context may be helpful in improving adherence. In addition, assessing how context may influence variability of experience, behavior, or glucose concentrations would increase our understanding of dynamic relationships.

Sociocultural and socioeconomic factors have also received insufficient attention in relation to daily variability in experience, behavior, and glycemic variability. Black and Hispanic individuals tend to have higher HbA1c values compared to non-Hispanic Caucasians (e.g., [21]). However, population-based survey data collected from US adults with T1D and T2D shows few ethnic differences in diabetes self-care [22]. Consistent potential racial or ethnic differences in variability in PROs, behavior and glycemic variability remain to be determined. Socioeconomic disadvantage does appear to be related to self-care and can be a significant barrier to diabetes technology use [23].

Insights for clinical care

Clinical assessment

The intensive longitudinal data collected using EMA methodology allows for the modeling of meaningful relationships within a single individual (i.e., an n-of-1 time series analysis), which can provide clinicians with a useful clinical picture of an individual patient. Clinicians can combine CGM and EMA-generated data to assess glycemic variability, related glucose metrics (e.g., % time in range), and daily experiences and behaviors to improve diabetes outcomes. There is a growing focus on integrating diabetes technology into electronic health records so that providers can directly access CGM and app-based data [24]. Such integration may improve provider decision-making, patient engagement in self-care, as well as health outcomes [24]. However, provider access to such data also creates new problems, including data privacy and how providers should respond to real- or near real-time data.

In addition, interpreting intensive longitudinal data (either from CGM or EMA) for a single person can be overwhelming, especially within the context of a brief doctor visit. Solutions to this problem will depend on the development of analytics that can create data summaries and identify centrally important information. One such approach uses the ambulatory glucose profile (AGP), which creates an aggregate visual for an average day from multiple days of CGM data and indicates the median level of the glucose concentration and glucose fluctuations [17]. Thus the AGP can facilitate quick identification of underlying patterns that affect clinical decisions, such as medication management.

The use of AGP as well as daily data on affect, symptoms, and self-care behaviors in clinical care can also be helpful in communicating the bidirectionality of these measures to people with diabetes and identify modifiable patterns. The visual nature of presented data such as AGP allows individuals to better understand their own glycemic patterns and could assist in engaging them with their diabetes care. For example, clinicians and individuals with diabetes can identify specific times of day, behaviors, or mood states that co-occur with or precede hypoglycemia, in order to modify future patterns.

Interventions and treatments

Interventions must account for an individual's changing internal and contextual states to be most effective. Thus understanding the relationship between experiences, behaviors, context, and various glucose parameters is valuable for informing the design of interventions and treatments. Greater insight into these relationships could allow clinicians and researchers to tailor interventions specific to the needs and behaviors of people with diabetes. In addition, the use of real-time data allows for opportunities to intervene in the moment, in a person's daily life through the development of technology-based algorithms that detect and respond to relevant behavioral patterns. Just-in-time adaptive interventions (JITAIs), which deliver in-the-moment interventions when needed in real-world settings [6,14], are growing in popularity. Algorithms based on an individual's history could tailor in-the-moment suggestions (e.g., coping or relaxation) based on what works for the individual. Predictive algorithms can also be used to anticipate challenges before they gain momentum and can allow for intervention before the maladaptive behavior occurs. Edge computing in a network, where decisions are made at the sensor level rather than on the cloud, is becoming increasingly established, and this paradigm will facilitate JITAI. Shiffman et al. reviewed several applications, such as treatment for addiction and eating disorders, but pointed out that JITAIs have received limited evaluation [8]. These interventions seem promising, but it is currently too early to identify how effective they will be compared to traditional interventions, or whether they can be effectively integrated with usual care.

Initial work involving app-based interventions support the idea that individualized feedback on tracked data holds the potential for improving adherence to self-care and glycemic control. For example, one study [19] found that viewing app feedback was negatively associated with missed mealtime SMBG among adolescents with T1D. The authors noted that the best interventional use of self-monitoring and feedback is likely to be the one that follows a cyclical pattern, is goal-focused, and involves problem-solving. In addition, it will be important to emphasize the timing of feedback in relation to self-care behaviors. This approach could contribute to the development of more contextually relevant feedback that can facilitate in-the moment self-care decision-making that is more impactful. Adherence to apps is also useful to consider. One study [19] showed generally high to moderate adherence to four app prompts over 30 days among adolescents with T1D and low app adherence was associated with male gender, higher HbA1c values, and missed SMBG. Promoting engagement in intervention-based apps is needed for these digital health tools to be effective.

New insights into the possibilities of diabetes technology to control glucose are also created by people with diabetes themselves. The "Do It Yourself" movement has been gaining momentum, with people creating their own "artificial pancreas" or "closed loop" systems out of existing diabetes technologies, and pushing the limits of gaining near-normal glucose control [25]. Many users make their data available to researchers, which creates an open-source culture that can be used to study glucose and its variability in large samples in real-life environments. Their experiences and data make it possible to analyze how diabetes technology, especially relating to insulin delivery, still requires adjustment and monitoring to minimize burden and maximize satisfaction.

Future directions

Developing the empirical basis for building dynamic models of the relations between experience, behavior, glucose concentrations, and context requires methodologies that utilize granular temporal data that can now be collected using technology. While technological advances have made it easier to collect complex psychological, contextual, behavioral, physiological, and glycemic data over time, the integration of these data is challenging because of the sheer amount of data and different temporal resolutions. Thus, when it comes to modeling dynamic relationships, more standards are needed for methodological best practices, data aggregation, and the selection of valid and reliable variables.

In addition, future work should continue to (1) examine the role of feedback in behavioral change when using technology as part of diabetes care and (2) characterize the benefits and burdens of feedback. For example, it is unknown whether the use of unblinded versus blinded CGM may influence self-care differently, and the assessment of the benefits and burdens of CGM feedback requires further attention. The impact of feedback from technology on dynamic relationships between PROs, self-care behavior, and glucose concentrations should also be examined. Previous studies have mainly relied on blinded CGM, meaning that individuals do not have real-time access to their glucose recordings, and the use of blinded versus unblinded CGM may have moderating effects on dynamic relationships. In addition, greater clarity is needed regarding (1) which glycemic parameters (e.g., variability, mean value, and % time in range) is most closely associated with variability in experience, behavior, and contexts; (2) which time-frames, if any, apply for different parameters; and (3) which directional pathway is strongest (e.g., glucose parameters influencing experience, or vice versa).

Behavioral and intervention theories that include temporal specificity and consider dynamic processes are needed for the successful development of JITAIs [14]. When existing theories acknowledge the dynamic nature of underlying mechanisms, these theories often do not specify how such mechanisms may change across time. Nahum-Shani et al. [14] point out that this need for temporal data can be illustrated with emotional distress. Emotional distress is known to be dynamic and change over time and contexts. Yet, current theories do not describe what the specific temporal dynamics of emotional distress may look like. For example, it is unclear what a meaningful change in distress would be and how much time such a change would take. Such detailed insights on timing and change are needed to better understand and model the dynamics of psychological processes to inform how and when interventions could intervene.

Conclusion

Technology has become increasingly central in diabetes care. The ability to assess variability in experiences, behavior, and contexts using technology, and examine these variability patterns concurrently, allows for nearly endless possibilities to assess the relation between glucose concentrations and self-management. This, in turn, provides clinicians with new treatment options and provides behavioral researchers with completely new perspectives and research questions. Studies are still rather scarce but pilot studies offer insights into the association between fluctuations in affect or mood, self-care behaviors, and glucose control [10]. Insights remain to be gained in the areas of (1) directionality of relationships, (2) individual patterns and trajectories, and (3) the impact of contextual factors on variability.

The ability to assess and model individual trajectories of experience, behavior, and glycemic variability goes hand in hand with a growing movement toward patient-centered care, and a growing acceptance that the experience of those affected is fundamental. With an ever-increasing capability to collect massive amounts of data, the process of managing and interpreting this data becomes more challenging. Future improvements will be needed to address the challenges that big data place on researchers, clinicians, and people with diabetes. Ultimately, interpretation of these data streams will inform the development of personalized and patient-centered psychological, behavioral, and public health interventions. This, in turn, may improve diabetes control and outcomes, as well as the physical and emotional functioning and quality of life of people with diabetes.

Grant support

This work was in part supported by the Einstein—Mount Sinai Diabetes Research Center (P30 DK020541) and the New York Regional Center for Diabetes Translation Research (P30 DK111022). In addition, J.S.G. is supported by grants R01 DK104845, R18 DK098742, R01 DK121298, and R01 DK121896 from the National Institutes of Health. C.J.H. and G.C.R. are supported by Drs. David and Jane Willner Bloomgarden Family Fellowship Fund.

References

[1]   Surwit RS, Feinglos MN, Scovern AW. Diabetes and behavior. A paradigm for health psychology. Am Psychol 1983;38:255—62.

[2]   Brownlee M, Hirsch IB. Glycemic variability: a hemoglobin A1c-independent risk factor for diabetic complications. JAMA 2006;295:1707—8.

[3]   Ayano-Takahara S, Ikeda K, Fujimoto S, Hamasaki A, Harashima S, Toyoda K, et al. Glycemic variability is associated with quality of life and treatment satisfaction in patients with type 1 diabetes. Diabetes Care 2015;38:e1-e2.

[4]   Polonsky WH, Fisher L, Guzman S, Villa-Caballero L, Edelman SV. Psychological insulin resistance in patients with type 2 diabetes: the scope of the problem. Diabetes Care 2005;28(10):2543—5.

[5]   Gonder-Frederick LA, Shepard J, Peterson N. Closed-loop glucose control: psychological and behavioral considerations. J Diabetes Sci Technol 2011;5(6):1387—95.

[6]   U.S. Food and Drug Administration. Guidance for industry: patient-reported outcome measures: use in medical product development to support labeling claims: draft guidance. Health Qual Life Outcomes 2006;4:1—20.

[7]   American Diabetes Association. 6. Glycemic targets: standards of medical care in diabetes—2018. Diabetes Care 2018;41(Suppl. 1):S55—64.

[8]   Shiffman S, Stone AA, Hufford MR. Ecological momentary assessment. Annu Rev Clin Psychol 2008;4:1—32.

[9]   Thompson RJ, Mata J, Jaeggi SM, Buschkuehl M, Jonides J, Gotlib IH. The everyday emotional experience of adults with major depressive disorder: examining emotional instability, inertia, and reactivity. J Abnorm Psychol 2012;121(4):819—29.

[10] Wagner J, Armeli S, Tennen H, Bermudez-Millan A, Wolpert H, Pérez-Escamilla R. Mean levels and variability in affect, diabetes self-care behaviors, and continuously monitored glucose: a daily study of Latinos with type 2 diabetes. Psychosom Med 2017;79 (7):798—805.

[11] Cox DJ, McCall A, Kovatchev B, Sarwat S, Ilag LL, Tan MH. Effects of blood glucose rate of changes on perceived mood and cognitive symptoms in insulin-treated type 2 diabetes. Diabetes Care 2007;30(8):2001—2.

[12] Hermanns N, Scheff C, Kulzer B, Weyers P, Pauli P, Kubiak T, et al. Association of glucose levels and glucose variability with mood in type 1 diabetic patients. Diabetologia 2007;50(5):930—3.

[13] Danne T, Nimri R, Battelino T, Bergenstal RM, Close KL, DeVries JH, et al. International consensus on use of continuous glucose monitoring. Diabetes Care 2017;40 (12):1631—40.

[14] Nahum-Shani I, Smith SN, Spring BJ, Collins LM, Witkiewitz K, Tewari A, et al. Just-in-time adaptive interventions (JITAIs) in mobile health: key components and design principles for ongoing health behavior support. Ann Behav Med 2017;52(6):446−62.

[15] Mulvaney SA, Rothman RL, Dietrich MS, Wallston KA, Grove E, Elasy TA, et al. Using mobile phones to measure adolescent diabetes adherence. Health Psychol 2012;31(1):43.

[16] Stone AA, Schwartz JE, Schkade D, Schwarz N, Krueger A, Kahneman D. A population approach to the study of emotion: diurnal rhythms of a working day examined with the day reconstruction method. Emotion 2006;6(1):139.

[17] Evans M, Cranston I, Bailey CJ. Ambulatory glucose profile (AGP): utility in UK clinical practice. Br J Diabetes 2017;17(1):26−33.

[18] Glooko [internet]. Annual diabetes report, Available from: <https://www.glooko.com/resource/2018-annual-diabetes-report-1/>; 2018 [accessed on 09.03.19].

[19] Mulvaney SA, Vaala S, Hood KK, Lybarger C, Carroll R, Williams L, et al. Mobile momentary assessment and biobehavioral feedback for adolescents with type 1 diabetes: feasibility and engagement patterns. Diabetes Technol Ther 2018;20(7):465−74.

[20] Borus JS, Blood E, Volkening LK, Laffel L, Shrier LA. Momentary assessment of social context and glucose monitoring adherence in adolescents with type 1 diabetes. J Adolesc Health 2013;52(5):578−83.

[21] Kirk JK, Passmore LV, Bell RA, Narayan KV, D'agostino RB, Arcury TA, et al. Disparities in A1C levels between Hispanic and non-Hispanic white adults with diabetes: a meta-analysis. Diabetes Care 2008;31(2):240−6.

[22] Johnson PJ, Ghildayal N, Rockwood T, Everson-Rose SA. Differences in diabetes self-care activities by race/ethnicity and insulin use. Diabetes Educ 2014;40(6):767−77.

[23] Tanenbaum ML, Adams RN, Hanes SJ, Barley RC, Miller KM, Mulvaney SA, et al. Optimal use of diabetes devices: clinician perspectives on barriers and adherence to device use. J Diabetes Sci Technol 2017;11(3):484−92.

[24] Kumar RB, Goren ND, Stark DE, Wall DP, Longhurst CA. Automated integration of continuous glucose monitor data in the electronic health record using consumer technology. J Am Med Inform Assoc 2016;23(3):532−7.

[25] Lee JM, Newman MW, Gebremariam A, Choi P, Lewis D, Nordgren W, et al. Real-world use and self-reported health outcomes of a patient-designed do-it-yourself mobile technology system for diabetes: lessons for mobile health. Diabetes Technol Ther 2017;19(4):209−19.

Chapter 7

Designing human-centered user experiences and user interfaces

Erin Henkel[1,2], Jessica Randazza-Pade[2,3] and Ben Healy[2,4,5]

[1]*Industrial Design, California College of the Arts, San Francisco, CA, United States,* [2]*IDEO, Chicago, IL, United States,* [3]*Communications Studies, University of Alabama at Birmingham, Birmingham, AL, United States,* [4]*Michener Center for Writers at the University of Texas at Austin, Austin, TX, United States,* [5]*American Studies, Brown University, Providence, RI, United States*

Abbreviations

AI	artificial/augmented intelligence
CDE	certified diabetes educator
GDPR	General Data Protection Regulation
HbA1c	hemoglobin A1c concentration
HCP	health-care professional
UI	user interface
UX	user experience

Key points

- Good UX/UI meets users where they are cognitively, physically, and emotionally.
- Create "give−get" loops that provide a good user experience and create a complete cycle of action when utilizing data from people.
- Do not be limited by the boundaries of digital experiences and the devices used when considering UX/UI.

The opportunity

Worldwide, the number of people living with diabetes continues to rise. Human-centered design can make a tremendous difference in creating digital experiences related to diabetes for all relevant stakeholders. This includes people with diabetes, physicians, diabetes educators, businesses working to improve standards of care, and organizations involved in paying for care.

Diabetes Digital Health. DOI: https://doi.org/10.1016/B978-0-12-817485-2.00007-9

Human-centered design considers how stakeholders can work more meaning-fully together to improve quality of life and outcomes and also reduce the cost of diabetes care. Thoughtfully designing user experiences (UXs) and user interfaces (UIs) requires (1) knowing what digital experiences are good for, (2) being thoughtful and intentional about context, and (3) recognizing the necessity of handling data responsibly. There also needs to be intentional thinking about the desired outcomes, as engagement is not necessarily the goal. Overall, we need to enable better health outcomes for people with diabetes by building self-efficacy so that they can express as much control as possible in the context of their care.

Diabetes and dimensions of design

Through relationships with industry stakeholders, design companies have explored and sought to address the challenges associated with diabetes through five dimensions of design. These include research, product design, interaction design, service design, and venture design.

Human-centered design, user experience, and user interface

Human-centered design is used to understand and solve complex problems. This means that for any kind of solution that is proposed, we first learn deeply from the people we are designing for and make room for them to describe their problems in their own voices. We are not talking about focus groups and surveys. Designers often need to spend time with the target audi-ence in their homes and day-to-day lives. We often design research activities to experience first-hand much of what these target users experience in their lives. For example, our designers have arranged to be admitted as patients in hospitals. There, they have tested their blood glucose levels, performed self-injections, tried unfamiliar diets, and subscribed to health coaching ser-vices—all to internalize and design in the context of what is being asked of the people we are designing for. Human-centered design requires empathy and a willingness to experiment, prototype, and iterate in the interest of inno-vation that is appropriate for those who need it.

Over decades of creating products, services, experiences, and ventures, we have seen how human-centered design can unlock real, lasting impact. We use the skills of design thinking, including desirability, viability, and fea-sibility [1] to apply what we learn about human needs and create solutions that are both technically feasible and economically viable. In order to help people with diabetes and support prevention, it is essential to learn from the people who are making daily trade-offs—and involve and empower them as active collaborators.

Ultimately, we are particularly concerned with UX and the ways in which people interact with the products and services we design. To achieve this, we need to consider some basic questions: is it clear how to navigate and find information? Does the design give people confidence by responding the way they expect? Does it transcend mere functionality and become something people enjoy?

The UI of an app or website is the outer layer of this experience—the most tangible representation of icons, buttons, photos, and text. But it is just the tip of the iceberg, representing a deeper set of decisions around the structure and behavior of the system. That is why these acronyms are often tied together: UX and UI are inextricably linked.

It is important to note that while we often talk about end users (i.e., people with diabetes), health-care professionals (HCPs) are also users of the diabetes digital products and services we design, so their needs must be considered as well. Too often the UX/UI for these professional users is deprioritized. This can have a doubly negative effect, frustrating not only the HCP but also trickling down to damage the connections these professionals have with people with diabetes. Human-centered design can help to maintain a holistic approach that considers all interactions among all relevant participants, not just the needs of individual users.

Lessons learned and principles for design

Grounding ourselves in human-centered design, we have identified several design principles to serve as guides for ongoing work. These principles can be applied in the design of any product or service intended for use by people with diabetes, and perhaps for people with other chronic diseases, as well.

Meet users where they are

Human-centered design means designing for a user's whole life context: income, employment, food preferences, emotional issues (e.g., shame, fear, and happiness), and the challenges of ongoing monitoring of any aspect of life, from children who are learning how diabetes affects them as they grow to older individuals living with diabetes-related complications, including neuropathy and impaired vision. Health-care providers are users too and as much as they might focus on their need for precision, data, and control as professionals, they also will respond to digital experiences that are clear, beautiful, and delightful, and also feel modern. We must consider the expectations, learned behaviors, and technological capabilities that each user brings to the experience. Users are often on their smartphones. It is noteworthy that racial and ethnic minorities and lower income Americans are more likely to rely solely on a smartphone (rather than a computer) for online access (Fig. 7.1) [2].

When designing a UX, we map out the full user journey to the extent that we are able. In that journey the user will likely interact with the digital

Mobile phone ownership over time

The vast majority of Americans – 96% – now own a cellphone of some kind. The share of Americans that own smartphones is now 81%, up from just 35% in Pew Research Center's first survey of smartphone ownership conducted in 2011. Along with mobile phones, Americans own a range of other information devices. Nearly three-quarters of U.S. adults now own desktop or laptop computers, while roughly half now own tablet computers and roughly half own e-reader devices.

% of U.S. adults who own the following devices

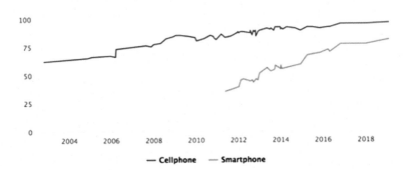

Source: Surveys conducted 2002-2019.

PEW RESEARCH CENTER

FIGURE 7.1   Growth of US Smartphone adoption—Pew 2017 [2].

product or service being designed in noncontiguous intervals. We must understand the user's emotional state as it may change through the different steps of a journey, and the role that established habits can play.

For example, in the course of designing a connected blood glucose meter, we observed that many people with diabetes do not test on a regular schedule. We also observed that certified diabetes educators (CDEs) asked individuals to log blood glucose values on a set schedule for 2 weeks before a scheduled in-person appointment. CDEs did this because they know it is unrealistic to expect people to adhere to a rigidly prescribed schedule of testing over a long period of time. Rather than deal with little to no information—or worse, false information created by people who feel guilty about not testing—they prefer to have at least 2 weeks of valid data in order to have a productive clinic visit. This work-around can be easily adapted into a digital application and is one of many examples where the practical wisdom of practitioners can be translated into a digital solution in order to amplify the benefit for patients who might not have access to a CDE.

The design of digital UX and UI enables a greater level of customization—because digital tools live in people's pockets and homes—allowing solutions to be tailored for the individual to a greater degree than is possible in the in-person clinical care environment. While skilled HCPs can certainly address the specific needs of a person with diabetes in the context of an in-person interaction, the disparity in health information available at that moment—and all the health information that exist about that individual—means that advice cannot always be as tailored the way the individual might need it. As an example of our approach, a design researcher recently interviewed an endocrinologist about the conversations she has with people with diabetes. This doctor told us that she had been inspired by the literature on the Mediterranean diet and was eager to introduce this into her clinical practice. She recommended the diet to a particular individual with a very high hemoglobin A1c concentration. The patient looked at her skeptically and said, "Lady, I'm a truck driver." That story exemplifies the opportunity to create solutions for people with diabetes that are human-centered. While the doctor was not wrong in her recommendation, for that particular individual, she was far away from his reality and design can help bridge that gap.

In short, we need to meet users where they are, especially if we hope to inspire meaningful behavior change over time. We need to recognize the human appetite for difficulty, as well as its limits. For example, Fogg's Behavior Model illustrates how the level of individual ability, motivation, and prompts must line up for a user to complete an activity (Fig. 7.2) [3]. If we make a task either too hard, or too time-consuming, then a majority of users will drop off.

For people with diabetes, we apply the tools of design to help them change their behavior. Meeting the user at the level of difficulty that they can sustain, and clearly acknowledging their threshold, is what can make both the design and the patient successful.

Create "give–get" loops

Imagine that a person with diabetes is introduced to a digital product or service by a health-care provider during a routine clinical visit. The user may

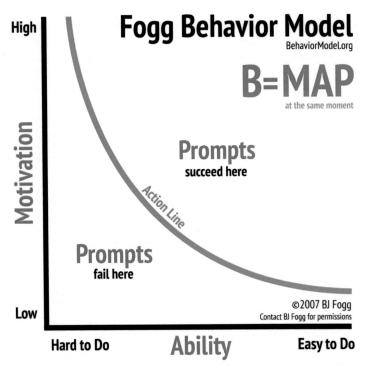

FIGURE 7.2 The Fogg Behavior Model shows that three elements must converge at the same moment for a behavior to occur: motivation, ability, and a prompt. When a behavior does not occur, at least one of those three elements is missing. *With permission from Fogg BJ. What causes behavior change. Fogg Behavior Model. [Internet]. Available from: <https://behavior-model.org>; 2009 [cited 25.07.19].*

then choose to search for the accompanying app and download it from the app store. They go through an onboarding process, create a username and passcode, give permission for data sharing, and decide whether to accept push notifications. They may also be asked to share sensitive health information or consent for the application to access it. All of these steps will generally happen before the user has gained any tangible value from the product or service. In the absence of clear benefit to users, it is not uncommon to lose many participants at this early stage.

One way we address early user drop-off is with a "give–get" loop that allows users to get value in return for the effort or data they contribute. This could be as simple as getting users to enter their weight in the app and in exchange giving them tailored suggestions about nutrition. Or we can give the user a Fitbit and they receive feedback for sharing data about their fitness routine. We must ask ourselves whether each request we make of the user is necessary in order to provide the experience, or whether there might be another way.

The give—get loop is a valuable model to keep in mind when trying to acquire user data [4]. Ultimately, good UX design incorporates that data to complete a cycle of action. When there are conditions for seamless and purposeful data gathering, we can then recognize patterns and help users discover insights that they could act upon by initiating new behaviors. For example, in the design of an app and paired digital blood glucose meter, a user pattern might surface of unusually high readings on Tuesdays. A user could benefit from actionable insight about why Tuesdays are problematic. Perhaps, the user has a weekly lunch with friends or family where indulgent food is the social norm. Understanding the conditions under which the meal occurs brings the user from a pattern detected through data analysis to an insight grounded in social and contextual input. Based on the insight that Tuesday lunches may cause a rise in the user's glucose readings, strategies for taking action can be created.

Getting through this entire cycle, from identifying patterns to articulating insights to taking new actions (and subsequently detecting new patterns), is what creates a holistic and valuable experience for the user [5]. The ability of digital platforms to share information across devices and applications while thoughtfully balancing "give" and "get" creates objective opportunities to support people with diabetes and those who care for them in developing new behaviors.

Data are the foundation of digital capabilities and the UXs they support. Advances in personal computing and mobile applications mean that today most people with diabetes can provide and receive data at any moment through their smartphones. Users often give others access to their data without understanding the purposes for which it will be used, which is a matter of particular concern when designing for people with diabetes, given the especially intimate data around lifestyle factors, geography, income level, family situation, physical activity, and mental health that is likely involved. The creators of a digital solution might be tempted to gather as much data as possible from the user in order to best meet their needs. However, both morally and ethically, as well as in regard to the General Data Protection Regulation legislation passed in the European Union [6], the onus is on the designer and creator to acquire informed consent and make sure that all personal data they collect can be protected.

At IDEO, we see data as a medium for design, one that creates great possibilities and equally great responsibilities. We often ask ourselves, "What is the worst thing that could happen if the data we collect were hacked?" Do we need to collect sensitive data in this case, or is there an alternate way to get to the same result? As a result of these conversations, we have created a set of data ethics cards (Fig. 7.3) [7] to help others navigate these questions.

We need to be mindful of not only the burden a digital solution might put on the user but also the role we might be creating for ourselves as recipients and holders of sensitive information. That is why we are careful to only collect the "minimally viable data" required to create the intended UX.

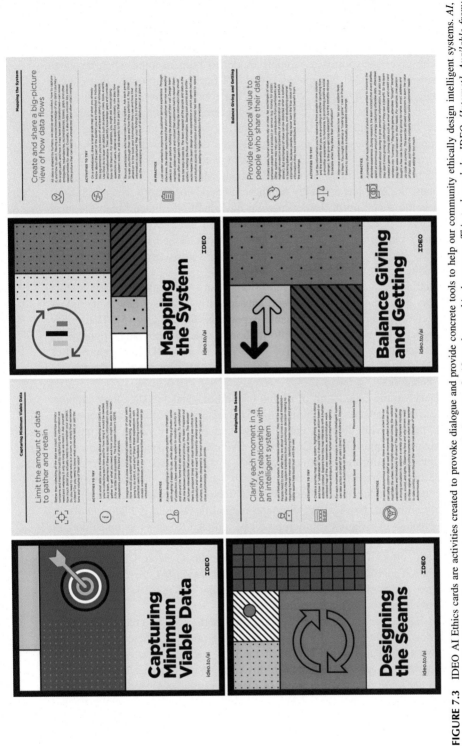

FIGURE 7.3 IDEO AI Ethics cards are activities created to provoke dialogue and provide concrete tools to help our community ethically design intelligent systems. AI, Artificial/augmented intelligence. *Image courtesy IDEO (Chapman M, Sampson O. AI needs an ethical compass. This tool can help. IDEO. [Internet]. Available from: <https://www.ideo.com/blog/ai-needs-an-ethical-compass-this-tool-can-help>; 2019 [cited 25.07.19]) [7].*

Design for relationships

UX design for people with diabetes is not solely about software and technology. Ultimately, it is about relationships. We need to consider people with diabetes and their entire network of care, including health-care providers, administrators, customer service agents, and even family members, as potential users. We need to always think of the UX in the context of a larger service ecosystem and be mindful of how the different components in that ecosystem intersect.

Returning to the original question, why do we need to create digital solutions for managing diabetes? The answer is simple, digital experiences can go beyond adherence with a prescribed treatment regimen: they can take people through to outcomes. At present, there is clearly still a way to go in delivering comprehensive outcomes. Pharmaceutical companies often use digital tools predominantly to drive adherence—to make sure that patients partake of their therapy as prescribed— at the right times and in the right ways. While there is certainly some value in this, we need to consider digital experiences and interactions as the ecosystems through which people with diabetes can live healthier lives. These ecosystems become agnostic of the particular therapies or regimens that circulate within them and can instead become real-time testing and validation systems for more comprehensive outcomes.

Do not be limited by the boundaries of "the device"

As an example, in 2006 we began working with a client on a novel approach to blood glucose testing. At that time, people with diabetes were able to access their own blood glucose data either by logging it themselves or by showing the meter to their doctor. This new meter opened up new opportunities for design, enabling people to plug the meter into a personal computer and transfer all readings to a single document. Once the meter launched, the next design challenge was to make it simpler and less expensive. We realized that the meter's color screen was adding unnecessary cost, without contributing enough benefit in return. While a color screen might seem like a great new opportunity to present rich information, the screen was only used for displaying simple information, including blood glucose values, meal markers, dates, and times. From a human-centered design perspective, it made more sense to eliminate the color screen and utilize users' smartphones instead, thereby opening the door for new possibilities in displaying, sharing, and storing information. At such a crossroads, making a bet on the future is often the way to go.

When designing applications for people with diabetes, it is critical to consider the needs of users with reduced or impaired vision, neuropathy, large fingers, or limited dexterity. We take these considerations into account, whether we are designing a digital or a physical product. When working with another client to redesign the insulin pen, the design team wanted to create an injection experience that felt unobtrusive and less "medical." The team created smaller, sleeker, and less noticeable physical prototypes that enabled more discreet injections and so addressed the issue of stigma. But as the surface area of the pen got smaller, it became more difficult to show users the dosing amount at a legible size. After more iteration and testing with users, the final design was equipped with a small magnifying glass over the dosage number. The design was still sleek and slim, and the dosage number was legible enough to address the real needs of the end user. To address dexterity issues and neuropathy, the designers also made sure that each incremental dosing adjustment made a meaningful click [8]. Adaptive design tactics like these can translate to the digital environment, where we can also use text-to-speech features, read content aloud, and use tools to judge appropriate contrast and color choice for color blindness as well as visual impairment.

Inspire the organization to evolve

As a rule, creating digital products and services will create the need for new capabilities and processes inside the organizations that deliver them. Digital UX are evolving systems, and so require organizational investment and structures ready to support near-constant change. As soon as we are "done" designing a digital experience, a software operating system might change, a new data privacy law might pass, or a content partner could change their rules of engagement, any of which would require additional refinement.

Today, many companies that deliver global offerings at scale work in silos are each oriented around different targets and metrics. There are several examples out in the world where organizations are recognizing this challenge and directly addressing it through new experimental ways of working. The corporate innovation lab model, internal incubators, and entirely separate new ventures are all ways to carve out a particular portion of the business to enable it to operate differently in the early stages, and then begin to transform organizational culture at scale once proof-of-concepts have been successful.

But even within the most nimble and flexible organizations, any digital product or service will need to continue to evolve and improve from day one. It is like the old adage about buying a car: once you drive it off the lot, then it immediately goes down in value. Once a digital solution is launched, then it is essential to start planning immediately for its next update.

To recap our design principles

1. Meet users where they are.
2. Create "give–get" loops.

3. Design for relationships.
4. Do not be limited by the boundaries of "the device."
5. Inspire the organization to evolve.

Key questions and opportunities

In the past few years, tremendous progress has been made in applying digital technologies to diabetes, and today we find ourselves at an interesting juncture. Digital transformation has changed the health-care landscape, but the effects of these changes are not yet mature. There are many unanswered questions and opportunities that we are eager to explore.

- How will augmented and artificial intelligence be applied in this space? These technologies are already embedded behind the scenes and in some new products and services, such as a sleep-coaching service for athletes [9]. As artificial/augmented intelligence becomes more ubiquitous in applications for people with diabetes, what will be the human-centered standards we apply to it, and what unintended consequences will need to be addressed?
- How do we design digital products and tools for the full age range of those affected by Type 2 diabetes? Type 1 diabetes has affected the young for quite some time, but now Type 2 diabetes is increasingly presenting in younger people. In addition, older adults with both Type 1 and Type 2 diabetes are living longer, which means we also need to design for comorbidities and other conditions that are prevalent in an aging population.
- How can mental and emotional well-being be more directly addressed in how we treat and manage diabetes? What new research in mood, sleep, and social relationships must be applied in the design of products and tools meant to prevent diabetes or slow disease progression (Fig. 7.4) [10,11]?
- How do larger societal, political, and cultural shifts change the landscape of design for people with diabetes [12]? The prevalence of sedentary jobs, changes in health insurance availability, issues of food access and quality, as well as the design of towns and cities to either encourage or discourage walking, biking, outdoor space, and public transportation use all greatly affect the people trying to make positive lifestyle changes.
- How might we commercialize and globally scale advances in the scientific understanding of the microbiome and metabolism? How will advances in physical augmentation—such as an artificial pancreas, biological therapeutics, or alternative ways to measure blood sugar—alter the landscape of which UXs and interfaces need to be designed?
- How will the changing business models for health-care delivery, payment, provider roles and incentives, and patient loyalty affect how and where care happens?

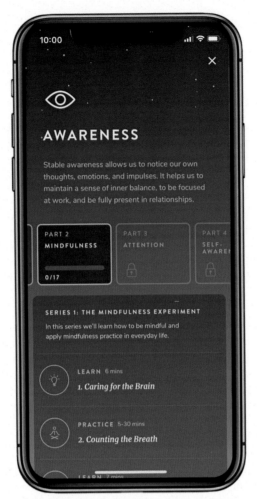

FIGURE 7.4   A well-being program for your mind, based on science and designed for life at work. *Image courtesy Healthy Minds Innovations, Inc (Center for Healthy Minds, University of Wisconsin—Madison. Health minds @ work. [Internet]. Available from: <https://hminnovations. org/hmi/products/healthy-minds-at-work>; 2019 [cited 25.07.19]) [10].*

Each of these questions present vast opportunities for the design—and in some cases redesign—of tools, products, and services. In the abundance of opportunities that lie ahead, the previously described design principles provide a foundation from which to approach these challenges while keeping the needs of people at the center, knowing that while technology may change, the human experience will remain universal.

References

[1] IDEO. Design thinking defined. [Internet]. Available from: <https://designthinking.ideo.com>; 2019 [cited 25.07.19].

[2] Pew Research Center Internet & Technology. Mobile fact sheet. [Internet]. Available from: <https://www.pewinternet.org/fact-sheet/mobile/>; 2019 [cited 25.07.19].

[3] Fogg BJ. What causes behavior change. Fogg behavior model. [Internet]. Available from: <https://behaviormodel.org>; 2009 [cited 25.07.19].

[4] IDEO. Balancing giving and getting, providing reciprocal value to people who share their data. [Internet]. Available from: <https://medium.com/ideo-stories/balancing-giving-and-getting-22c5b0b3387b>; 2018 [cited 25.07.19].

[5] Ascensia Diabetes Care. Contour next one. App patterns day of the week High_v1.1; 2019.

[6] European Parliament and The Council of the European Union. On the projection of natural persons with regard to the processing of personal data and on the free moment of such data, and repealing directive 95/46/EC (General Data Protection Regulation). Off J Eur Union 2016;   <https://eur-lex.europa.eu/legal-content/EN/TXT/?uri = CELEX:32016R0679> [cited 25.07.19].

[7] Chapman M, Sampson O. AI needs an ethical compass. This tool can help. IDEO. [Internet]. Available from: <https://www.ideo.com/blog/ai-needs-an-ethical-compass-this-tool-can-help>; 2019 [cited 25.07.19].

[8] Becker S. Specs. [Internet]. Available from: <https://specs.design>; 2016 [cited 25.07.19].

[9] IDEO. A game changing approach to sleep for athletes. [Internet]. Available from: <https://www.ideo.com/case-study/a-game-changing-approach-to-sleep-for-athletes>; 2016 [cited 25.07.19].

[10] Center for Healthy Minds, University of Wisconsin—Madison. Health minds @ work. [Internet]. Available from: <https://hminnovations.org/hmi/products/healthy-minds-at-work>; 2019 [cited 25.07.19].

[11] van Son J, Nyklíček I, Pop VJ, Blonk MC, Erdstjeck RJ, Spooren PF, et al. The effects of a mindfulness-based intervention on emotional distress, quality of life, and HbA1c in outpatients with diabetes. Diabetes Care J [Internet] 2013;. Available from: <https://care.diabetesjournals.org/content/36/4/823> [cited 25.07.19].

[12] IDEO. A new way to vote for the people of Los Angeles. [Internet]. Available from: <https://www.ideo.com/case-study/a-new-way-to-vote-for-the-people-of-los-angeles>; 2015 [cited 25.07.19].

Section 2

Clinical aspects of digital health for diabetes

Chapter 8

Using social media to support type 1 diabetes management and outcomes for adolescents and young adults: areas of promise and challenge

Elissa R. Weitzman[1,2,3] **and Lauren E. Wisk**[1,3,4]
[1]Division of Adolescent/Young Adult Medicine, Boston Children's Hospital (BCH), Boston, MA, United States, [2]Computational Health Informatics Program, Boston Children's Hospital (BCH), Boston, MA, United States, [3]Department of Pediatrics, Harvard Medical School (HMS), Boston, MA, United States, [4]Division of General Internal Medicine & Health Services Research, David Geffen School of Medicine, University of California, Los Angeles (UCLA), Los Angeles, CA, United States

Abbreviations

AYA adolescents and young adults
T1D type 1 diabetes

Key points

- Adolescents and young adults (AYA) have unique needs for psychosocial and disease management support around type 1 diabetes (T1D).
- Engaging AYA with T1D in social media spaces may provide opportunities for increased information and support relevant to better disease management and outcomes.
- Issues related to ensuring quality, safety, connectedness to care, and accessibility are central to optimal use of diabetes social media for AYA and are complex, requiring attention to technical, policy, market development, and oversight mechanisms.

Diabetes Digital Health. DOI: https://doi.org/10.1016/B978-0-12-817485-2.00008-0

Introduction

Psychosocial needs of adolescents and young adults (AYA) are often poorly met in healthcare settings despite evidence that intensive, patient-centered care can improve glycemic control and reduce risks for complications [1]. Gaps in healthcare coverage and constraints on accessing care are acute for AYA. The mobile and digitally oriented nature of AYA makes them an ideal group for considering whether and how it may be possible to harness social media to engage them in disease management and self-care. The diabetes online community involved in social media could provide AYA with access to peer and expert guidance, feedback, and the contextualization of personal experiences, helping to alleviate isolation and distress and motivating disease management, supporting favorable outcomes. This chapter provides an overview of this opportunity in the context of the developmental epidemiology of type 1 diabetes (T1D) among AYA and identifies challenges inherent in using social media for these purposes.

Developmental epidemiology of type 1 diabetes for adolescents and young adults

Living with T1D places high demands on effective disease self-management to achieve target blood sugar control, avoid diabetes complications, and reduce the economic costs of treatment nonadherence and lost productivity [2]. These efforts may be particularly challenging for AYA, who typically have worse glycemic control than both older and younger T1D patients [3]. Adolescence and emerging adulthood are critical periods during which health outcomes may be imperiled as delays in care, declines in self-management, and adoption/escalation of risk behaviors all pose acute health threats and jeopardize present and future outcomes. Few clinical interventions have been able to produce sustained improvements in glycemic control during this time, highlighting the need to develop new strategies to engage and support AYA. Such strategies may include interventions that are specifically designed for their unique psychosocial needs. AYA with diabetes experience rates of depression or anxiety nearly three times that of the general population [4], much of which goes un-/undertreated. Many experience high levels of diabetes distress—the fears, worries, and sense of being overwhelmed that persons living with diabetes often experience on a daily basis, which have been shown to lead to decreased self-management and poor glycemic control [4]. Adolescence and young adulthood are periods when AYA gain autonomy and transition from the roles and settings typical of childhood into those that mark adulthood. AYA transition from pediatric- to adult-focused care, and from their childhood home to independent living arrangements, can include moving from high school to college and community settings. Glycemic control can plummet in this time and social and clinical supports may attenuate.

The opportunity

In the United States the average adult spends nearly half of each day online or viewing a screen [5] and AYA likely mirror or exceed this level. The online world reflects a rapidly expanding ecosystem of social media platforms and environments that enable sharing of content and information. For AYA with T1D, social media may provide opportunities to obtain and exchange information, support, and encouragement from peers or experts. As a group, AYA are very willing to share personal health information, to help others and improve care, and they value online interactions as sources of information and support [6]. Standards of care for AYA with T1D [7] include a quarterly healthcare visit plus meetings with a nurse educator and nutritionist, often totaling not more than 3 of the 8760 annual hours that persons living with diabetes spend on self-management. Social and informational support gleaned from online interactions could help AYA remain engaged in self-care and disease management.

Defining social media

The term "social media" indicates a host of online spaces in which individuals have the potential to interact with friends (e.g., Facebook), colleagues (e.g., LinkedIn), strangers (e.g., reddit), information (e.g., Wikipedia), visual content (e.g., Instagram), and more. Several taxonomies have emerged to classify this digital environment by function [8,9] and this chapter focuses on several types of social media that are most popular among AYA (Box 8.1).

Many platforms share common features, such as the ability for messaging between users and tools to create formalized connections (friends or followers). Sites may overlap in nearly all aspects of the user-interface. Yet, even within the same social media site, users may have extremely different experiences based on their desired functionalities and settings. For instance, individuals on networking sites who set their profile to "private" may only allow a curated group of "friends" or "followers" to view their posted content, while others may have a "public" profile while curating individuals' posts.

According to the Pew Research Center, in 2018 around 70% of the US adults use at least one social media site, up from only 5% in 2005 [10]. AYA have always had the highest rates of social media use with nearly 90% of young adults and 97% of adolescents using social media in 2018; over 80% visit each platform on a daily basis. AYA point to the increased connectedness to friends, exposure to diverse groups of people, and potential to receive support during tough times as to why they use social media so frequently [11]. There are benefits and risks for adolescents of using social media and studies point to constructive as well as destructive effects, including declining social skills, extreme and unhealthy patterns of engaging in the

---

BOX 8.1 Taxonomy of social media platforms germane to adolescents and young adults.

There are many categories of social media and taxonomies continuously developing as the ecosystem changes. *Social networking sites* have a focus on building and maintaining social relationships among individuals who may interact in real life or share common interests, and these sites may be thematically focused, advancing of professional ties (e.g., LinkedIn), or designed for more general interactions (e.g., Facebook). *Micro- and general blogging platforms* (blog is short for "web log") are services that chronicle user-generated posts (e.g., Twitter) that are often opinion but may also be used as a source of information dissemination. *Media sharing platforms* are sites that nearly exclusively host visual content such as photos (e.g., Instagram), and videos (e.g., YouTube). *Curation sites* allow users to form collections of images or articles on topics of interest (e.g., Pinterest) but may also thematically organize discussion-based content (e.g., reddit). *Micro-media sites* have become a favorite of AYA as these platforms combine aspects of social networking, media sharing, and curation applications (apps) and appeal to users through offering ephemeral posting (e.g., Snapchat), and limiting content to short-form media (e.g., TikTok).

---

virtual rather than "brick and mortar" world, and heightened sense of disconnection and depression among AYA growing up in the social media age [12,13]. Most scholars agree that further research is needed.

The developing evidence base

As general social media platforms have expanded, so too have diabetes-specific ones [14]. Research is proliferating on the potential for using these systems to support diabetes management and outcomes (see Fig. 8.1).

Online communities for AYA with T1D can enable social and observational learning, support ties among persons or groups with shared problems or interests, provide access to peer- and professionally generated content and resources, and afford opportunities to share personal health information and participate in research [15]. These factors may help alleviate isolation and distress and motivate daily disease management, supporting favorable outcomes. Engagement with diabetes online communities that foster peer-to-peer exchange and psychosocial support has been associated with improved disease management and, in some cases, better glycemic control [14,16–18]. Nevertheless, rigorous evaluations of the effects of such engagement on health outcomes and well-being among AYA with T1D are limited. To date, many studies use small self-selecting adult samples, raising questions about the suitability and fit of these approaches across a more representative/diverse population of AYA. Rigorous research is needed to characterize use patterns

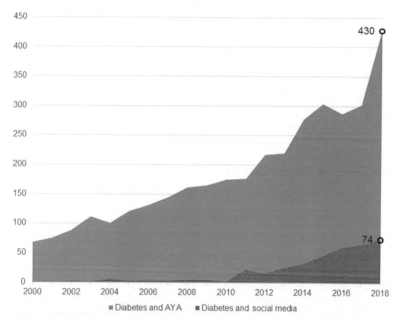

Diabetes and AYA [Title/Abstract] search string included [(("diabetes" OR "diabetes mellitus" OR "type 1 diabetes" OR "type 2 diabetes")) AND ("adolescence" OR "adolescent" OR "young adult" OR "emerging adult" OR "teen" OR "teenager" OR "young adulthood" OR "emerging adulthood")].
Diabetes and Social Media [Title/Abstract] search string included [(("diabetes" OR "diabetes mellitus" OR "type 1 diabetes" OR "type 2 diabetes")) AND ("social media" OR "social network" OR "social networking" OR "Facebook" OR "Twitter" OR "Instagram" OR "online forum")].

FIGURE 8.1   PubMed search results since 2000.

by social media features, and the impacts of specific engagement patterns on all relevant outcomes, including experience of informational and emotional support, psychosocial well-being, disease management and adherence, glycemic control, and health status/complications.

Challenges

Efforts to advance the use of social media to support improved disease management and outcomes among AYA with T1D are challenged by lack of evidence regarding efficacy, and limited control over key practice features. These features reflect 1) quality and alignment with diabetes science, 2) safety, 3) connectedness to care, and 4) accessibility and suitability to the developmental needs of AYA.

Verifying quality

Across social media tools and environments, a range of quality metrics can be applied, including alignment of content with diabetes science and clinical practice recommendations. As the diabetes social media landscape gains complexity, interactive tools and applications are diffusing that have social features and may include tools for self-tracking and data sharing among peer networks and others (i.e., behavioral health providers). As such, quality control may include verification of tracking and sharing practices for alignment with user permissions. Social media platforms may also promote tools that afford self-tracking and personal feedback. Transparency (or "white boxing") of algorithms can facilitate accuracy checks but is inconsistent with the goals of tools that are privately owned or proprietary. Additional quality criteria may include practices for external auditing and sourcing of content including to check that content reflects clinical guidelines and diabetes science; and support for moderation of user-generated content and peer-to-peer communications. Sites and tools can be evaluated for the extent to which they reflect high standards of user-centeredness, features that extend to readability and accessibility of privacy policies, and control over privacy risks; this includes provision of clear and accessible communications around the sharing of personal data by sites or systems, and implementation of clear and effective user controls over information sharing.

Formal quality rating systems are diffusing [19]. However, it is unclear whether these rating systems reflect the unique needs, legal status, and engagement patterns of AYA. Furthermore, rating systems may imperfectly apply to many social media that AYA use and only loosely fit the model of centrally operated diabetes-related online communities, which host and publish extensive amounts of user-generated content.

Using a comprehensive set of indicators, investigators have found that online diabetes social networking sites often employ practices in support of some, but rarely all, features signifying quality [15,20]. There are acute gaps in guaranteeing the accuracy of content, and transparency or validation of algorithms that may serve content to users. Protection against low-quality/inaccurate information is especially challenging around user-generated materials, given their volume, and there are important open questions about who has authority or responsibility to oversee accuracy. Health behaviors may be affected by content transmitted through social media making it especially important to identify solutions or mechanisms to ensure safety and flag inaccurate, misleading, or malignant content. Models to support quality review may require new mechanisms that account for gaps and disparities in regulatory policies across geographic boundaries given that social media transcend traditional geographies.

Safety

Safety issues are central concerns for all social media use and need careful consideration when engaging and supporting AYA around diabetes management. Foremost are issues related to complying with standards for protecting privacy and taking steps to ensure that AYA understand and protect themselves from risks related to permissioned and predatory information sharing.

In the United States, the Children's Online Privacy Protection Act applies only to children younger than 13; hence, adolescents are without privacy protections in online environments [21]. While concern for privacy increases with age, even among young cohorts [21] proportionately few adolescents report high levels of such concern albeit many report having been contacted by others online in a way that makes them feel uncomfortable or having been served online advertisements that they deem inappropriate [22].

Safety concerns may also arise from exposure to misinformation or distressing materials. Because AYA experience high levels of diabetes distress, depression, anxiety, and risk behaviors, all of which may be impacted by exposure to others' reports of these problems, safety monitoring of content may be especially important. Absent scalable and effective automated monitoring, encouraging providers to ask AYA about their social media use, including in relation to their diabetes management and distress, may serve as an important strategy for monitoring safety. Provider education about these issues is therefore crucial but also largely lacking.

In some cases, social media may offer an advantage for monitoring AYA safety: individuals in users' networks may notice when a user posts troubling content or publicly reaches out for support—active surveillance and attention to these concerns may be required. Many sites are working on implementing machine learning and artificial intelligence approaches for automated processing of user-generated content to identify and respond to safety concerns discerned in real time. For example, these automated methods have been used for postmarket pharmaceutical safety surveillance and are identified as having the potential to identify rare adverse events earlier than traditional systems [23]. In the context of diabetes care, safety/efficacy of medications and devices, acute disease exacerbations, and general and diabetes-specific distress could all be monitored on social media with the potential for integration into clinical care or to facilitate safety reporting to regulatory bodies [24,25].

Social media sites are experiencing growing pains as they figure out how to navigate nascent regulatory environments that are still more reactive than proactive regarding user protections and data ownership. As technical solutions are developed, there is a need for formal guidance from policy-makers and regulators about what level of monitoring is appropriate (active without being invasive) and what level of response is warranted (protective without stifling innovation). For researchers and healthcare providers interacting with AYA on social media, the practicality of individualized responses to every potentially worrisome post across multiple platforms is unclear if not unlikely—which is a reason for caution.

Connectedness to care

Advocacy groups and professional societies are attending to the potential for integrating social media into diabetes care to provide psychosocial support [26]. At present, the potential to utilize social media for direct communication between patients and providers and as a space to host educational information are at the forefront of potential models. However, most of this integration is ad hoc and has not yet been advanced for wide-scale use. For meaningful connectedness to occur, all relevant stakeholders (patients, providers, policy-makers/regulators, and technologists) need to understand and address potential privacy and safety concerns and answer challenging implementation questions: How do providers obtain access to useful data without inadvertently obtaining access to other personal information that may be irrelevant to care but sensitive for patients, or without disclosing disease/treatment status on these platforms? What are the legal risks to providers from integrating social media into care, and how can risks be managed? And, regarding confidentiality: Are social media–sourced data to be stored in the medical record and are these data subject to the same protections that govern information obtained during a clinical encounter? What happens to this information when a clinical relationship ends, or a platform or tool becomes outmoded or inactive, including when platforms are commercial? These issues are acutely important for AYA who, as a group, are especially likely to adopt social media tools, experience changes in care and insurance status, be highly mobile, and risk tolerant.

Connection, integration, and complementarity of social media with care offer a potential opportunity for a rich and important new avenue to increase support and engagement of AYA around diabetes management, However, workable models that offer equipoise are as yet elusive [14].

Accessibility

As diabetes social media proliferate, issues related to accessibility arise, including those centered on whether they will be made available for all populations or only to select or insured populations (some platforms offer social media tools and support through insurance and employee programs)—which raises questions of equity and justice. AYA without insurance, stable employment, or adequate understanding of the evolving information and healthcare marketplaces may be less able to benefit from diabetes programs or initiatives that use social media. Low-literacy AYA may be less able to navigate terms of use and privacy policies, with resultant risks to privacy and confidentiality [27,28]. Studies have found that privacy policies and administrative content about social media applications may be written at very high reading levels [20]. On the other hand, peer-to-peer communications may employ simpler language and short texts that are more accessible to AYA [29]. Consideration of equipoise is needed, including by addressing access/accessibility issues, quality/safety, scale and sustainability, and by advancing reimbursement for delivering evidence-based interventions and treatments that include social media components [30].

Summary

Diabetes social media are expanding in an evolving marketplace of health information technologies and healthcare delivery. Growth in this area represents enormous potential for helping to address acute AYA needs for psychosocial support. The "digital phenotype" of AYA makes them an ideal fit for developing models — on average, AYA are highly mobile, appreciative of online connectedness, and are tech savvy and established users of social media. They are yet developing an attunement for risk and the self-restraint needed to protect them from unhealthy, impulsive, or risky influences. While AYA generally have strong relationships with social media, they may have weak ties to self-care and disease management practices and shifting clinical relationships. As such, harnessing social media to support disease management and health outcomes makes sense. However, considerable work is needed to advance workable and effective models that reflect values of quality, safety, clinical connectedness, and accessibility. Ongoing conversations about key questions (see Table 8.1) are needed as is continued development, testing, and thoughtful oversight to optimize the dynamic diabetes social media space to best serve AYA needs.

TABLE 8.1 Key questions related to the advancing use of social media to support diabetes management and outcomes among adolescents and young adults, for stakeholder groups.

Stakeholder	Issues to consider
AYA	Are social media tools/platforms suitable for AYA developmental, psychosocial, and healthcare needs? AYA may discount privacy and safety risks, experience heightened diabetes distress, have intermittent care patterns, and experience transitions in clinical relationships and settings
	What information sharing practices and privacy protections apply best to AYA? Do policies and practices allow for parental supervision when developmentally appropriate and needed? How are these permissions explained and modified as an adolescent ages?
	Can social media bridge pediatric and specialty care, subspecialty and internal medicine? Home, clinic, and college or employment?
	Are AYA skills adequate for navigating the online world, that is, media literacy, health literacy, and numeracy? What resources are suitable for supporting those skills? Can diabetes advocacy groups or clinicians support skill development?

(Continued)

TABLE 8.1 (Continued)

Stakeholder	Issues to consider
Clinicians	How available and adequate are training opportunities for clinicians regarding social media relevant to AYA with T1D? Do professional organizations have a role in advancing training? Are there are mechanisms to support CME credit for training?
	What are the next steps for advancing tools and platforms for integration with care to support patient and panel management?
	Can tools be developed that resolve quality, safety, and privacy/confidentiality issues around connectedness with clinicians?
	What are the reimbursement models for evidence-based applications/uses of social media–supported tools?
	What is the role of professional medical societies in advancing policies and guidelines around "friending and following" practices with patients, viewing shared information, overseeing the safety and efficacy of developing social media?
	What is the role of clinicians in advocating for rigorous evidence to guide integration and use of social media within healthcare?
Technologists, developers	How can technologists ensure readability and accessibility of content including around information sharing and disclosure for AYA?
	What features are needed to support tools that can interoperate and integrate across sites and settings of care or geographies recognizing the mobility of AYA?
	What mechanisms exist to support scalable quality and safety controls over centrally generated content, user-generated content, and interactive content that diffuses through social media?
	Can design features be developed to facilitate information sharing between platforms and clinicians? Would these features be tunable to AYA preferences around how much information to share, with whom, and when?
Regulators/policy-makers	What business models exist for integrating evidence-based social media tools and systems within care? Are there quality/performance metrics that can be developed that are evidence-based to support reimbursement?
	Who is accountable for monitoring the quality and safety of diabetes social media including around protecting minors online?
	What are the relevant regulatory frameworks or existing laws that can inform and accelerate this work (e.g., European GDPR)?
	How can we advance discussion around challenging issues such as promulgation of quality/safety practices across geographies given that social media transcend national borders?

AYA, Adolescents and young adults; *CME*, continuing medical education; *GDPR*, General Data Protection Regulation.

References

[1] Ellis DA, Frey MA, Naar-King S, Templin T, Cunningham P, Cakan N. Use of multisystemic therapy to improve regimen adherence among adolescents with type 1 diabetes in chronic poor metabolic control: a randomized controlled trial. Diabetes Care 2005;28 (7):1604−10.

[2] American Diabetes Association. Economic costs of diabetes in the U.S. in 2017. Diabetes Care 2018;41(5):917−28.

[3] Foster NC, Beck RW, Miller KM, Clements MA, Rickels MR, DiMeglio LA, et al. State of type 1 diabetes management and outcomes from the T1D exchange in 2016−2018. Diabetes Technol Ther 2019;21(2):66−72.

[4] Kreider KE. Diabetes distress or major depressive disorder? A practical approach to diagnosing and treating psychological comorbidities of diabetes. Diabetes Ther 2017;8 (1):1−7.

[5] Nielson. Time flies: U.S. adults now spend nearly half a day interacting with media. 2018.

[6] Vaala SE, Lee JM, Hood KK, Mulvaney SA. Sharing and helping: predictors of adolescents' willingness to share diabetes personal health information with peers. J Am Med Inf Assoc 2018;25(2):135−41.

[7] American Diabetes Association. 13. Children and adolescents: standards of medical care in diabetes-2019. Diabetes Care 2019;42(Suppl. 1):S148−64.

[8] Grajales 3rd FJ, Sheps S, Ho K, Novak-Lauscher H, Eysenbach G. Social media: a review and tutorial of applications in medicine and health care. J Med Internet Res 2014;16(2):e13.

[9] Patel R, Chang T, Greysen SR, Chopra V. Social media use in chronic disease: a systematic review and novel taxonomy. Am J Med 2015;128(12):1335−50.

[10] Smith A, Anderson M. Social media use in 2018. Washington, DC: Pew Research Center; 2018. March 1.

[11] Anderson M, Jiang J. Teens' social media habits and experiences. Washington, DC: Pew Research Center; 2018. November 28.

[12] Orben A, Dienlin T, Przybylski AK. Social media's enduring effect on adolescent life satisfaction. Proc Natl Acad Sci USA 2019.

[13] Turkle S. Reclaiming conversation: the power of talk in a digital age. New York: Penguin Press; 2015. 436 pages p.

[14] Hilliard ME, Sparling KM, Hitchcock J, Oser TK, Hood KK. The emerging diabetes online community. Curr Diabetes Rev 2015;11(4):261−72.

[15] Ho YX, O'Connor BH, Mulvaney SA. Features of online health communities for adolescents with type 1 diabetes. West J Nurs Res 2014;36(9):1183−98.

[16] Litchman ML, Edelman LS, Donaldson GW. Effect of diabetes online community engagement on health indicators: cross-sectional study. JMIR Diabetes 2018;3(2):e8.

[17] Gabarron E, Arsand E, Wynn R. Social media use in interventions for diabetes: rapid evidence-based review. J Med Internet Res 2018;20(8):e10303.

[18] Colorafi K. Connected health: a review of the literature. Mhealth 2016;2:13.

[19] Boyer C. Accessing quality online health information: what is the solution? Stud Health Technol Inf 2016;225:718−20.

[20] Weitzman ER, Cole E, Kaci L, Mandl KD. Social but safe? Quality and safety of diabetes-related online social networks. J Am Med Inf Assoc 2011;18(3):292−7.

[21] Montgomery KC, Chester J, Milosevic T. Children's privacy in the big data era: research opportunities. Pediatrics 2017;140(Suppl. 2):S117−21.

[22] Costello CR, McNiel DE, Binder RL. Adolescents and social media: privacy, brain development, and the law. J Am Acad Psychiatry Law 2016;44(3):313–21.

[23] Tricco AC, Zarin W, Lillie E, Jeblee S, Warren R, Khan PA, et al. Utility of social media and crowd-intelligence data for pharmacovigilance: a scoping review. BMC Med Inf Decis Mak 2018;18(1):38.

[24] Mandl KD, McNabb M, Marks N, Weitzman ER, Kelemen S, Eggleston EM, et al. Participatory surveillance of diabetes device safety: a social media-based complement to traditional FDA reporting. J Am Med Inf Assoc 2014;21(4):687–91.

[25] Weitzman ER, Kelemen S, Quinn M, Eggleston EM, Mandl KD. Participatory surveillance of hypoglycemia and harms in an online social network. JAMA Intern Med 2013;173(5):345–51.

[26] Warshaw H, Edelman D. Building bridges through collaboration and consensus: expanding awareness and use of peer support and peer support communities among people with diabetes, caregivers, and health care providers. J Diabetes Sci Technol 2019;13 (2):206–12.

[27] Osborn CY, Cavanaugh K, Wallston KA, Rothman RL. Self-efficacy links health literacy and numeracy to glycemic control. J Health Commun 2010;15(Suppl. 2):146–58.

[28] White RO, Wolff K, Cavanaugh KL, Rothman R. Addressing health literacy and numeracy to improve diabetes education and care. Diabetes Spectr 2010;23(4):238–43.

[29] Hoedebecke K, Beaman L, Mugambi J, Shah S, Mohasseb M, Vetter C, et al. Health care and social media: what patients really understand. F1000Res 2017;6:118.

[30] Brown LL, Lustria ML, Rankins J. A review of web-assisted interventions for diabetes management: maximizing the potential for improving health outcomes. J Diabetes Sci Technol 2007;1(6):892–902.

Chapter 9

Social media for adults

Elia Gabarron[1], Meghan Bradway[1,2] and Eirik Årsand[1,3]

[1]*Norwegian Centre for E-health Research, University Hospital of North Norway, Tromsø, Norway,* [2]*Faculty of Health Sciences, Department of Clinical Medicine, UiT The Arctic University of Norway, Tromsø, Norway,* [3]*Faculty of Science and Technology, Department of Computer Science, UiT The Arctic University of Norway, Tromsø, Norway*

Abbreviations

DIY do-it-yourself
HbA1c glycated hemoglobin
T1D type 1 diabetes
T2D type 2 diabetes

Key points

- Adults with diabetes increasingly use social media for sharing and obtaining diabetes-related information and also for giving and receiving support.
- Health-care professionals could participate more on social media channels to provide validated health information.
- Higher interaction between stakeholders and future approaches using social media might be useful both to prevent diabetes and improve individuals' health outcomes.

Introduction

The commercial use of the Internet is more than 30 years old. In the early years the World Wide Web was based on static data that could only be read or downloaded. However, during the 1990s, a new type of dynamic web was developed, enabling individuals with very little computing skills to develop their own websites. At the same time the first social media emerged (Sixdegrees.com). The novelty of this website was that it allowed its users to interact with each other—making it very popular very quickly—achieving more than 3.5 million registered users in only 2 years. Since the creation of this first online social network, the number of individuals registered on different

Diabetes Digital Health. DOI: https://doi.org/10.1016/B978-0-12-817485-2.00009-2

social media has grown dramatically in both developed and developing countries. To date (beginning in 2020) there are almost 3 billion active social media users worldwide, with over 2 billion of them on Facebook alone.

But what is social media today? Social media refers to democratized Internet-based services that allow their users to generate content, create their own profiles, and connect and interact with other users [1]. Social media includes online networking platforms, that is, Facebook, YouTube, Instagram, and other file-sharing sites; forums; instant-messaging platforms (i.e., Skype, Telegram, Snapchat, and WhatsApp); blogs and microblogging (i.e., Twitter); and also wikis (i.e., Wikipedia) [1].

These channels present several advantages. They are highly usable; very easy to reach through smartphones, tablets, and computers; accessible at any time; and free of charge in the majority of cases. Although younger generations have typically been the most frequent users of these channels, the online presence of older generations has increased in recent years. In developed countries, where the Internet is ubiquitous, almost 90% of adults use social media to seek out and share health information [2].

This trend is especially true for people with diabetes. The dangers of elevated blood glucose levels are well established and include kidney disease, loss of vision, damage to the circulation and nerves, and a greater risk of developing cardiovascular disease and stroke prematurely [3]. To reduce the personal risk of developing these serious complications of diabetes, individuals with diabetes must undertake frequent monitoring of glucose levels in relation to physical activity, medication, diet, stress, and other lifestyle factors. These daily, sometimes hourly, tasks can become overwhelming. Therefore these individuals often use medical and commercial technology, such as blood glucose monitors and mobile health apps, respectively, to help keep track of all of these factors. Individuals with diabetes are now more empowered by the amount of information available on the Internet as well as these new technologies to help them answer some of the questions about how to best manage this complicated disease. However, while the health-care system has resources, such as structured education programs, informative websites, and consultations with health-care providers, it unfortunately does not have the capacity to respond to the detailed questions that people with diabetes may have about their data (including real-time information) that they are gathering or learning from their health apps, medical devices, and the Internet [4]. Therefore individuals with diabetes are turning toward the Internet, and especially social media—their new resource, and sometimes haven—for diabetes information and support by others living with diabetes.

In 2011 one of the first articles was published that analyzed how social media was being used in relation to diabetes. Greene et al. reviewed Facebook groups' posts and discussions around diabetes and found that two-thirds of the content dealt with users' personal experiences with self-management, while one-third of the posts provided emotional support [5]. Authors of this study highlighted (1) the importance of online social networking to support and educate others with similar conditions and (2) the risks of an unregulated environment supporting substantial promotional and data-gathering activities [5]. These features of social media remain true today.

In this chapter, we will present an overview of how social media is being used in relation to diabetes for adults, by both people affected by diabetes and health-care professionals. We will point to some of their advantages and challenges and refer to current examples.

Social media and its use by people affected by diabetes

So, how is social media being used by people affected by diabetes, their relatives, and their loved ones?

There are several reasons why people search for diabetes information. They may need, or have interest in, knowing more about treatments, health-care services, self-management, to share information, or to give and receive emotional support. This is known as health information-seeking behavior. Information-seeking behavior is an intentional and planned behavior that is related to wanting better health [6]. With the advent of social media, these channels have become the leading sources for health information seekers. This appears to follow a weekly pattern; information seekers seem to search more actively for diabetes-related information early in the workweek (mostly on Mondays and Tuesdays) and are less active on Saturdays [7] (see Fig. 9.1). This temporal pattern follows under the "fresh start effect" hypothesis that associates temporal landmarks or calendar events (i.e., beginning of a week or month, New Year, or birthday) with increases in aspirational activities, in this case, with increases in diabetes-related information-seeking behavior.

Type, quality, and tone of diabetes-related information on social media

A simple search using the term "diabetes" on Facebook, Twitter, Instagram, or any other social media will show results related to thousands of users, groups, and pages specifically dealing with this topic.

The type of diabetes-related information on social media is heterogeneous and differs depending on users, groups, and channels. For example, it has been reported that health information seekers searching for diabetes-related contents in open social media channels will find a higher proportion of posts on diabetes awareness, whereas the same search on closed social media groups will result in contents related mainly to diabetes self-management [8,9] (see Fig. 9.2).

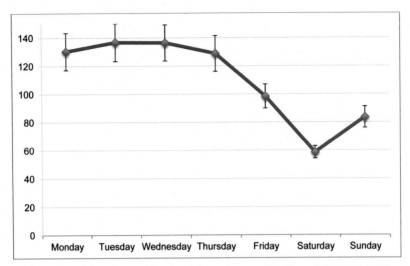

FIGURE 9.1 Weekly average of online information searches about diabetes on Wikipedia (period: January 1, 2013–June 30, 2015). Error bars indicate 95% CI. ANOVA tests, $P < .001$. *Data from Gabarron E, Lau AYS, Wynn R. Is there a weekly pattern for health information searching and is the pattern unique to health topics? J Med Internet Res 2015;17(12):e286.*

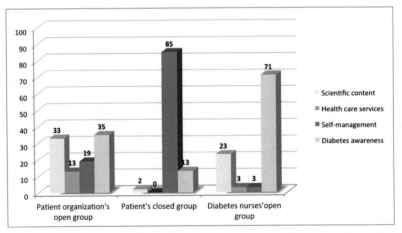

FIGURE 9.2 Visual representation of the percentage of the main topics posted among three various groups: patient organization's group, patients' group, and diabetes nurses' group. *Modified from Årsand E, Bradway M, Gabarron E. What are diabetes patients versus healthcare personnel discussing on social media? J Diabetes Sci Technol 2019;12:2499–506.*

Health-related content published on social media can have a substantial impact on individuals in their decision-making [10,11]. Therefore it is important that the information posted on social media is trustworthy. Reports about the quality of diabetes contents in online networking sites is inconsistent—differing from site to site and from user to user. For example, one recent study reported that most of the diabetes-related health information that can be found on the Internet and social media is of good quality, and individuals tend to trust in the advice they found there [12]. However, when another study used a questionnaire to ask social media users to rate their satisfaction with the quality of diabetes-related information on social media, the respondents rated the quality as just slightly better than mediocre [13].

Because social media contents can be published or edited by anyone, one often finds incorrect or imprecise diabetes-related information, which is potentially harmful. This means a potential risk of misinformation leading to misunderstandings. The accuracy and reliability of diabetes-related content on social media is often unknown and unverified, and therefore must be considered a potential danger to individuals [14].

Correct and appropriate information is the basis for optimal self-management. Diabetes self-management is defined as the individual's ability to manage the symptoms, treatment, physical and psychological consequences, and lifestyle changes inherent to living with diabetes. As in other chronic conditions, the trend is that the responsibility for the daily management of diabetes is shifting from clinicians to the individuals affected by the disease. Therefore those affected need to develop a diverse skill set to maintain a satisfactory quality of life [15]. Social media provides unprecedented opportunities for enhancing health communication and health care, including diabetes self-management.

However, individuals are not influenced only by the quality and accuracy of the contents; the tone, or how these contents are expressed, can also impact individuals. In fact, a study found that social media posts specifically mentioning type 2 diabetes (T2D) had a more negative tone than the ones focusing on type 1 diabetes (T1D) [16]. As emotions can spread on social media, and positive emotions are linked to a more cooperative behavior and better decision-making, more diabetes-related posts with a positive tone on social media are needed [16].

Social or peer support in relation to diabetes

There are many reasons that people with diabetes seek out social or peer support on social media. These reasons include feelings of isolation and stigma due to the personal demands of the condition and the exhausting requirements of self-management [17]. In a recent study, members of the Nightscout project (a project that allows patients and relatives to access real-time blood glucose data by sharing this data in the cloud) were interviewed. Respondents remarked that they interacted with other patients on social media by giving and receiving technical, emotional, and medical support [18].

This finding is in line with the results from other studies, which found that one of the main reasons, why people use diabetes social media channels, is to offer support or encouragement to other individuals affected by the disease [9,18], and also for sharing personal experiences [18]. However, just as with the quality of social media contents, not all interactions with other social media users are supportive or emotionally beneficial [14].

A positive correlation between using diabetes social media channels and having a better lifestyle has been reported in the literature [17]. The perception of having good social support affects individuals' perceived self-efficacy by encouraging the adoption of healthier lifestyles. In the online Big Blue Test (a program that reinforces the importance of exercise in managing diabetes), it was even found that the perception of having social support had positive impacts on improving blood glucose levels [15].

Do-it-yourself and technology on social media

Social media has had a significant impact on the spread of do-it-yourself (DIY)-activities for people with diabetes in the last 5 years. The best example is the Nightscout project, with their closed Facebook group "CGM in the cloud" attracting more than 30,000 members. On Twitter, this project also uses the hashtag #WeAreNotWaiting. This hashtag is used to echo the general trend that those with diabetes are no longer waiting for the health-care system to give them the answers and tools for their daily self-management challenges. Instead, this message encourages members to share challenges and technological solutions with one another using DIY. This hashtag has become so well-known that a Google search returns thousands of results, thereby demonstrating the widespread dissemination of this rather technical disease-specific theme. From an even more technical perspective, the #OpenAPS hashtag represents DIY efforts related to building an artificial pancreas for T1D. Through social media, more than 1300 people have now used this advanced and complex procedure to construct a closed loop system or an artificial pancreas. There are many other examples of how social media is used to spread information on innovative ways of using technologies for diabetes self-management, either from users' own ideas or adapting industry products (sometimes referred to as "hacking")—most often a combination of these two.

Social media for diabetes and its use by health-care professionals

The characteristics of social networks, such as their ubiquity and high accessibility, suggest that these channels can be considered a valuable resource for health-care professionals, public health promoters, researchers, authorities, and other stakeholders working with diabetes. These channels are beginning to be used for the monitoring of behavior and content related to diabetes, for health promotion, and to enhance other types of interventions.

Since participants' activities, that is, their interactions, on social media can be logged and accessed, the users' behaviors can be monitored, which could be especially valuable resources for public health surveillance. Monitoring diabetes-related contents and online behaviors on social media offers the potential for the right actors to identify diabetes-related concerns, interests, misinformation, attitudes, or information-seeking patterns within online communities. In doing so, they have the potential to react accordingly.

Health promotion in diabetes

It has been proposed that social media platforms could be effective educational channels to promote healthier lifestyles in order to prevent or reduce the effects of the disease. In general, social media users are interested in finding health promotion content on these channels, and they have expressed the need to see more contents on research and innovation [12].

Because of their cost-effectiveness, potential for precise evaluations of campaign success, and increased sustainability, social media can also offer a powerful means of encouraging secondary prevention measures and behavior change to people already affected with diabetes—for example, for preventing foot-related complications [19]. When using social media for health promotion purposes, the contents could be posted according to the weekly patterns (Fig. 9.1) of diabetes-related information-seeking behavior, in order to enhance its impact.

Interventions including social media

There is evidence that using social media in interventions, to provide health education to those with diabetes, is beneficial, especially to young adults with T1D [20]. Most of the studies that have used social media as a communication tool or to provide health education, reported significant improvements in patients' glycated hemoglobin concentrations [20,21]; while the impact of social media interventions on other patient outcomes such as hypoglycemic episodes, blood pressure, or quality of life is inconsistent across the different studies [20]. So far, no studies have reported that patients' health worsened as the result of a social media intervention. This suggests that interventions based on these channels are mostly beneficial for improving patient outcomes [20]. Social media interventions could be especially valuable for improving outcomes among people affected with gestational diabetes and T2D, since these diseases' prevalence has been increasing rapidly in the past few decades.

Challenges for more use

The use of social media for diabetes by health-care professionals and other stakeholders should be monitored. Currently, both the pharmaceutical and medical devices industries' strategies for advertising their products include using social media. When targeting people affected with any health condition on social media, keeping the privacy, confidentiality, and anonymity of the target population is especially relevant. Furthermore privacy policies might change at any time on social media, so what was private at some point could be public later.

An important challenge for health-care professionals who want to use social media is the fact that being active on these channels is time-consuming, and in most of today's clinical settings, such activities cannot be conducted during working hours. Health-care professionals might also feel insecure about the quality of the content, as well as how to use social media as part of their job, because this is not usually taught in medical, nursing, or other health-care education programs.

New trends and opportunities

Social media channels can be very useful for recruiting participants for research, because they allow for targeting of specific populations quickly and with a minimum of costs. In addition, the use of online social networks provides secondary advantages for research, such as individual interactions and lower study dropout rates [1].

The use of big data and artificial intelligence—combining data from medical devices, sensors, mobile phones, and social media—could be very valuable in the prevention of diabetes and improving related health outcomes in the near future. The creation of real-world data sets could, for example, help to predict diabetes onset, or to prevent severe hypoglycemia [20]. However, utilization of these technologies is still in their infancies, and there are many risks and methodological challenges to overcome. This includes ensuring the quality of the data, incorporating both quantitative and qualitative data, language limitations, and standardization processes [22].

It has been indicated that the future use of social media for diabetes may also include the use of fully automated self-help interventions integrated in chatbots and connected to sensors. Social media chatbots are based on statistical learning, statistical analysis, and educational theories aiming at simulating a human conversation by text or voice message. The use of social media chatbots for health-related purposes, that is, computer programs that simulate conversation with human users on social media, is an emerging field that could bring health benefits.

Discussion

The main power of social media, that is, enhancing communication between individuals, does not seem to be working optimally between different diabetes-affected stakeholders. Despite the increased use of social media for diabetes, those with diabetes and their health-care personnel discuss diabetes very differently, and they do not seem to frequently interact with one another on social media platforms. A recent study illustrated how different stakeholder groups on social media have different agendas, evident through the messages that are shared and discussed regarding diabetes-related information. For example, while social media users in closed patient groups mainly discuss diabetes self-management, in open social media groups administrated by patient organizations and health-care professionals, the main topic was diabetes awareness [9].

This nonoptimal interaction between people with diabetes and health-care professionals today is a difficult challenge, because of the enormous amount of information that is shared on social media and the lack of sufficient resources to devote to these activities. At the moment, only a few medical associations, such as the American Medical Association and the British Medical Association, have proposed guidelines advising clinicians on how they should use social media to avoid or reduce risk [23,24]. More guidelines and standard procedures are needed, including the addition of social media use as a topic within medical curricula. Subsequently, this could also result in better communication between health professionals and people with diabetes.

In addition, although it seems like most of the health information available on social media is of reasonably good quality, nevertheless, social media users are subject to risks associated with misleading or inadequate information, as well as their own misunderstanding of the content [25]. Health-care professionals, public health institutions, and other stakeholders need to have a greater presence on social media. They have the potential for interacting with individuals, delivering trustworthy information, correcting misinformation, and providing the correct responses to personal and public concerns.

The use of social media has escalated recently, and it is establishing itself as platform for health information and communication—transforming our views of the health domain and the optimal types of communication between different stakeholders. We expect to see increasing online interactions between stakeholders, and the use of new approaches for social media. In the future, social media tools for diabetes will likely incorporate software algorithms that can combine data from multiple sources, such as sensors, mobile phones, and social media itself. Furthermore, chatbots will be increasingly used. These developments in social media will likely be important factors in both preventing T2D, and improving the health of those affected with all forms of diabetes.

References

[1] Syed-Abdul S, Gabarron E, Lau AYS. Participatory health through social media. Elsevier; 2016. p. 2016.
[2] Tennant B, Stellefson M, Dodd V, Chaney B, Chany D, Paige S, et al. eHealth Literacy and Web 2.0 health information seeking behaviors among baby boomers and older adults. J Med Internet Res 2015;17(3):e70.

[3] NIH, National Institute of Diabetes and Digestive and Kidney Diseases. Diabetes overview, Available from: <https://www.niddk.nih.gov/health-information/diabetes/overview/what-is-diabetes>; 2019.

[4] Eng DS, Lee JM. Mobile health applications for diabetes and endocrinology: promise and peril? Pediatr Diabetes 2013;14(4):231−8 10.1111.

[5] Greene JA, Choudhry NK, Kilabuk E, Shrank WH. Online social networking by patients with diabetes: a qualitative evaluation of communication with Facebook. J Gen Intern Med 2011;26(3):287−92.

[6] Hone T, Palladino R, Filippidis FT. Association of searching for health-related information online with self-rated health in the European Union. Eur J Public Health 2016;26 (5):748−53.

[7] Gabarron E, Lau AYS, Wynn R. Is there a weekly pattern for health information searching and is the pattern unique to health topics? J Med Internet Res 2015;17(12):e286.

[8] Gabarron E, Bradway M, Årsand E. What are diabetes patients discussing on social media? Int Integr Care 2016;16(5):S14.

[9] Årsand E, Bradway M, Gabarron E. What are diabetes patients versus healthcare personnel discussing on social media? J Diabetes Sci Technol 2019;12:2499−506.

[10] Oyeyemi SO, Gabarron E, Wynn R. Ebola, Twitter, and misinformation: a dangerous combination? BMJ 2014;349:g6178.

[11] Bode L, Vraga EK. See something, say something: correction of global health misinformation on social media. Health Commun 2018;33(9):1131−40.

[12] White K, Gebremariam A, Lewis D, Nordgren W, Wedding J, Pasek J, et al. Motivations for participation in an online social media community for diabetes. J Diabetes Sci Technol 2018;12(3):712−18.

[13] Gabarron E, Dorronzoro E, Bradway M, Rivera-Romero O, Wynn R, Årsand E. Preferences and interests of diabetes social media users regarding a health-promotion intervention. Patient Prefer Adherence 2018;12:2499−506.

[14] Reidy C, Klonoff DC, Barnad-Kelly KD. Supporting good intentions with good evidence: how to increase the benefits of diabetes social media. J Diabetes Sci Technol 2019;13(5), 1932296819850187.

[15] Gómez-Zúñiga B, Pousada M, Hernandez MM, Colberg S, Gabarron E, Armayones M. The online big blue test for promoting exercise: health, self-efficacy, and social support. Telemed J E Health 2015;21(10):852−9.

[16] Gabarron E, Dorronzoro E, Rivera-Romero O, Wynn R. Diabetes on Twitter: a sentiment analysis. J Diabetes Sci Technol 2019;13(3):439−44.

[17] Gavrila V, Garrity A, Hirschfeld E, Edwards B, Lee JM. Peer support though a diabetes social media community. J Diabetes Sci Technol 2019;13(3), 1932296818818828.

[18] Nelakurthi AR, Pinto AM, Cook CB, Jones L, Boyle M, Ye J, et al. Should patients with diabetes be encouraged to integrate social media into their care plan? Future Sci OA 2018;4(7):FSO323.

[19] Abedin T, Al Mamun M, Lasker MAA, Ahmed SW, Shommu N, Rumana N, et al. Social media as a platform for information about diabetes foot care: a study of Facebook groups. Can J Diabetes 2017;41(1):97−101.

[20] Gabarron E, Årsand E, Wynn R. Social media use in interventions for diabetes: rapid evidence-based review. J Med Internet Res 2018;20(8):e10303.

[21] Petrovski G, Zivkovic M. Are we ready to treat our diabetes patients using social media? Yes, we are. J Diabetes Sci Technol 2019;13(2):171−5.

[22]   Kerr D, Klonoff DC. Digital diabetes data and artificial intelligence: a time for humility not hubris. J Diabetes Sci Technol 2019;13(1):123–7.

[23]   American Medical Association. AMA policy: professionalism in the use of social media, Available from: <https://mededu.jmir.org/article/downloadSuppFile/4886/28296>; 2012.

[24]   British Medical Association. Doctors' use of social media, Available from: <https://www.gmc-uk.org/-/media/documents/doctors-use-of-social-media_pdf-58833100.pdf>; 2013.

[25]   Cole J, Watkins C, Kleine D. Health advice from Internet discussion forums: how bad is dangerous? J Med Internet Res 2016;18(1):e4.

Chapter 10

Using diabetes technology in older adults

Nancy A. Allen and Michelle L. Litchman
University of Utah College of Nursing, Salt Lake City, UT, United States

Abbreviations

apps applications
FGM flash glucose monitoring
HbA1c hemoglobin A1c
mHealth mobile health
PWD people with diabetes
RT-CGM real-time continuous glucose monitoring
T1D type 1 diabetes
T2D type 2 diabetes

Key points

- Older adults with diabetes may have changes in cognitive abilities, physical abilities, perception, and motivation that affect their use of technology.
- There are unique facilitators and barriers to the use of technology in older adults with diabetes compared to younger age groups.
- Diabetes technology can improve quality of life in older adults as they age and their diabetes becomes more difficult to manage.

Background

Almost one-third of adults over 65 years of age in the United States have diabetes, approximately half of whom are undiagnosed [1]. An additional one-third of older adults have prediabetes [1]. Approximately 366,000 people aged 65 years or older are newly diagnosed with diabetes every year [1]. Overall, the number of older adults with type 1 diabetes (T1D) and type 2 diabetes (T2D) has been increasing in the United States since 1958 with a serious increase since 2000 [2]. Because of improved clinical care involving

Diabetes Digital Health. DOI: https://doi.org/10.1016/B978-0-12-817485-2.00010-9

complex insulin and monitoring regimens, the life span of people with T1D has been increasing; these individuals are now living approximately 15 years longer than individuals diagnosed in 1950−80 [3]. The life expectancy for males with T2D 5 years after diagnosis varies from 13 years with high risk factors to 21 years with low risk factors, including smoking, hypertension, and elevated hemoglobin A1c (HbA1c) concentrations [4]. Adults with an earlier onset of T1D generally have a longer duration of diabetes because they are diagnosed earlier and are more likely to exhibit micro- and macro-vascular complications and other comorbidities [5].

Glucose management in older adults with diabetes can be challenging. In particular, older patients have an increased risk of severe hypoglycemia secondary to their reduced ability to detect low blood glucose and produce counterregulatory hormones to prevent hypoglycemia [6]. Hypoglycemia in older adults is associated with an increased risk of falls with injury, myocardial infarction, arrhythmias, temporary or permanent cognitive impairment, and death [6]. Furthermore, older adults with diabetes have an elevated likelihood of frailty, mortality, lower extremity complications, polypharmacy, depression, and functional (e.g., vision and hearing) impairment [6]. Polypharmacy is particularly problematic because drug metabolism differs between older adults and people less than 60 years of age [7]. Older adults with T2D also have a twofold higher incidence of dementia than those without diabetes that is in part related to insulin resistance [8].

Currently, the American Diabetes Association recommends glycemic goals [e.g., HbA1c < 7.5% (58 mmol/mol)] for healthy older adults with few coexisting chronic illnesses, intact cognitive function, and high functional status [9]. Less stringent goals (e.g., HbA1c < 8.0%−8.5% [64−69 mmol/mol]) are recommended for those with multiple coexisting chronic illnesses, cognitive impairment, or functional dependence. Avoiding hyperglycemia is important for preventing acute complications of high blood glucose levels, such as dehydration, poor wound healing, urinary incontinence, and hyperglycemic hyperosmolar coma. Technology can help people with diabetes (PWD) meet their glycemic goals while avoiding hypoglycemia.

Safe and comprehensive diabetes management is a priority in older adults with diabetes to reduce complications and poor outcomes, as well as to optimize quality of life. The aforementioned factors commonly found in older adults with diabetes can affect their ability to engage in diabetes self-management and the use of technology. In the past, many studies regarding diabetes-related technology have excluded older adults. However, this trend is changing because of the rising number of older adults with diabetes and increased recognition of the difficulties that older adults experience when managing their diabetes. Diabetes technology (e.g., continuous glucose monitoring and insulin pumps) and mobile health (mHealth) technology (e.g., digital health, mobile applications [apps], and telehealth) can assist PWD to manage their glucose levels, decrease their risk of diabetes-related complications, and improve their quality of life. In the Diamond trial designed to determine the effectiveness of real-time continuous glucose monitoring (RT-CGM) in adults ≥ 60 years of age, there was a high usage rate of RT-CGM [10]. Ninety-seven percent of participants with T1D and T2D wore an RT-CGM ≥ 6 days/week over 6 months indicating the usefulness of this technology to older PWD.

The American Diabetes Association also recommends that prior to initiating any complex technology such as an insulin pump, mobile apps, in older adults, a geriatric assessment should be conducted for PWD who are older than 65 years [9]. Technology use may require tailoring to account for physical and cognitive functioning, comorbidities, and family or social support. An older adult with diabetes can benefit from more technology training time, having a care partner educated with them, setting alarms such that they are safe but not bothersome, using bigger screens such as an iPad and tailoring alarms to alert the user by hearing, feeling, or seeing. Depending on the type of technology, clinicians should consider administering tests to assess cognition (e.g., Mini Cog, Montreal Cognitive Assessment) [11,12], depression (e.g., geriatric depression scale) [13], and functional ability (e.g., activities of daily living, instrumental activities of daily living) [14]. The results of these assessments can provide a framework to determine targets and therapeutic approaches.

Cognitive decline can increase the risk of medication errors that can lead to severe hypoglycemia. Older adults with cognitive impairment who are taking insulin may make unrecognized errors in doses, timing of injections, or timing and content of meals. Moreover, cognitively impaired PWD may forget to eat, experience a change in taste, or develop a lack of interest in shopping for food and preparing meals. Cognitive impairment is common among older adults. Memory aids, such as electronic pill dispensers or alarms, can remind individuals to take their medications. Memory features in some insulin pens and all insulin pumps, allowing individuals to see whether an insulin dose was taken. However, cognitively impaired older adults may have difficulty using electronic medication delivery units if they are confused by the terminology [15]. RT-CGM and Bluetooth-enabled insulin pens may serve as a memory aid and increase insulin safety [16]. These devices can thereby increase the safety of living with diabetes and accompanying age-related changes. Technology decreases the likelihood of severe hypoglycemia when used effectively.

Older adults interact with technology differently

Older adults interact with technology differently than younger people related to the use of diabetes technology [15]. There are several barriers related to the use of diabetes technology. These barriers can be classified into four categories: (1) cognitive function, (2) physical ability, (3) perception (vision and hearing), and (4) motivation [15]. Understanding technology barriers in older adults can assist in developing and improving PWD's acceptance of technology, as well as inform teaching strategies.

Cognitive function

Cognitive barriers can affect several types of memory (e.g., working, prospective, semantic, procedural) and attention. This can, in turn, affect a person's ability to process and recall information [15]. For example, remembering to take insulin 4 hours later can be difficult because this is a future- and time-based task. When teaching older adults, it is important to recognize that they need more time to learn new skills. They can have difficulty with mental imagery, which can impair their ability to complete tasks on a computer [15]. Older adults may also have a decline in numeracy and the ability to organize and process complex concepts, which can affect their ability to understand content specific to technology interventions. Reduced numeracy and representational fluency may decrease their ability to read and interpret tables and charts on measures related to health information. In general, PWD who have T1D are most likely to have a decreased ability to switch from one concept to another (mental flexibility) and slowing of mental speed; learning and memory are less likely to be impaired [16]. The ability to learn and memorize information improves an older adult's ability to use technology such as how to complete the multiple steps necessary in using an insulin pump to bolus for a meal. However, slowing of mental speed may result in a longer learning curve and longer times to complete tasks. This may lead to a decrease in task completion such as using mHealth apps designed to assist in diabetes self-management. Older adults with T2D typically exhibit a decline in executive function, memory, learning, attention, and psychomotor efficiency [16]. These cognitive changes may make it difficult to learn, remember, and make decisions such as required in using an insulin pump, RT-CGM, and mHealth apps. Recent studies have also shown a higher prevalence of cognitive dysfunction in older adults with T1D, compared with individuals without diabetes, although T1D appears to have less impact than T2D on cognitive dysfunction [16].

Physical abilities

Physical abilities may affect the ability to use software. Arthritis (which affects 60% of the US population) and diabetes-related neuropathy may lead to difficulties with clicking on small buttons in computer website interfaces or other technologies [16]. These conditions can also limit the ability to hold a device in one hand. Older adults often have slower movements and reflexes, stiff muscles and joints, and hand tremors, all of which are potential concerns when developing or using technology. Thus technology use may be hampered by impairments in learning time, speed of performance, error rate, retention time, and self-reported satisfaction [15].

Diabetes-related tasks that require fine-motor movements of the hands can be particularly challenging for older PWD. These include checking glucose levels, removing insulin from a vial, using an insulin pen, inserting an insulin pump infusion cannula, and using RT-CGM or flash glucose monitoring (FGM). Other technology difficulties may include pressing buttons on diabetes technology devices. Older adults with physical challenges may require assistance from their care partners, such as a spouse, to support the use of diabetes technology.

Perception

Diabetic retinopathy is a leading cause of vision loss. Of an estimated 285 million PWD worldwide, approximately one-third have signs of diabetic retinopathy, which is vision threatening in one-third of those with retinopathy [17]. Visual abilities that decrease with age are the ability to resolve details, focus on close objects, discriminate between colors (especially violet, blue, and green), detect contrast, and adapt to darker conditions [15]. Older adults are likewise more susceptible to glare, leading to vision impairment with direct and reflective light. In general, older people require more light to see images sharply, have reduced peripheral vision (i.e., tunnel vision), and are less able to detect motion [15].

An estimated 34.5 million with diabetes have some type of hearing loss [18]. This can affect their ability to perceive audible alarms and video content. Older adults with moderate-to-severe hearing impairment have lower computer desktop and Internet use than those without hearing difficulties [15]. PWD with hearing impairment may compensate by using vibration or visual cues (e.g., flashing lights).

Motivation barriers

Older adults have reported lower acceptance of technology in terms of motivation that is subsequently linked to the usage and adoption of mHealth apps [15]. Motivation can be affected by attitudes and perceptions of technology and by cognitive issues such as concentration issues and learning disabilities [15]. However, little research has been done to determine usage and adoption rates in this population. Recent estimates of technology use in middle-age adults from the T1D exchange report that among individuals ≥ 50 years, 62% use insulin pumps, 34% use CGM, and 28% use self-monitoring of blood glucose [19]. More study is needed in the older adult population with diabetes to determine the types of technology and the amount of technology adoption.

One possible explanation of motivation barriers is an insufficient consideration of older adults' usability requirements. Other technology factors have been identified in a review of older adults' adoption of technology [20]. They include (1) usability—perception of user-friendliness and ease of learning, (2) affordability—perception of cost savings, (3) accessibility—knowledge of existence and availability in the market, (4) technical support—availability and quality of professional assistant throughout use, (5) social support—support from family, peers, and community, (6) emotion—perception of emotional value and psychological value, (7) independence—perception of social visibility or how technology makes the look to others, (8) experience—relevance with their prior experiences and interactions, and (9) confidence—empowerment without anxiety or intimidation [20]. Technology that addresses these benefits can increase older adults' motivation to use technology.

MOLD-US framework

The MOLD-US framework (Fig. 10.1) provides a visual overview summarizing the potential barriers of older adults, including those with diabetes, that limit their ability to use mobile technology [15]. This model shows the anticipated effects of age-related changes and medical conditions. The MOLD-US framework was developed from a synthesis of the literature regarding the use of mHealth apps (Fig. 10.1) [15].

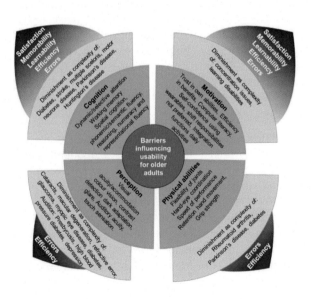

FIGURE 10.1 MOLD-US framework [15].

Digital health technology in older adults with diabetes

Blood glucose monitors

There are many blood glucose monitoring options for older adults experiencing age-related changes. Some blood glucose monitors have audio capabilities that can assist individuals with hearing loss. Many blood glucose monitors have features to help PWD with impaired vision, including background lights, lighted ports for glucose strip insertion, large screens, contrasting screen backgrounds, and selectable fonts. Some blood glucose monitor can store several strips, which is useful for PWD with reduced hand dexterity. This feature reduces the number of times a person must open the strip containers and insert test strips into the monitor. Indeed, care partners can preload the strips for them, allowing PWD to maintain their independence during glucose testing. Other features can aid individuals with cognitive difficulties. For example, blood glucose monitors can save data to the cloud, which not only eliminates the need to manually enter glucose values in a logbook but also transfers the values into a data management system that displays glucose trends. Data management systems facilitate the interpretation of glucose trends, although some people with PWD may be unable to take full advantage of this, depending on the nature of their cognitive impairment. For older adults using insulin pumps, some blood glucose monitors communicate glucose readings automatically to the pumps, thereby preventing errors associated with manually entering blood glucose values. Unfortunately, most blood glucose monitors with features assisting older adults are expensive and not covered by Medicare.

Continuous glucose monitoring and remote data sharing

A systematic review revealed that among older adults, RT-CGM systems are useful for detecting hypoglycemia unawareness, improving HbA1c concentrations, and improving well-being and diabetes-related distress [21]. FGM demonstrated HbA1c reduction without significant hypoglycemia events in people with increased glycemic variability, although the effects are less clear among individuals older than 65 years [22]. In addition, it is unknown whether FGM is useful for detecting hypoglycemia unawareness which is more common with advanced diabetes duration.

RT-CGM technology is a good example of a technology that has been shown to improve the quality of life in older PWD. Quality of life is the perception of physical, emotional (happiness), social, and cognitive (satisfaction) well-being [23]. RT-CGM can increase quality of life by improving confidence with (1) keeping glucose levels in range, (2) increasing safety from a hypoglycemia perspective, and (3) improving relationships with family and friends. This may be at least partially because older adults have a higher frequency of viewing their RT-CGM readings than other age groups

[10]. Older adults also have an increased sense of independence when using RT-CGM, especially with respect to their ability to self-manage hypoglycemia, which may otherwise require support by care partners or others. This is because most RT-CGMs provide a 20-minute trend alarm allowing alerting the user to hypo- or hyperglycemia.

Older PWD appreciate the ability to track the effects of food and physical activity on blood glucose levels, thus allowing them to learn more about their diabetes [23]. Moreover, older adults desire the ability to function better, with fewer episodes of hypoglycemia, in daily activities by viewing glucose trend graphs before activities, such as driving, exercising, traveling, and just before sleeping. In addition, older adults feel that they are being supported by using a technology that may allow them to live longer, have fewer hypoglycemia-related injuries (i.e., falling), and experience fewer diabetes-related complications. [23] Quality of life in older adults with diabetes may drive the future of technology development as this population continues to increase in number and demands this type of support for managing their diabetes. However, access to insurance coverage is seen as a major barrier to RT-CGM in the older population. Until recently, older adults have not had access to CGM because of lack of Medicare coverage, thereby necessitating reliance on multiple blood glucose checks throughout the day. Medicare began covering RT-CGM in 2017 and this has decreased this barrier to using RT-CGM among older adults [24].

Data sharing is available for both RT-CGM and FGM systems, although the literature regarding this in older adult populations is limited. Among the general population, RT-CGM data sharing can enhance feelings of safety [25]. However, data sharing can also produce tensions between PWD and the people they share data with unless boundaries are established to avoid judgment [25]. Another benefit of RT-CGM is remote monitoring in which health-care providers can view RT-CGM data and assist individuals with dosing changes between visits, as needed.

RT-CGM benefits are dependent on device accuracy, ease of operability, and trust in one's own ability to make use of RT-CGM data [26]. To minimize barriers to RT-CGM use, educational interventions that improve confidence in using their RT-CGM data may help older adults to have reasonable expectations and use. Education could focus on potential fact there may be discrepancies between blood glucose values and RT-CGM readings [26]. Furthermore, training may take more time in an older adult population and should focus on how to initiate CGM (site selection, sensor insertion, entering glucose data following a warm-up period, linking a smartphone for FGM or RT-CGM for trend graph viewing, initiate RT-CGM sharing, sharing RT-CGM viewing codes with health-care providers), CGM maintenance (adhesive management, FGM scanning, RT-CGM viewing on receiver or smartphone), and CGM decision-making (how to make insulin adjustments based on trend graphs).

Insulin pumps

Insulin pumps are desired by all age groups and should be considered an option for older adults with diabetes requiring multiple daily injections. Although insulin pumps are less commonly initiated in older adults than in younger individuals, health-care providers must consider that younger adults using insulin pumps may wish to continue to do so as they age.

When initiating pump therapy, in any population, safety is critical. There may be instances when an insulin pump must be discontinued, if it is no longer considered safe. Insulin pumps can be used safely— independently or with support—in older adults. Compared to younger PWD, additional training is often required when initiating pump therapy or upgrading to a newer device [27], which may require increased time of clinic visits or multiple visits. For safety reasons it may be appropriate to use saline when initiating pump therapy to determine whether the pump features are being used correctly. The ability to properly use the insulin pump should be routinely reassessed, and additional support systems should be established to deal with safety concerns, such as those related to pump site changes, entering information into the pump (e.g., carbohydrate count and glucose level), or insulin dosing. Additional support could include family, friends, or home health services.

Mobile apps

The majority of mobile apps are used with cell phones. Today, approximately 50% of older adults over the age of 65 years who own cell phones have a smartphone. [28] Smartphone ownership among older adults declines with age: 59% of 65- to 69-year olds own smartphones, whereas the percentage falls to 49% among 70- to 74-year olds [28]. Approximately 41% of people between 65 and 69 years of age have tablet computers, while this percentage is 20% in people aged 80 years and older [28]. However, only 26% of Internet users aged 65 years and over report feeling very confident when using computers, smartphones, or other electronic devices to accomplish online tasks. [28] This low level of confidence has implications when considering the use of apps in this population. Nevertheless, many older adults have a positive outlook about technology and the benefits it can provide, and once they become familiar with using technology many will engage deeply with online content and activities [28].

Smartphones provide an opportunity for older adults to use a large number of available diabetes apps. According to a recent systematic review, many diabetes apps offer similar functionalities and are primarily used for logging glucose levels, diet, and exercise [29]. Findings from this review show the majority of diabetes apps offer only one or two functions, such as logging glucose levels and/or diet information, which is beneficial for older adults, as the usability of diabetes apps in PWD over the age of 50 years is higher when apps offer a small range of functions. The review also noted that several apps exhibit a lack of suitability and usability for older adults with diabetes, the main target group [29]. Overall, there were moderate to good evaluations on usability criteria with one exception: "fault tolerance." Fault tolerance refers to the acceptability of inaccuracies or failures within apps. Older adults with diabetes generally benefit from easy, understandable language. They likewise prefer images that are simple to understand and interpret, primarily because older adults often have limited experience with mobile devices and apps. Interestingly, apps with documentation and analysis functions perform worse in terms of usability in this age group [29]. Many older adults prefer using a conventional diary for documentation; they find apps too complicated and time-consuming for this purpose.

Telehealth

There are no current estimates of the usage of telehealth in older adults with diabetes. Telehealth is the use of electronic information and telecommunications technologies to support and promote long-distance clinical health care as well as patient and professional health-related education. Older adults with diabetes may benefit from telehealth coaching. One of the benefits is when older adults with diabetes have difficulty seeing their health-care provider on a regular basis for various reasons, such as physical impairment, transportation problems, and geographic limitations. The features of telehealth coaching vary by system but may include a blood glucose monitor, automatic coaching when glucose levels fall outside a certain range, and scheduled coaching by telephone, text messages, or video communications. Coaching can cover a range of diabetes self-management behaviors, such as glucose measurements, healthy eating, physical activity, and risk reduction. In a systematic review addressing telemedicine and telecare for older patients, the majority of studies showed a trend toward better results for behavioral endpoints (e.g., adherence to medication or diet, and self-efficacy) compared to results from clinical outcomes (e.g., blood pressure), quality of life, and economic outcomes (e.g., costs or hospitalization) [30]. In another systematic review, facilitators and barriers were identified to using telehealth in older adults [31]. The identified telehealth facilitators were feelings of safety, security, and aging in place. Moreover, telehealth use increases when an individual's autonomy is considered. Barriers include devices that do not work outside the home, a misfit between technology and user's needs, and a perception that they are seen as being frail and helpless by using the telehealth technology. Overall, older adults must see the value of the telecare in order to use it [31].

Summary

Many important issues exist when considering technology use in older PWD. These individuals may have reduced cognitive abilities, physical abilities, perception (e.g., sight and hearing), and motivation. These changes should not limit the use of technology in older PWD but rather inform providers and clinicians to consider adaptions for providing education and the use of the technology in light of these aging changes. Also, technology can assist with several of these age-related changes. Digital health technology provides many options to manage diabetes in older PWD and their changing abilities and can increase their feelings of safety. However, there is a lack of research in older adults with diabetes on specific features of these technologies and how they enhance or hinder their ability to provide self-care. Currently, older PWD are increasingly using insulin pumps and continuous glucose monitoring. Some older PWD may have low confidence using the Internet that affects the adoption of mHealth apps. To increase acceptance, integration of diabetes technology into care plans must incorporate user-centered design, developmental needs of each population, and a possibility of enhancing quality of life. As older PWD are now living longer than in the past, quality of life has become an important consideration. Several existing technologies can improve quality of life, and future technological discoveries will have the potential to further minimize the effects of diabetes on the lives of older adults.

References

[1] Center for Disease Control. National diabetes statistics report 2017, Available from: <https://www.cdc.gov/diabetes/pdfs/data/statistics/national-diabetes-statistics-report.pdf>; 2017.

[2] CDC's Division of Diabetes Translation. United States Diabetes Surveillance System. Long term trends in diabetes, Available from: <https://www.cdc.gov/diabetes/statistics/slides/long_term_trends.pdf>; 2017.

[3] Diabetes Control and Complications Trial (DCCT)/Epidemiology of Diabetes Interventions and Complications (EDIC) Study Research Group. Mortality in type 1 diabetes in the DCCT/EDIC versus the general population. Diabetes Care 2016;39(8):1378−83.

[4] Leal J, Gray AM, Clarke PM. Development of life-expectancy tables for people with type 2 diabetes. Eur Heart J 2009;30(7):834−9.

[5] Dhaliwal R, Weinstock RS. Management of type 1 diabetes in older adults. Diabetes Spectr 2014;27(1):9−20.

[6] Abdelhafiz AH, Rodriguez-Manas L, Morley JE, Sinclair AJ. Hypoglycemia in older people—a less well recognized risk factor for frailty. Aging Dis 2015;6(2):156−67.

[7] Sherifali D, Bai JW, Kenny M, Warren R, Ali MU. Diabetes self-management programmes in older adults: a systematic review and meta-analysis. Diabetes Med 2015;32 (11):1404−14.

[8] Mayeda ER, Whitmer RA, Yaffe K. Diabetes and cognition. Clgeriatric Med 2015;31 (1):101−15.

[9] American Diabetes Association. 12. Older adults: standards of medical care in diabetes—2019. Diabetes Care 2019;42(Suppl. 1):S139—47.

[10] Ruedy KJ, Parkin CG, Riddlesworth TD, Graham C. Continuous glucose monitoring in older adults with type 1 and type 2 diabetes using multiple daily injections of insulin: results from the DIAMOND trial. J Diabetes Sci Technol 2017;11(6):1138—46.

[11] Borson S, Scanlan J, Brush M, Vitaliano P, Dokmak A. The mini-cog: a cognitive 'vital signs' measure for dementia screening in multi-lingual elderly. Int J Geriatr Psychiatry 2000;15(11):1021—7.

[12] Abd Razak MA, Ahmad NA, Chan YY, Mohamad Kasim N, Yusof M, Abdul Ghani MKA, et al. Validity of screening tools for dementia and mild cognitive impairment among the elderly in primary health care: a systematic review. Pub Health 2019;169:84—92.

[13] Sheikh JI, Yesavage JA. Geriatric Depression Scale (GDS). Recent evidence and development of a shorter version. In: T.L. Brink (Ed.), Clinical Gerontology: A Guide to Assessment and Intervention. NY: The Haworth Press, Inc. 1986;165—73.

[14] Lawton MP, Brody EM. Assessment of older people: self-maintaining and instrumental activities of daily living. Gerontologist 1969;9:179—86.

[15] Wildenbos GA, Peute L, Jaspers M. Aging barriers influencing mobile health usability for older adults: a literature based framework (MOLD-US). Int J Med Inform 2018;114:66—75.

[16] Munshi MN. Cognitive dysfunction in older adults with diabetes: what a clinician needs to know. Diabetes Care 2017;40(4):461—7.

[17] Lee R, Wong TY, Sabanayagam C. Epidemiology of diabetic retinopathy, diabetic macular edema and related vision loss. Eye Vision (London, Engl) 2015;2:17.

[18] American Diabetes Association. Diabetes and hearling loss. American Diabetes Association; 2017. Available from: <http://www.diabetes.org/living-with-diabetes/treatment-and-care/seniors/diabetes-and-hearing-loss.html>.

[19] Foster NC, Beck RW, Miller KM, Clements MA, Rickels MR, DiMeglio LA, et al. State of type 1 diabetes management and outcomes from the T1D exchange in 2016—2018. Diabetes Technol Ther 2019;21(2):66—72.

[20] Lee C, Coughlin JF. Older adults' adoption of technology: an integrated approach to identifying determinants and barriers. J Prod Innov Manage 2015;32(5):747—59.

[21] Mattishent K, Loke YK. Detection of asymptomatic drug-induced hypoglycemia using continuous glucose monitoring in older people—systematic review. J DiabetComplications 2018;32(8):805—12.

[22] Anjana RM, Kesavadev J, Neeta D, Tiwaskar M, Pradeepa R, Jebarani S, et al. A Multicenter real-life study on the effect of flash glucose monitoring on glycemic control in patients with type 1 and type 2 diabetes. Diabetes Technol Ther 2017;19(9):533—40.

[23] Litchman ML, Allen NA. Real-time continuous glucose monitoring facilitates feelings of safety in older adults with type 1 diabetes: a qualitative study. J Diabetes Sci Technol. 2017;11(5):988—95.

[24] Centers for Medicaid and Medicare Services. Current coverage of diabetes supplies, Available from: <https://www.cms.gov/Outreach-and-Education/Medicare-Learning-Network-MLN/MLNMattersArticles/Downloads/SE18011.pdf>; 2018.

[25] Litchman ML, Allen NA, Colicchio VD, Wawrzynski SE, Sparling KM, Hendricks KL, et al. A qualitative analysis of real-time continuous glucose monitoring data sharing with care partners: to share or not to share? Diabetes Technol Ther 2018;20(1):25—31.

[26] Polonsky WH, Hessler D. What are the quality of life-related benefits and losses associated with real-time continuous glucose monitoring? A survey of current users. Diabetes Technol Ther 2013;15(4):295–301.

[27] Matejko B, Cyganek K, Katra B, Galicka-Latala D, Grzanka M, Malecki MT, et al. Insulin pump therapy is equally effective and safe in elderly and young type 1 diabetes patients. Rev Diabetes Stud: RDS 2011;8(2):254–8.

[28] World Economic Forum. Think older people are technophobes? Think again, Available from: <https://www.weforum.org/agenda/2017/05/think-older-people-are-technophobes-think-again>; 2019.

[29] Arnhold M, Quade M, Kirch W. Mobile applications for diabetics: a systematic review and expert-based usability evaluation considering the special requirements of diabetes patients age 50 years or older. J Med Internet Res 2014;16(4):e104.

[30] van den Berg N, Schumann M, Kraft K, Hoffmann W. Telemedicine and telecare for older patients—a systematic review. Maturitas 2012;73(2):94–114.

[31] Karlsen C, Ludvigsen MS, Moe CE, Haraldstad K, Thygesen E. Experiences of community-dwelling older adults with the use of telecare in home care services: a qualitative systematic review. JBI Database Syst Rev Implement Rep 2017;15(12):2913–80.

Chapter 11

Socioeconomic factors: access to and use of diabetes technologies

Samantha A. Barry-Menkhaus[1], David V. Wagner[2], Maggie Stoeckel[3] and Michael A. Harris[2,4]

[1]*University of California, San Francisco, San Francisco, CA, United States,* [2]*Oregon Health & Science University, Portland, OR, United States,* [3]*The Children's Program, Portland, OR, United States,* [4]*Harold Schnitzer Diabetes Health Center, Portland, OR, United States*

Abbreviations

CGM	continuous glucose monitor
EHR	electronic health record
mHealth	mobile health
P-LSES	people of lower socioeconomic status
SES	socioeconomic status
T1D	type 1 diabetes
T2D	type 2 diabetes

Key points

- Digital health advancements across proximal (e.g., pump and continuous glucose monitor) and distal (e.g., telehealth and mobile applications) technologies offer exciting opportunities to reduce health inequalities in diabetes care for individuals of lower socioeconomic status (SES).
- The vast majority of the literature does not consider SES in evaluations of diabetes technologies, a subgroup of technology evaluations includes SES as a variable of interest, and a very small number of studies specifically target this group, address their unique barriers, and evaluate their distinct user-profiles.
- Future diabetes technology development and evaluation must focus on designing technologies for and thoughtfully delivering services to people of lower SES in order to appropriately address the needs of this high-risk group.

Diabetes Digital Health. DOI: https://doi.org/10.1016/B978-0-12-817485-2.00011-0

Adults and youth with type 1 and type 2 diabetes (T1D and T2D) often experience complex self-management expectations with high risk for complications and exorbitant health-care costs. It is generally the case that, regardless of lifespan stage and diabetes diagnosis, socioeconomic status (SES; i.e., educational attainment, financial security, and perception of social status and class) accounts for significant variability in diabetes outcomes. Indeed, people of lower SES (P-LSES) with T1D or T2D, hereafter referred to as "diabetes" unless otherwise specified, are more likely than those of higher SES to have poorer glycemic control, worse diabetes self-management, lower quality of life, more frequent hospital admissions, higher mortality risk, and more long-term (e.g., cardiovascular disease) and short-term (e.g., diabetic ketoacidosis) complications [1,2]. While racial or ethnic minority status, level of English proficiency, and insurance status are individually associated with diabetes outcomes, SES demonstrates strong associations with glycemic control and quality of life above and beyond these factors [1].

Contributing to this population health concern is the current diabetes care model and its inherent incompatibility with the needs of socially disadvantaged groups. P-LSES are more likely to have difficulty attending outpatient visits during regular clinic hours, often because of unreliable transportation, long travel times from rural areas, difficulty taking time off of work and/or the burden of associated lost wages, and troubles accessing childcare [3]. P-LSES also experience longer wait times, fewer referrals to specialty care, less access to diabetes self-management education programs, and greater difficulty affording out-of-pocket costs for necessary supplies and treatments [4]. While current care models struggle to address these distinctive challenges, digital health advancements provide a unique opportunity to reduce health inequities for those in greatest need. However, technologies not purposefully designed for and thoughtfully delivered to P-LSES threaten to increase the divide in diabetes outcomes across socioeconomic groups.

This review addresses digital health interventions, including access to and use of these interventions by P-LSES, with a specific focus on interventions exhibiting the greatest potential to address health disparities. We include discussions of (1) proximal technologies, by which we mean those worn on the body that offer a technology-mediated intervention, such as insulin pumps, continuous glucose monitors (CGMs), closed-loop and artificial pancreas systems and (2) distal technologies, by which we mean those that provide services remotely, such as telehealth and mobile health (mHealth). We cover the quality and breadth of research on specific technologies and SES, present limitations in the literature, and conclude with recommendations for future directions.

Proximal technologies and socioeconomic status

Disparities in access exist for several proximal diabetes technologies, including insulin pumps and CGMs, which are associated with improved glycemic control and accessed at lower rates by P-LSES [5,6]. In the United States, individuals with private health-care insurance demonstrate higher rates of pump [7] and CGM [8] use. Historically, public insurances have approved CGMs at lower rates, partially because of concerns related to maintenance of technology use by P-LSES [9]. Although insulin pumps for individuals with T1D are similarly covered across private and public insurances, families report that financial concerns (e.g., supply costs, copayments, and deductibles) interfere with decisions to initiate pump therapy [10]. P-LSES are more likely to have lower health literacy and education, which may create difficulties in successfully obtaining and utilizing these technologies [10]. Inappropriate "gatekeeping" by health-care professionals may also play a role, with providers often relying on their perceptions of the personal and psychological attributes needed to make optimal use of technology when prescribing insulin pumps, which may disproportionately impact already vulnerable groups [11].

While proximal technologies demand health literacy, time-intensive trouble-shooting, and substantial health engagement that may present barriers to effective participation for socially disadvantaged groups, as proximal technologies advance (e.g., increased accuracy, lower reliance on calibrations, and more user-friendly data-sharing), P-LSES may still be precluded from accessing these technologies. Furthermore, new technology (e.g., artificial pancreas) trials requiring previous experience with proximal technologies for enrollment exacerbate existing disparities, although many trials do seek out subjects without previous experience with these technologies. This can be especially unfortunate, given evidence of similar continuation rates for newer CGM models across socioeconomic groups [9] and worse diabetes outcomes for P-LSES when using multiple daily injections, but similar outcomes when utilizing insulin pumps [12]. If accessed equally across groups, these technology advancements could help to alleviate some of the socioeconomic differences in glycemic control rather than exacerbate them, driving efforts to improve adoption rates, identify technology shortcomings, and reduce access disparities for P-LSES [e.g., JDRF No (Type) One Left Behind].

Telehealth and socioeconomic status

Telehealth, which is the use of technology to facilitate live interactions between health-care providers and patients, may address access barriers often reported by P-LSES, decrease the burden of diabetes appointments, and increase access to quality care across SES. As the current national shortage of board-certified pediatric and adult endocrinologists [13] impedes access to specialty care for individuals with diabetes (i.e., long wait times for and travel times to appointments) and disproportionately impacts individuals without flexible schedules or reliable transportation and/or living in rural or underserved areas, there is a call for feasible alternatives to clinic-based diabetes care that does not sacrifice access to tailored treatment.

Fortunately, telehealth use is associated with improved appointment attendance, with families of young adults reporting saving an average of 6 hours of work/school per virtual visit compared with in-person clinic-based appointments [14]. A variety of telehealth strategies (e.g., group-based teleconference, telemonitoring, and teleconsultation) also appear equivalent to in-person diabetes visits in maintaining glycemic control, improving psychosocial variables, and fostering therapeutic alliance [15—17]. Strong evidence demonstrates that telehealth addresses important barriers to diabetes care, including distance, time, and cost; however, few studies have specifically recruited P-LSES. Those studies that have investigated the feasibility and impact of telehealth explicitly for P-LSES with diabetes have demonstrated similar telehealth interest, satisfaction, utilization decreases, cost savings, and improvements in treatment outcomes (e.g., HbA1c) across SES groups [18—20].

While Internet access for adults in the United States (89%) is quite high [21], there continue to be individuals and families with unreliable access to both high-speed Internet and a compatible device. In fact, 43% of Americans without Internet in their homes cite cost as the barrier [22], and 60% of those in rural areas report that high-speed Internet access is a problem in their community [23]. Furthermore, privacy and confidentiality concerns may exist for those accessing Internet in public (e.g., a friend's home or a library) or who have few spaces in their home wherein sessions can be completed with only the intended parties. Finally, the current health-care system and fee-for-service model continue to present financial challenges for clinics and patients, with ongoing difficulties in obtaining reimbursement for telehealth [24] threatening its sustainability within diabetes clinics and its affordability for individuals that could most benefit. While telehealth parity laws mandate commercial insurers to reimburse telehealth visits in some states, Medicare requires that select telehealth visits occur with the patient at a local clinic or facility in order to be reimbursable [24], potentially reducing travel times for individuals in rural areas, but failing to eliminate nongeographic barriers (e.g., transportation, employment, and childcare). Furthermore, state laws require that providers be licensed and credentialed in the place of service, making the delivery of services across state lines a barrier, which is particularly troubling for individuals living in rural states with very few board-certified endocrinologists and diabetes specialists [13] and even fewer behavioral health providers with relevant expertise [25]. In summary, telehealth is an effective and feasible alternative to clinic-based medical care for some [15] that appears to have the potential to address barriers impacting P-LSES; however, further research is needed to ensure that telehealth meets the needs of those that could most benefit.

Mobile health and socioeconomic status

Mobile technology may also be a feasible method for reaching previously underserved populations, as the availability and adoption of mobile phones is growing significantly and cell phone ownership does not differ by income or race/ethnicity for adult users [26]. However, adults of higher SES are more likely to own smartphones (i.e., with Internet access and an operating system) than adults of lower SES [26], potentially making voice communication and text-messaging favorable over other mHealth interventions requiring cellular data (e.g., health applications, apps, and social media) to avoid increasing the health disparities associated with the digital divide.

Text messaging

Currently, text-messaging rates are high among adults and youth, and there are no disparities in the use of cellphones for text messaging across racial and socioeconomic groups. Text interventions have shown promise, with interventions that use messaging to facilitate data recording and personalized clinician feedback having more compelling empirical support than automated or untailored interventions [15]. Recent findings suggest that P-LSES demonstrate satisfaction, engagement, and improved targeted outcomes (e.g., diabetes self-management) with text interventions [27,28]. However, when compared to individuals of higher SES, P-LSES may be less engaged in text interventions [28]. While this literature is promising, the overwhelming majority of available text interventions for P-LSES have targeted adults with T2D, and the heterogeneity of outcomes measured (e.g., self-reported health behaviors and HbA1c) and texting protocols (e.g., live-texting, automated tailored two-way texting and automated untailored one-way texting) make it difficult to determine the comparative success of these programs, the program features driving change, and their generalizability to other lower SES groups.

Portals

Despite disparities in ownership of smartphones, there are a considerable number of individuals who rely solely on smartphones for accessing online content, the majority of whom identify as nonwhite, less educated, and lower income. In fact, approximately 30% of individuals with a yearly income of <$30,000 indicated that they use only a smartphone to access online content [29]. Thus when choosing between platforms for an Internet-based intervention, mHealth programs, compared to computer-based programs, may reach more P-LSES. This is particularly relevant data when considering the recent push from Centers for Medicare & Medicaid Services toward sharing the electronic health record (EHR), with requirements for providing patients with access to their EHR and tailored patient education via a patient portal [30]. However, these portals are not required to provide mobile device accessibility [30], which is unfortunate given that computer access has explained most of the variation by race/ethnicity and income in the use of secure messaging patient portals. Furthermore, when offering a mobile platform version to individuals with diabetes, P-LSES are significantly more likely to access EHR technology than when the EHR is available via a computer-based portal alone [31]. It is important to consider, however, that lower health literacy has been associated with requiring more assistance and time to perform standard EHR portal tasks [32]. Thus portals that are easily accessible and user-friendly via both computer and mobile phone are preferable, and assistance should be offered to aid those with lower literacy in their use.

Mobile apps

Few health apps have been specifically developed for and/or evaluated with P-LSES. However, the available research does suggest that P-LSES are less likely to download health-related apps than people of higher SES [33] and that the complexity of available apps may interfere with prolonged use by P-LSES and/or limited health or technology literacy [34]. The social platform landscape also suggests that app trends differ for P-LSES. However, while lower income, less education, and rural community residence are associated with less social media use [35], the number of US adults using social media apps across all groups has increased significantly over the course of the last decade, making these social platforms increasingly practical when trying to reach diverse groups and overcome geographic and other barriers. Importantly, the types of apps and use of these apps may vary across SES groups. For example, while teen use of social media has shifted away from Facebook and toward several other apps (e.g., Instagram and Snapchat), teens from lower income households continue to predominantly use Facebook [35], suggesting that general trends in social media use may not be applicable across demographic groups.

Discussion

While proximal and distal technologies offer the diabetes community many tools to improve self-management, it is unclear whether these technologies are effective for P-LSES with diabetes. Practitioners and researchers envisioned that proximal and distal technologies would "level the playing field" for P-LSES by overcoming many of the barriers differentially impacting this group, increasing access to quality care for those at greatest risk, and engaging a technologically-savvy generation in their health. However, the extant literature indicates that technologies as currently designed are often suboptimal tools for P-LSES. To fulfill the immense potential that technologies offer, developers, researchers, clinicians, and policy makers must modify current approaches to better fit P-LSES with diabetes.

Limitations to current design

Existing technologies appear to be designed by and piloted on technophilic individuals with reliable high-speed Internet access, above-average reading skills, and the financial stability to purchase needed components. Inherent trade-offs may exist between device accessibility, usability, and efficacy, suggesting the need for a broad range of options. However, current technology design approaches seem to predominantly favor profit and efficacy for select groups over health equity, signaling a preference to reach and treat those of higher SES while, at best, hoping that broader systems (e.g., education and insurance industry) and policy changes will someday make such devices accessible to and effective for P-LSES.

Research status and recommendations

Investigators have much room for growth in effectively studying access to and impact of technology for P-LSES [36]. Individuals with diabetes in greatest need are also those least likely to engage and be retained in research studies [37,38]. Researchers would benefit from using recommended techniques (e.g., partnering with community clinics and local organizations serving P-LSES, providing access to participation on evenings and weekends, and conducting assessments in settings convenient for participants) to recruit and retain those in greatest need both in cross-sectional studies and intervention trials [39]. In particular, investigators should consider how to address barriers often encountered by this population (e.g., unreliable transportation and inconsistent phone/Internet service), such as providing necessary mobile devices, services plans, hotspots, and/or other logistical tools upon which these apps rely. While this may not simulate the real-world experiences of P-LSES with diabetes, such results could be used to advocate for access to the needed technologies that support these interventions. While these recommended research changes may be less convenient and more costly to implement, relying upon methods seemingly designed for those in middle- to upper-income brackets does a disservice to both our field and the populations in greatest need of our expertise.

Clinical implications and recommendations

Given existing literature gaps regarding which technologies are most effective for various diverse groups, clinical decisions should be individually tailored, based on relevant patient-, health-care system-, and technology-specific factors. Because systematically screening out P-LSES from accessing technology (i.e., "gatekeeping") is both poor care and unethical, providers, health-care institutions, and payers should perform quality improvement projects to identify whether and how they contribute to disparities in technology access, and adjust accordingly. Regardless of patient SES, when providers consider recommending a specific technology, they or a member of their team should be both knowledgeable enough and able to dedicate adequate time to thoroughly discussing pertinent technology logistics (e.g., recurring out-of-pocket costs of insulin pumps and CGMs, Internet access, and data requirements for web-based resources or apps) as well as inform patients of local and national resources available to attempt to address such costs and other potential barriers. The combination of maintaining current technology-specific expertise, tailoring recommendations to individuals, and dedicating ample time to engage in explicit conversations with patients will not entirely address the issues highlighted throughout this chapter. However, these practices should contribute to ameliorating existing technology and health disparities.

Health-care system status and recommendations

At the broader systemic level, health-care institutions and systems should similarly discontinue use of "one size fits all" approaches to clinical services and take responsibility for the health of their *entire* patient population. They should provide a range of engagement and treatment modalities (e.g., satellite clinics in low SES communities, in-home providers, or in-school providers) and consider integrating behavioral health clinicians with expertise in diabetes management and hiring engagement specialists whose primary role is building relationships with families and ensuring that service delivery across providers is tailored to individual and family characteristics. While a recent metaanalysis suggested that physician practices and health-care systems may actually lose money when interventions reduce utilization [40], it is clearly in the financial (if not moral) interest of local and national governments for their respective populations to be healthier. Furthermore, interventions that specifically improve health for P-LES represent an opportunity for cost savings for all stakeholders given the limited reimbursement associated with public insurance.

At the payer level, insurers should increase monetary incentives that reward reaching and effectively caring for those who are most vulnerable, possibly with reimbursement structures that provide rising payments associated with a patient's social determinants of health. To date, however, there has been little data on outcomes of programs emphasizing racial and ethnic diversity in translational efforts organized by government and academic partnerships [41]. From a policy-making perspective, technology that effectively engages with and creates improvements for P-LSES should be incentivized, as should provider engagement in helping individuals use and access technology reliably. Such initiatives may require upfront costs to institutions and payers; however, given the disproportionate health-care costs attributed to a relatively small percentage of the broader population [42], investing in the health and well-being of P-LSES should decrease long-term economic costs associated with absenteeism, complications/disability, and premature death.

One promising example of partnering with payors to serve a high-risk population in diabetes care is Novel Interventions in Children's Healthcare (NICH), an intensive, multicomponent program, which includes innovative uses of technology specifically designed for the vulnerable population being served [43]. Insurers contract to make a partially capitated prospective payment in order to direct resources to patient's unique needs and ultimately, decrease health-care utilization and costs longer term [44,45]. Although warranting future study before definitive conclusions can be drawn, NICH preliminary findings suggest the viability of alternative payment structures to simultaneously engage key health-care system stakeholders while also addressing the unique needs of P-LSES. Other research has similarly demonstrated the economic benefits associated with technology [46] when willing to abandon more traditional, often shortsighted metrics and evaluate beyond upfront costs. It is likely the case that with continued thoughtful implementation of alternative payment models, efforts to evaluate and document economic benefit of otherwise costly technologies, and innovative programming that challenges the boundaries of the conventional system, we will be better able to impact change for a currently underserved group.

Conclusion

Given the role that SES plays in perpetuating health disparities and the promise of technology to succeed where office-based care has not, clear potential exists to reach and effectively treat the socially vulnerable, thereby reducing or eliminating health disparity. However, despite continued emphasis from influential organizations (e.g., American Academy of Pediatrics and Society of Pediatric Psychology) to address social risk, proximal and distal tools continue to be underutilized with those in greatest need. This is extremely unfortunate, because technology has a unique potential to address all three phases of Kilbourne et al.'s [47] health disparity framework. Regarding phase one (i.e., detection), technology offers the potential to reach those unable to regularly access office-based research and care, thereby increasing our ability to truly capture the extent of health disparities experienced by those with diabetes. For phase two (i.e., understanding), the ability of technology to provide real-time monitoring and 24/7 information sharing overcomes many of the barriers to typical research and clinical practice, increasing our odds of truly understanding the mechanisms by which health disparities are perpetuated for broad populations and on an individual level. For phase three (i.e. dissemination of effective interventions), technology can also improve our ability to both detect and understand health disparity. This dissemination role of technology is likely unmatched, with a few standout programs, such as the Extension for Community Healthcare Outcomes

(Project ECHO) [48], demonstrating this potential. Project ECHO is a program for P-LSES, which uses video conferencing technology to connect academic specialists with a network of rural primary care clinicians; no economic data has been reported to date for this project.

Taken together, optimal technology use could plausibly advance the field's ability to effectively detect, understand, and reduce health disparities on an unparalleled level—thus highlighting the irony of disparities in both current tech-related research recruitment and access to tech-related interventions. From a pragmatic sense, some may argue that local and national governments should shoulder the majority of financial investment in technologies demonstrated to improve the health and daily functioning of their populations, especially those at greatest risk of other costly outcomes (e.g., homelessness, substance addiction, and incarceration) and most likely to be dependent on public insurance. Ideally, the onus for change would be borne across systems, with particular need for technology developers and companies, researchers and funding agencies, health-care systems and service providers, and policy makers at all levels to contribute to effectively maximizing the value of technology to address health inequities.

References

[1] Hassan K, Loar R, Anderson BJ, Heptulla RA. The role of socioeconomic status, depression, quality of life, and glycemic control in type 1 diabetes mellitus. J Pediatr 2006;149 (4):526−31.

[2] Grintsova O, Maier W, Mielck A. Inequalities in health care among patients with type 2 diabetes by individual socio-economic status (SES) and regional deprivation: a systematic literature review. Int J Equity Health 2014;13:43.

[3] Ahmed SM, Lemkau JP, Nealeigh N, Mann B. Barriers to healthcare access in a non-elderly urban poor American population. Health Soc Care Community 2001;9(6):445−53.

[4] Dunlop S, Coyte PC, McIsaac W. Socio-economic status and the utilisation of physicians' services: results from the Canadian National Population Health Survey. Soc Sci Med 2000;51(1):123−33.

[5] Wong JC, Foster NC, Maahs DM, Raghinaru D, Bergenstal RM, Ahmann AJ, et al. Real-time continuous glucose monitoring among participants in the T1D Exchange clinic registry. Diabetes Care 2014;37(10):2702−9.

[6] O'Connor RM, Carlin K, Tumaini C, Zierler B, Pihoker C. Disparities in insulin pump therapy persist in youth with type 1 diabetes despite rising overall pump use rates. J Pediatr Nurs 2019;44:16−21.

[7] Cortina S, Repaske DR, Hood KK. Sociodemographic and psychosocial factors associated with continuous subcutaneous insulin infusion in adolescents with type 1 diabetes. Pediatr Diabetes 2010;11(5):337−44.

[8] Tanenbaum ML, Adams RN, Hanes SJ, Barley RC, Miller KM, Mulvaney SA, et al. Optimal use of diabetes devices: clinician perspectives on barriers and adherence to device use. J Diabetes Sci Technol 2017;11(3):484−92.

[9] Prahalad P, Addala A, Buckingham BA, Wilson DM, Maahs DM. Sustained continuous glucose monitor use in low-income youth with type 1 diabetes following insurance

coverage supports expansion of continuous glucose monitor coverage for all. Diabetes Technol Ther 2018;20(9):632−4.

[10] Commissariat PV, Boyle CT, Miller KM, Mantravadi MG, DeSalvo DJ, Tamborlane WV, et al. Insulin pump use in young children with type 1 diabetes: sociodemographic factors and parent-reported barriers. Diabetes Technol Ther 2017;19(6):363−9.

[11] Lawton J, Kirkham J, Rankin D, White DA, Elliott J, Jaap A, et al. Who gains clinical benefit from using insulin pump therapy? A qualitative study of the perceptions and views of health professionals involved in the Relative Effectiveness of Pumps over MDI and Structured Education (REPOSE) trial. Diabet Med 2016;33(2):243−51.

[12] Senniappan S, Hine P, Tang W, Campbell J, Bone M, Sankar V, et al. The effect of socio-economic deprivation on efficacy of continuous subcutaneous insulin infusion: a retro-spective paediatric case-controlled survey. Eur J Pediatr 2012;171(1):59−65.

[13] Stewart AF. The United States endocrinology workforce: a supply-demand mismatch. J Clin Endocrinol Metab 2008;93(4):1164−6.

[14] Raymond JK, Berget CL, Driscoll KA, Ketchum K, Cain C, "Fred" Thomas JF. CoYoT1 Clinic: innovative telemedicine care model for young adults with type 1 diabetes. Diabetes Technol Ther 2016;18(6):385−90.

[15] Duke DC, Barry S, Wagner DV, Speight J, Choudhary P, Harris MA. Distal technologies and type 1 diabetes management. Lancet Diabetes Endocrinol 2018;6(2):143−56.

[16] Gentry MT, Lapid MI, Clark MM, Rummans TA. Evidence for telehealth group-based treatment: a systematic review. J Telemed Telecare 2019;25:327−42.

[17] Lee SWH, Chan CKY, Chua SS, Chaiyakunapruk N. Comparative effectiveness of tele-medicine strategies on type 2 diabetes management: a systematic review and network meta-analysis. Sci Rep 2017;7(1):12680.

[18] Flores Garcia JJ, Reid MW, Raymond J. Feasibility of shared telemedicine appointments for low SES adolescents and young adults with T1D. Diabetes 2018;67:1325.

[19] Malasanos TH, Burlingame JB, Youngblade L, Patel BD, Muir AB. Improved access to subspecialist diabetes care by telemedicine: cost savings and care measures in the first two years of the FITE diabetes project. J Telemed Telecare 2005;11(Suppl. 1):74−6.

[20] Shea S, Kothari D, Teresi JA, Kong J, Eimicke JP, Lantigua RA, et al. Social impact anal-ysis of the effects of a telemedicine intervention to improve diabetes outcomes in an eth-nically diverse, medically underserved population: findings from the IDEATel study. Am J Public Health 2013;103(10):1888−94.

[21] Hitlin P. Internet, social media use and device ownership in U.S. have plateaued after years of growth. Washington, DC: Pew Research Center; 2018.

[22] Horrigan J, Duggan M. Barriers to broadband adoption: cost is now a substantial chal-lenge for many non-users. Washington, DC: Pew Research Center; 2015.

[23] Anderson M, Jingjing J. Teens, social media & technology 2018. Washington, DC: Pew Research Center; 2018.

[24] Mehrotra A, Jena AB, Busch AB, Souza J, Uscher-Pines L, Landon BE. Utilization of telemedicine among rural Medicare beneficiaries. JAMA 2016;315(18):2015−16.

[25] Barry SA, Harlan DM, Johnson NL, MacGregor KL. State of behavioral health integration in U.S. Diabetes care: how close are we to ADA recommendations? Diabetes Care 2018;41(7):e115−16.

[26] Mobile Fact Sheet. Washington, DC: Pew Research Center; 2018.

[27] Holtz B, Lauckner C. Diabetes management via mobile phones: a systematic review. Telemed J E Health 2012;18(3):175−84.

[28] Nelson LA, Mulvaney SA, Gebretsadik T, Johnson KB, Osborn CY. The MEssaging for Diabetes (MED) intervention improves short-term medication adherence among low-income adults with type 2 diabetes. J Behav Med 2016;39(6):995−1000.

[29] Internet/Broadband Fact Sheet. Washington, DC: Pew Research Center; 2018.

[30] Medicare and Medicaid Programs; Electronic Health Record Incentive Program-Stage 3 and Modifications to Meaningful Use in 2015 Through 2017; Corrections and Correcting Amendment. Centers for Medicare & Medicaid Services (CMS); 2016.

[31] Graetz I, Gordon N, Fung V, Hamity C, Reed ME. The digital divide and patient portals: Internet access explained differences in patient portal use for secure messaging by age, race, and income. Med Care 2016;54(8):772−9.

[32] Tieu L, Schillinger D, Sarkar U, Hoskote M, Hahn KJ, Ratanawongsa N, et al. Online patient websites for electronic health record access among vulnerable populations: portals to nowhere? J Am Med Inform Assoc 2016;24(e1):e47−54.

[33] Krebs P, Duncan DT. Health app use among US mobile phone owners: a national survey. JMIR Mhealth Uhealth 2015;3(4):e101.

[34] Sarkar U, Gourley GI, Lyles CR, Tieu L, Clarity C, Newmark L, et al. Usability of commercially available mobile applications for diverse patients. J Gen Intern Med 2016;31 (12):1417−26.

[35] Social Media Fact Sheet. Washington, DC: Pew Research Center; 2018.

[36] Rose M, Aronow L, Breen S, Tully C, Hilliard ME, Butler AM, et al. Considering culture: a review of pediatric behavioral intervention research in type 1 diabetes. Curr Diab Rep 2018;18(4):16.

[37] Harris MA. Your exclusion, my inclusion: reflections on a career working with the most challenging and vulnerable in diabetes. Diabetes Spectr 2018;31(1):113−18.

[38] Klonoff DC, Gabbay RA, Kerr D. Barriers and solutions to a recently noted failure of diabetes care outcomes to improve from 2005 to 2016 in the United States. J Diabetes Sci Technol 2020;14:189−90.

[39] Whittemore R, Jaser SS, Faulkner MS, Murphy K, Delamater A, Grey M. Type 1 diabetes eHealth psychoeducation: youth recruitment, participation, and satisfaction. J Med Internet Res 2013;15(1):e15.

[40] Nuckols TK, Keeler E, Anderson LJ, Green J, Morton SC, Doyle BJ, et al. Economic evaluation of quality improvement interventions designed to improve glycemic control in diabetes: a systematic review and weighted regression analysis. Diabetes Care 2018;41 (5):985−93.

[41] Yi SS, Chamany S, Thorpe L. Academic and government partnerships to address diabetes in the USA: a narrative review. Curr Diab Rep 2017;17(9):75. Available from: https://doi. org/10.1007/s11892-017-0895-y.

[42] American Diabetes Association. Economic costs of diabetes in the U.S. in 2017. Diabetes Care 2018;41(5):917−28.

[43] Wagner DV, Barry SA, Stoeckel M, Teplitsky L, Harris MA. NICH at its best for diabetes at its worst: texting teens and their caregivers for better outcomes. J Diabetes Sci Technol 2017;11(3):468−75.

[44] Harris MA, Teplitsky L, Nagra H, Spiro K, Wagner DV. Single (aim)-minded strategies for demonstrating value to payers for youth with medical complexity. Clin Pract Pediatr Psychol 2018;6(2):152.

[45] Barry SA, Teplitsky L, Wagner DV, Shah A, Rogers BT, Harris MA. Partnering with insurers in caring for the most vulnerable youth with diabetes: NICH as an integrator. Curr Diab Rep 2017;17(4):26.

[46]   Wan W, Skandari MR, Minc A, Nathan AG, Winn A, Zarei P, et al. Cost-effectiveness of continuous glucose monitoring for adults with type 1 diabetes compared with self-monitoring of blood glucose: the DIAMOND randomized trial. Diabetes Care 2018;41 (6):1227—34.

[47]   Kilbourne AM, Switzer G, Hyman K, Crowley-Matoka M, Fine MJ. Advancing health disparities research within the health care system: a conceptual framework. Am J Public Health 2006;96(12):2113—21.

[48]   Bouchonville MF, Paul MM, Billings J, Kirk JB, Arora S. Taking telemedicine to the next level in diabetes population management: a review of the Endo ECHO model. Curr Diab Rep 2016;16(10):96.

Chapter 12

The autonomous point-of-care diabetic retinopathy examination

Michael D. Abràmoff[1,2]

[1]*The Robert C Watzke Professor of Ophthalmology and Visual Sciences at the University of Iowa, Retina Service, UI Hospital Clinics, Iowa City, IA, United States,* [2]*Founder and Executive Chairman, IDx, Coralville, IA, United States*

Abbreviations

A1C	or HbA1C, a measure of the beta-*N*-1-deoxy fructosyl component of hemoglobin, used to measure medium-term metabolic control in diabetes
AI	artificial intelligence or augmented intelligence. Autonomous AI is a form of augmented intelligence
CMOS	complementary metal−oxide semiconductor, a form of widely available low-cost image sensor
DR	diabetic retinopathy
DRCR	Diabetic Retinopathy Clinical Research (Network)
DRS	Diabetic Retinopathy Study
ETDRS	Early Treatment of Diabetic Retinopathy Study
FDA	US Food and Drug Administration
HEDIS	Healthcare Effectiveness Data and Information Set
OCT	optical coherence tomography
QMS	quality management system
SEE	Safety efficacy and equity, three criteria for autononomous AI
WFPRC	Wisconsin Fundus Photograph Reading Center

Key points

- The autonomous point-of-care retinal examination allows people with diabetes to receive a eye examination during their diabetes wellness visit within minutes, with an immediate diagnostic result without a specialist involved in the diagnosis.
- The autonomous point-of-care retinal examination has the potential to improve three key health-care barriers for people with diabetes—cost, access, and quality.

Diabetes Digital Health. DOI: https://doi.org/10.1016/B978-0-12-817485-2.00012-2

- Clinical acceptance and payments require rigorous validation and adherence to the three criteria of safety, efficacy, and equity.

Introduction

The benefits of early detection of diabetic retinopathy (DR) are well established [1,2]. Traditionally, early detection was performed through a dilated retinal examination by an ophthalmologist, retina specialist, or optometrist, and thus many practice guidelines refer to this method as the standard of care [3]. In the 1990s evidence showed that telemedicine for DR, where retinal images are taken and then evaluated remotely, has at least a similar safety profile as the dilated retinal examination [4,5]. While improving access, traditional telemedicine does not allow point-of-care diagnosis. There is a delay of typically days between when the patient is imaged, and the ophthalmologist is available to read the images and make a diagnosis. In many cases, low image quality requires calling the patient back for another examination. Therefore, adherence to any form of regular retina examination can be challenging, primarily caused by lack of access and convenience. Furthermore, recent research shows that in the United States, adherence to a regular documented retinal examination remains as low as 15.3%, even though all practice guidelines and standards recommend regular eye examinations [3,6,7].

Point of care diagnostics have been shown to improve access, compared to testing at a remote laboratory, such as with point-of-care A1C testing [8,9], and improve outcomes [10]. At the same time, for a number of reasons, such as the introduction of electronic health records, physician productivity in healthcare, has been declining, which leads to rising costs for healthcare, including the retinal examination [11,12]. Finally, consistency of clinicians performing the eye examination is limited, and studies show that compared to the most rigorous patient outcome-based reference standard, clinician accuracy is as low as 33% or 34% [13,14].

An autonomous point-of-care diagnostic retinal examination that uses artificial intelligence to diagnose DR has the potential to address these five problems of (1) delay, (2) adherence, (3) access, (4) productivity, and (5) consistency. Allowing the diagnosis for DR to be performed in real time, at the point of care, within minutes can improve higher adherence, access, lower cost, and increased accuracy and diagnosability. The first autonomous AI system was cleared by the US Food and Drug Administration (FDA) in 2018, enabling a noneye care provider to administer a DR examination in their office without needing a specialist or telemedicine to interpret the images. This chapter will discuss the risks and benefits of such autonomous AI systems, the broader implications for clinical practice, and how such AI systems can be evaluated and their clinical studies can be interpreted.

Background, and difference between assistive and autonomous AI

The term AI—for Augmented Intelligence or Artificial Intelligence—is used in this chapter to describe systems that make decisions of high cognitive complexity, and that only a few humans are capable of performing. For example, only a small percentage of the US population (ophthalmologists and optometrists, as well as some other experts, account for only 0.02% of the US population) are capable of making a DR diagnosis with at least a reasonable degree of accuracy.

It is useful to clarify some widely used terms. *Autonomous* (or alternatively automatic or automated) AI refers to AI systems—rigorously validated—that provide a direct diagnostic or treatment recommendation without physician interpretation. The distinction between a "locked" or "continuous learning" AI system is that a locked system, once validated, does not automatically update based on new inputs, while a continuous learning system automatically updates as it processes new inputs. Thus the safety, efficacy, and equity of an AI system that is locked are known and persist. An autonomous point-of-care diagnostics system described in this chapter is a locked system, meaning that it is fixed at the point where the validation and clinical studies remain applicable to the continued use of the AI system.

There is a long history of attempting to use artificial intelligence for medical diagnostic purposes, starting in the 1960s with Mycin, an AI that helped physicians prescribe antibiotics [15]. This continued through the 1980s with new AI algorithms such as the perceptron [16] and multilayer neural network learning using backpropagation [17]. However, the performance of these AI systems was limited, largely because of a lack of high quality maximally objective input data. Input consisted of physicians interpreting the patient's symptoms and signs and then typing them in, a process with an inherently low signal-to-noise ratio. Thus, much of the foundational methodology for modern AI had been developed over the past decades. The recent introduction of affordable digital retinal cameras with high-quality complementary metal−oxide semiconductor (CMOS) image sensors is a pivotal moment that led to the introduction of the first autonomous diagnostic AI in the United States in 2018: an autonomous point-of-care digital DR examination [18]. These CMOS image sensors make it possible to acquire retinal images of high fidelity and consistency and thus provide highly objective input data for AI algorithms. Multilayer neural network algorithms and faster graphics processing units for parallel processing have also been helpful.

It should not come as a surprise that the first autonomous AI cleared by FDA was for DR. Developing AI is relatively straightforward when both high-quality digital inputs and a corresponding high validity disease state—called reference standard or truth, such as patient outcomes—are available, as well as widely accepted associations between the disease state and clinical management and practice. Where diabetes is concerned, this includes decades of scientific research on the diagnosis and management of diabetes and DR, through the Diabetes Control and Complications Trial, the Epidemiology of Diabetes Interventions and Complications study, the Diabetic Retinopathy Study (DRS), the Early Treatment of Diabetic Retinopathy Study (ETDRS), and the Diabetic Retinopathy Clinical Research (DRCR) studies [19–22]. In addition, the widely accepted surrogate (or proxy) for patient outcome, the ETDRS severity scale [19,23], was an invaluable factor that made DR well suited for diagnosis with an autonomous AI. A number of clinical studies demonstrating high algorithm performance at detecting DR have been published in recent years [24,25]. However, most of these applications were tested in laboratory settings, not real-world primary care settings, with different methodologies, datasets, and reference standards that do not clinically validate an autonomous indication for use outside of eye care specialty clinics. Only in 2018 was the first preregistered prospective clinical trial of autonomous AI performed, in a real-world clinical setting, with primary care operators [26].

The benefits and potential benefits of autonomous point-of-care retinal examination

The introduction section explained how autonomous point-of-care retinal examination has the potential to improve three key health-care issues for people with diabetes: cost, access, and quality. These benefits derive from autonomous AI's immediacy and scalability—once it has been developed and validated, the marginal cost of the AI diagnosing additional patients is low.

For years, ophthalmologists have attempted to improve the low adherence to regular retina examinations by people with diabetes [27]. Nonetheless, a recent study showed that in the United States, adherence to the regular documented retinal examination is as low as 15.3% in the Medicare population [6]. Past efforts to educate physicians and patients have proven unsuccessful, highlighting the importance of new strategies to improve accessibility to eye care for people with diabetes [27,28]. A major factor in low adherence to the retinal examination for people with diabetes is limited access to eye care specialists. In fact, patient adherence for diabetes management itself is 96%, because access, in the diabetes doctor's office, is so much better [29,30]. Thus, enabling patients to complete a retinal examination while they are already in that diabetes doctor's office (with an established adherence of 96%) has the potential to increase adherence with the retinal examination to similar levels. When A1C testing was introduced at the point of care for people with diabetes during their diabetes wellness visit, this led to better patient outcomes than when patients were sent to a lab for A1C testing, which had been the traditional way [8]. In fact, point-of-care A1C testing caused documentation of A1Cs in the medical record to increase to 95%, 6 months after its introduction [10]. Thus, the autonomous point-of-care retinal examination promises to improve adherence in a similar fashion by increasing patient access. The examination can now be performed wherever there is an outlet and a few square feet of space, because a human specialist is not needed for the procedure and diagnosis. Furthermore, the need for reimaging can decrease because of the immediacy of the diagnostic result. Following a DR diagnosis, not all patients that need treatment end up receiving it [31]. The immediacy of the result allows a system of coordinated DR care, where a care coordinator is notified automatically following a positive diagnosis of DR, to improve follow-through, the continuum of care, and ultimately outcomes [32].

US health-care expenditures are among the highest in the world and continue to rise, even when correcting for improvements in medical services [33]. More concerning is that in the US outpatient, productivity (measured as output per hour) has been declining rather than increasing over the past two decades [11]. This decrease in productivity is in large part due to the introduction of efficiency-decreasing electronic health records [34−41]. Increased productivity leads to lower costs, all else being equal, and conversely, decreasing productivity leads to higher costs, all else being equal. In other sectors of the economy, productivity has been increased by automation [42]. Thus, for healthcare, it is essential to increase productivity, and autonomous AI promises to do so.

Depending on the AI use case—assistive or autonomous—the impact on productivity gains differs greatly. First, assistive AI relies on physician interpretation to guide patient care. Because assistive AI still requires a physician who is trained to make the clinical decision, to be involved in the clinical decision-making, productivity gains are limited. In contrast, autonomous AI provides direct clinical care and/or treatment decisions without specialist interpretation. Because autonomous AI is replacing what a physician does on narrowly defined tasks, it significantly reduces or eliminates the physician workload [11]. Thus, using an autonomous AI for the point-of-care digital retinal examination stands to lower costs and improves physician productivity, allowing eye care providers to focus more on treatment rather than diagnosis. While autonomous AI promises to yield significant benefits to healthcare over assistive AI, it also brings additional legal considerations because it does not require a human to review its diagnostic output for accuracy. While the AI does not have legal standing as a "person," there are at least two legal implications that do not exist for assistive AI, which measures or in other ways helps physicians make clinical decisions. These legal implications will be discussed later in this chapter.

Finally, AI offers the potential for better quality of care. More patients with DR can be evaluated at increasing diagnostic accuracy. Multiple studies have shown that AI can outperform human experts on retinal diagnostic tasks for such diseases as macular degeneration [43] and DR [44]. In fact, in three separate populations of patients with diabetes, autonomous AI has been shown to be substantially more sensitive (87%) [26] than board-certified ophthalmologists (33% and 34%) [13,14]. In these studies the AI system and the ophthalmologists' diagnostic examinations (consisting of indirect ophthalmoscopy and slit lamp biomicroscopy) were all compared to the same standard, a surrogate for patient outcome. The standard in these three studies was the ETDRS severity scale applied by retinal experts at the Wisconsin Fundus Photograph Reading Center (WFPRC). The two aforementioned ophthalmologist diagnostic sensitivity studies are the only two studies that have measured human expert accuracy against this WFPRC standard. A reading center, such as the WFPRC, consists of multiple independent experts that have processes to ensure consistency over time and minimize intra- and interobserver variability, often over decades. Furthermore, consistency among and between ophthalmologists diagnosing DR is limited: repeatability, where consistency is measured by comparing ophthalmologists against themselves on the same patient but on different days, is 60%−80% [45]. The autonomous AI point-of-care retinal examination achieves 99.6%, when the same patient is diagnosed by the same AI operated by the same operator [46]. Reproducibility, where consistency is measured between ophthalmologists on the same patient, is 83% [45], while the autonomous AI point-of-care retinal examination achieves 99.2% when the same patient is diagnosed but the AI is operated by different operators [46].

Thus the high-level benefits include better access, lower cost, and higher quality, but beyond that there are secondary effects: eye care providers benefit from an improved patient mix that includes more patients that need their expertise; primary care physicians are enabled to provide more comprehensive diabetes care in their office; and patients benefit from the increased convenience of immediate results, eliminating the need to come back when image quality is not sufficient. Clear, well-defined standards for determining whether an image is high enough quality to make a diagnosis is important for both human readers and AI solutions. If image quality is insufficient, then signs of disease may go undetected, resulting in vision loss. Automated screening solutions address this problem by providing a consistent, repeatable determination of whether an image is sufficient quality, whereas humans vary in their assessment.

Risks and concerns with autonomous point-of-care retinal examination

Ultimately, new technology such as autonomous AI should not increase the risk of harm to the patient. Specifically, for autonomous AI, the SEE criteria: safety—first, do no harm; efficacy—that efficiency and thereby cost savings result; and finally equity—that the autonomous AI works on the vast majority of patients for which it is indicated, not just a subgroup, and that safety and efficacy are similar in subgroups. This is also addressed in the new American Medical Association Policy on AI [47].

Safety, efficacy, and equity are criteria, whereas sensitivity, specificity, diagnosability, and nonsignificant differences are (trial) end points. The concept of equity may need more explanation because it is an additional end point for autonomous AI validation. Equity for autonomous AI is linked to safety and efficacy, and all three (safety, efficacy, and equity) require accountability and transparency. The concept of AI equity emphasizes that the AI needs to be safe and efficient for the vast majority of patients for which it is intended for use, not just a specific subset of patients, including across races, ethnicities, sex, and ages. Furthermore, all three criteria, equity, safety, and efficacy, need to be safeguarded during the design, development, validation, and clinical use of AI.

Here is an example of how the end points for these criteria work in the autonomous point-of-care retinal examination. Safety is measured using the sensitivity metric: how many patients with disease it diagnoses correctly, as any time a patient with disease is missed there may be patient harm. Efficacy is measured with the specificity metric: how many patients without disease (normals) it diagnoses correctly, as any time a patient without disease is misdiagnosed, it increases resource use without patient benefit. Equity is measured by both a diagnosability metric and a statistical analysis. The diagnosability metric measures: how many patients receive a valid diagnostic result—rather than some form of a "don't know" result. If only a small subset of all patients with the disease can be adequately diagnosed, then equity is diminished. The statistical analysis determines the magnitude of performance biases, because these may lead to clinical outcome disparities. This analysis includes a stratification of sensitivity, specificity, and diagnosability by race, ethnicity, sex, age, and any other relevant group characteristics so that potential effects of performance bias of the AI system can be brought to light. If we want a diagnostic AI that is 100% sensitive, then we could just program it to always output a diseased diagnosis for any patient: the AI is 100% sensitive but this would be useless (because the specificity would be 0%). Similarly, if we want a diagnostic AI that is 100% specific, then we could program it to always output a normal diagnosis for any patient, but this would also be useless (because the sensitivity would be 0%). The challenge has always been to build an AI with both high sensitivity and high specificity. Equity now adds a third requirement to the balance. Not only do we want an AI with high sensitivity and specificity, but we also want this AI to be safe and effective on the vast majority of patients for which it is indicated and to have minimal performance bias in safety and efficiency. In other words, it is good to minimize differences in safety and efficacy for different groups.

In addition to ensuring that an autonomous AI meets these essential SEE criteria, there are other risks and concerns with autonomous point-of-care retinal examinations. For diagnostic AI, addressing safety and efficacy quickly leads to well defined and narrow indications for use. Rigorously validating safety, efficacy, and equity for the diagnosis of a single disease requires a certain study size, involving real-world workflow and concomitant resources and funds. The importance of rigorous validation of the AI system in the actual workflow setting (rather than in a modeled laboratory setting) was first shown by Fenton et al. [48]. In their randomized clinical trial patients who were diagnosed by radiologists assisted by an FDA-cleared assistive, AI had worse outcomes than those diagnoses made by a radiologist without the assistive system. This study was significant because it showed that AI-powered software can be safe when it is tested in an in silico setting, but when it is introduced to a real-world setting, then unexpected problems can arise. Adding any additional disease to be diagnosed under SEE necessarily must lead to algebraic growth of the study size. Therefore, autonomous AI diagnostics will likely be narrow in the near future. The autonomous point-of-care retinal examination currently detects DR and is neither designed nor validated to diagnose other diseases. This means that autonomous AI cannot serve as a replacement for a complete eye examination either now or for the foreseeable future. Currently, the indications for using autonomous point-of-care diabetic eye examination are specifically to diagnose moderate or greater DR according to the ETDRS severity scale, and/or clinically significant or center-involved macular edema [26]. This type of eye examination is also only indicated for people with diabetes not previously known to have DR and who do not have visual symptoms that require the attention of a specialist.

So-called incidental findings, that potentially can be discovered in a general eye examination, such as glaucoma or macular degeneration, may be missed by the autonomous AI. While there is widespread evidence for the effectiveness and cost-effectiveness of early detection of DR [49], this is not the case for glaucoma [50], macular degeneration [51], and many other eye diseases. Therefore, clinical trials for a specific AI will typically not be designed or powered to analyze diagnostic accuracy on other retinal abnormalities or other eye abnormalities in people with diabetes. However, it is important to note that little good data exists as to know how accurately clinicians can diagnose these incidental findings, because their performance has not been evaluated in formal studies. In fact, such studies might be logistically impossible to power and may never be performed because of the enormous number of subjects required. For example, at a prevalence of 5 per million, evaluating the diagnostic performance of either ophthalmologists or autonomous AI for choroidal melanoma diagnosis would require a clinical trial with approximately 40 million subjects [52].

When the safety, efficacy, and equity of the autonomous AI are proven under specific conditions, these need to be maintained or improved in accordance with regulatory oversight. These conditions include specific digital retina cameras, specific operator training, and specific clinical settings, such as primary care, depending on the validation trials. For example, the diagnostic accuracy of autonomous AI in a primary care setting with primary care operators may seem to be lower than that of the same AI in an ophthalmology clinic with highly experienced operators and specific environmental conditions, while actually, the latter conditions led to overestimation. It should be noted that at present, there is no corresponding requirement for validation of safety, efficacy, and equity of telemedicine for an ophthalmologist's or optometrist's clinical examination. Furthermore, when images are used, their quality is neither overseen nor regulated for (1) telemedicine or (2) the clinical examination. However, image quality still needs to be high and sufficient for safe performance for all three of these assessments.

There are additional, societal concerns: fear of job loss and human replacement, legal concerns with respect to who is liable for any errors of the AI, and concerns about whether the output of an autonomous AI is a medical record in the legal sense. In fact, the first autonomous AI authorization by FDA in 2018 encountered many hurdles in the health-care system that required human oversight for medical tasks—and these hurdles are now being overcome one by one. Another example is that this author was nicknamed "The Retinator" in 2010 because of his scientific work on AI in ophthalmology and the concern that this technology would lead to job loss among his colleagues or lower quality care of patients [53]. Only through a relentless focus on transparency and accountability can such barriers be overcome.

Legal considerations of autonomous point-of-care retinal examination

As mentioned earlier in the chapter, autonomous AI systems, such as the autonomous point-of-care retinal examination, make a clinical decision without a physician being involved in the diagnostic decision. This type of decision-making raises at least three new legal considerations.

First, the creator of the autonomous AI, which is typically the company selling it, must assume medical liability, which is a principle recently endorsed by the American Medical Association (AMA) in its 2019 AI policy [47]. Just as a physician, grading an examination would be held responsible for the diagnosis given, companies and other groups developing autonomous AI products can obtain medical malpractice insurance in case issues of liability arise. This paradigm for responsibility shifts medical liability for the medical diagnostic from the provider managing the patient's diabetes—who orders the autonomous point-of-care retinal examination—to the AI manufacturer. This seems appropriate because that provider does not have the proficiency to make the clinical decision. These liability concerns also make continuous learning AI systems problematic, because these have unknown safety, efficacy, and equity, after continuous learning is started, even though they were previously validated. An important reason is that in most use cases, the additional input data in medical continuous learning AI does not have an adequate reference standard (see next), given the enormous resources required to create such a reference standard. This is especially the case for chronic diseases, such as DR, where adding the collection of high-quality surrogate outcome data, for each patient input, would eliminate the efficacy and cost savings that are the goal of autonomous AI.

Second, the output of the autonomous point-of-care retinal examination, while valid as a diagnostic record from a regulatory perspective, is not currently defined as a medical record. What is, and what is not, and who can and who cannot create, a medical record is determined by the state medical boards; but most state medical boards do not currently consider an autonomous AI output to be the same as a physician documentation. The legal status of reports generated by AI is currently being considered by the Federation of State Medical Boards.

Third, care process quality measures, such as HEDIS (Healthcare Effectiveness Data and Information Set) in the United States, are intended to increase adherence to the diabetic eye examination, support point-of-care autonomous AI, provided strict workflow and supervision criteria are met. HEDIS is administered by the National Committee for Quality Assurance and is one of healthcare's most widely used performance improvement tools [54].

The SEE criteria apply during the entire autonomous AI life cycle: design, development, validation, deployment, and postmarket monitoring. This life cycle for the autonomous point-of-care retinal examination is presented in detail next.

AI system design: safety, efficacy, and equity considerations for autonomous AI

During the autonomous AI design phase, the following aspects need to be considered:

1. The indications for use, which describe its task.
2. How the task fits in with clinical practice and evidence.
3. Whether it is locked before validation.
4. How this system benefits patients.
5. Which patient groups it is designed for.
6. The environment and context where it will be used.
7. Who the operator will be.
8. What the inputs will be.
9. What the outputs will be.

Many of these design aspects are not considered in a vacuum—rather they depend on what can and cannot be proven in the clinical validation studies. Specifically, it is crucial that the AI system be explainable, meaning we must understand how it works and follow how it arrives at its clinical decision. This understanding is important not only for AI to gain the trust of physicians and patients but also to improve AI safety. The increased safety associated with understanding the basis for AI has been demonstrated for AI algorithms, which analyze a retinal image for biomarkers in a similar manner as the visual cortex of a retina specialist who performs an analysis. The author, as well as others, have shown that explainable AI algorithms (such as these biomarker-based AI algorithms), compared to nonexplainable algorithms, are significantly more robust to small perturbations in the input, or unexpected catastrophic failure [55−57].

Explainable biomarker-based algorithms have the additional advantage that these biomarkers are often supported by clinical evidence and are known to be invariant at the racial, ethnic, and other levels, thus addressing the equity principle at the design phase. Specifically, the autonomous point-of-care retinal examination has detectors for the different indicators of DR, such as hemorrhages, microaneurysms, and neovascularization, which have been known for over 150 years to consistently indicate DR [58,59]. If a design that aligns with the biomarkers associated with clinical evidence and outcome-based preferred practice recommendations is not prespecified in the design phase, then the design should revalidate that the AI will ultimately align with the same outcomes, which would typically necessitate a prospective study.

For the autonomous point-of-care retinal examination, its design involved aligning (1) the diagnostic output, (2) the evidence for patient outcomes [19], and (3) the corresponding clinical management. Specifically, alignment with the American Academy of Ophthalmology's preferred practice pattern ensures that the output is clinically relevant and actionable [3]. There are multiple partially overlapping severity scales for DR, but only the ETDRS severity scale is directly associated with patient outcomes. In some cases, clinical patterns and guidelines are built on a different DR scales such as Eurodiab [60] or UK NHS [61]. Because these grading scales do not completely map to each other, this issue needs to be considered when deploying the AI system in clinic [62].

The environment and context in which the autonomous system is intended to be used also play a major role in the design. The autonomous point-of-care retinal examination is designed for the primary care environment, where proficiency in taking retinal photos does not exist, and there typically is no space for a darkened room. Thus patient-friendly, easy-to-use retinal cameras are required that can typically take high-quality images without pharmacologic dilation. This allows desk staff with minimal training to operate the AI. In addition, an assistive AI was designed to guide the operator take high-quality images of the correct part of the retina that are required for the AI to make a diagnosis. If the quality of the image just taken is insufficient, or the wrong area of the retina is imaged, then this problem will be reported to the operator in near real-time, allowing the retaking of that specific image while the patient is still in the examination chair. In a small number of cases, the operator may need to use pharmacologic dilation if the patient is difficult to image. If the AI had been designed for a different use case, such as dilation by an optometrist, then many of these requirements would not have been specified and the design of the system would have been simpler.

It is critical that AI system validation requirements also include ongoing monitoring of real-world performance after deployment. Typically, this is achieved by instituting a comprehensive quality management system (QMS), such as that under 21 CFR 820, that accommodates user feedback, complaints, reportable events, and ongoing product monitoring. Performance data monitored under the QMS should include a predefined protocol for determining whether the AI system results remain within the specified performance range that aligns with safe, effective, and equitable use of the AI system. In addition, ongoing monitoring of real-world performance includes all other quality responsibilities that remain within developers' control such as usability, user experience, product performance (which include uptime, bugs, and issues), and necessary safety controls (which include a comprehensive framework for cybersecurity, data protection, and data privacy).

AI system training: safety, efficacy, and equity considerations

For the highest diagnostic performance, autonomous AI uses machine learning. Machine learning requires large amounts of training data. This is a challenge for health-care AI applications, because medical data requires plentiful resources, and the acquisition of training data can harm patients or create privacy risks.

In addition, training data is not only the medical data itself but also the truth—the clinical outcome associated with it. We want this truth, technically known as reference standard, to be the best predictor of the patient's health outcome. However, in chronic disease, such as DR, clinical outcome may not be apparent for years or even decades, and in addition, it may be unethical to wait this long without offering treatment that affects this outcome. Therefore in the case of DR, surrogate outcomes for clinical outcomes are the second-best alternative reference standard. Clinician agreement is typically less good at predicting clinical outcomes, especially when there is no evidence that the clinicians' estimates correspond to clinical outcomes, as is often the case. For initiating development of many types of AI software, the normal process is that a patient image is first taken and evaluated by a single clinician, for clinical purposes. There is often no data available whatsoever about how this evaluation relates to a clinical outcome. Later, AI developers come in, acquire the images with the clinician evaluation in the medical records, and then train the AI with that data. Given that the AI's training is optimized on agreeing with that clinician, not with clinical outcomes, the AI safety, efficacy, and equity will very likely disappoint when the AI is then compared to true clinical outcomes.

Given these differences, a hierarchy of validity of the reference standard is as follows:

Level A reference standard: A reference standard that either is a clinical outcome or an outcome that has been validated to be equivalent to patient-level outcome—that is—a surrogate for a specific patient outcome. This reference standard is derived from an independent reading center, (where the clinicians or experts performing the reading are not otherwise involved in performing the study) with validated published protocols, and with published reproducibility and repeatability metrics. An A level reference standard is based on at least as many modalities as the test and ideally more.

Level B reference standard: A reference standard derived from an independent reading center, with validated published reading protocols, and with published reproducibility and repeatability metrics. A B level reference standard has not been validated to correlate to a patient-level outcome.

Level C reference standard: A reference standard created by adjudicating or voting of multiple independent expert readers, documented to be masked, with published reproducibility and repeatability metrics. A C level reference standard has not been derived from an independent reading center and has not been validated to correlate with a patient-level outcome.

Level D reference standard: All other reference standards, including single readers and nonexpert readers. A D level reference standard has not been derived from an independent reading center and has not been validated to correlate with a patient-level outcome, and readers do not have published reproducibility and repeatability metrics.

The surrogate for DR outcome is the ETDRS severity scale, combined with clinically significant macular edema determination, as performed by the Wisconsin Reading Center. However, this older outcome surrogate did not include the presence or absence of center-involved macular edema, which is defined by DRCR and determined from macular optical coherence tomography (OCT). The optimal surrogate for DR outcome is currently felt to be a combination of DR per ETDRS, the presence of clinical significant macular edema, and the presence of center-involved macular edema according to DRCR [63]. The management of DR has used these metrics in various combinations for over 40 years [19,20,64,65].

In contrast, other DR scales, such as Eurodiab or the UK NHS DR, are based on clinician agreement, or agreement between multiple clinicians. Such a reference standard is much less appropriate given intra- and interobserver variability, lack of evidence for association with clinical outcomes, and the phenomenon of diagnostic drift. The term diagnostic drift refers to clinicians deviating diagnostically over time and across training programs meaning that truth is not normally distributed. Clinicians cluster depending on where they were trained, and so their average is not Gaussian but multimodal [26,66,67]. Reading centers, on the other hand, have quality control systems to prevent diagnostic drift [26,66,67].

All of these considerations underscore why AI in healthcare will always be more limited in the amount of training data that can be available. This limitation is not seen with other autonomous AI applications, such as autonomous cars, where obtaining vast amounts of characterized data is generally quite effortless. To illustrate the difficulty in obtaining health-care data for AI, retinal image acquisition for an autonomous point-of-care examination confers a small but definite risk of harm from (1) the flashes, (2) pharmacologic dilation, (3) Health Insurance Portability and Accountability Act and privacy considerations, and (4) cost. In addition, achieving the desired surrogate clinical outcome-based reference standard (ETDRS) (compared to clinician agreement) requires certified WFPRC retinal photographers, additional high-quality, high-cost retinal cameras and OCT for diagnosing diabetic macular edema reliably.

Various approaches to deal with these data limitations have been developed and require careful choices for how to approach training when resources are limited. Some AI developers acquire vast amounts of data, using minimal truth (for example a level D reference standard). Other developers use smaller amounts of data, with a more expensive, level A reference standard [24,25]. Furthermore, unanticipated biases can occur in the training data. For example, some ethnic groups with more severe DR than others may be overrepresented, which may result in undesirable biases in accuracy that affect the equity of the AI.

For all of the abovementioned reasons, transparency and accountability about the characteristics of the training data and reference standards is important. Developers should aim for the highest amount of traceability of the training data. If possible, the training data should be traceable back to individual patients and reference standards, where allowed by law.

AI system validation: safety, efficacy, and equity considerations

Finally, transparency and accountability for the SEE criteria is achieved primarily by system design and scientific evidence from clinical trials, measuring respectively, sensitivity, specificity, and equity as defined earlier. The level of rigor of such studies should be commensurate with the risk of patient harm. In the case of autonomous AI, where perceived and real risk is great, we list important considerations. An important consideration is an alignment between validation study design and actual clinical use. As Fenton et al. [48] showed, validation of AI should be maximally aligned with the intended use of the autonomous AI. Thus clinical trial design for autonomous diagnostic AI systems should consider the intended use for the autonomous AI, and the following four factors should be considered during the design of a validation study:

1. Disease level: the precise disease severity level(s) that the autonomous AI diagnoses.
2. Patient level: the patient population for which it was designed and validated.
3. Clinical context: the indicated clinical context, including physician role, imaging hardware and environment, operator qualifications, and imaging workflow.
4. Locked AI: The training of the autonomous AI system as well as the specific thresholds for disease level(s) is completed and finalized before the start of the trial so that the diagnostic performance will be validated on that version of the AI system. Thus, such trial designs do not allow validation of continuous learning AIs, which can be retrained during deployment, after the validation study has been completed—it is not possible to know whether such a trained AI is still safe, efficient, and equitable, without redoing a validation trial.

For example, the clinical trial for validating the first autonomous point-of-care DR diagnostic AI system had such a design [26]:

A *(disease level)*: AI designed to diagnose moderate or worse DR and or center involved, or clinically significant macular edema (disease severity).

B *(patient population)*: AI designed to diagnose all people with diabetes over the age of 21, not previously diagnosed with DR, who visiting primary care clinic for their diabetes management.

C *(clinical context)*: AI designed to be autonomous, without physician oversight of the clinical diagnosis, performed in primary care clinics, with a specified type of robotic retinal camera, in-room light with no special requirements for dimming the light, and operated by existing clinic staff requiring no more than high school graduation.

D *(deterministic AI)*: a completely developed and finished AI system documented and with fixed thresholds, locked before inclusion of the first subject.

If instead of the prespecified protocol, the validation trial will be performed in ophthalmology clinics with experienced ophthalmic photographers, in darkened rooms, and with subjects that had experience with having undergone retinal imaging before, then this protocol is likely to lead to an overestimation of its underlying diagnostic accuracy. Because of this misalignment between intended use and validation, when the autonomous AI is deployed in a true primary care environment as described earlier, then safety, efficacy, and equity cannot be guaranteed.

Other considerations are related to good clinical practice [68]. These include preregistration of the clinical trial to avoid replication issues [69], a hypothesis-testing design with predefined end points, a predefined method for statistical analysis, predefined inclusion and exclusion criteria, a predefined sampling protocol, a plan for handling of the trial data by an Independent Contract Research Organization or a third party, and prohibition of access by the researchers to the subject level results before finalizing the statistical analysis.

Summary

The autonomous point-of-care retinal examination has the potential to improve three key health-care issues for people with diabetes: (1) cost, (2) access, and (3) quality. This technology allows primary care providers to administer an examination, taking up to 10 minutes, during a diabetes wellness visit and to receive an immediate diagnostic result, without a specialist or telemedicine interpreting the images. Autonomous AI has enormous potential, but clinical acceptance and payments require both rigorous validation as well as adherence to the three core criteria of safety, efficacy, and equity. Safety means to first do no harm. Efficacy means to make sure there is a benefit to using the AI. Equity means to make sure the intervention benefits the vast majority of patients, and that ethical norms are abided by across all subgroups of patients. These three criteria of safety, efficacy, and equity must be safeguarded during the design, development, validation, and clinical use of AI, which requires transparency and accountability from AI developers.

References

[1] Bragge P, Gruen RL, Chau M, Forbes A, Taylor HR. Screening for presence or absence of diabetic retinopathy: a meta-analysis. Arch Ophthalm 2011;129(4):435–44.
[2] Fong DS, Aiello LP, Ferris III FL, Klein R. Diabetic retinopathy. Diabetes Care 2004;27 (10):2540–53.
[3] American Academy of Ophthalmology Retina/Vitreous Panel, Hoskins Center for Quality Eye Care. Preferred practice patterns: diabetic retinopathy. In: American Academy of Ophthalmology Retina Panel, editor. Updated 2016 ed. San Francisco, CA: American Academy of Ophthalmology; 2016.
[4] Ahmed J, Ward TP, Bursell SE, Aiello LM, Cavallerano JD, Vigersky RA. The sensitivity and specificity of nonmydriatic digital stereoscopic retinal imaging in detecting diabetic retinopathy. Diabetes Care 2006;29(10):2205–9.

[5] Aiello LM, Bursell SE, Cavallerano J, Gardner WK, Strong J. Joslin Vision Network Validation Study: pilot image stabilization phase. J Am Optom Assoc 1998;69 (11):699−710.

[6] Benoit SR, Swenor B, Geiss LS, Gregg EW, Saaddine JB. Eye care utilization among insured people with diabetes in the U.S., 2010-2014. Diabetes Care 2019;42(3):427−33.

[7] Solomon SD, Chew E, Duh EJ, Sobrin L, Sun JK, VanderBeek BL, et al. Diabetic retinopathy: a position statement by the American Diabetes Association. Diabetes Care 2017;40 (3):412−18.

[8] Cagliero E, Levina EV, Nathan DM. Immediate feedback of HbA1c levels improves glycemic control in type 1 and insulin-treated type 2 diabetic patients. Diabetes Care 1999;22 (11):1785−9.

[9] Lian J, Liang Y. Diabetes management in the real world and the impact of adherence to guideline recommendations. Curr Med Res Opin 2014;30(11):2233−40.

[10] Egbunike V, Gerard S. The impact of point-of-care A1C testing on provider compliance and A1C levels in a primary setting. Diabetes Educ 2013;39(1):66−73.

[11] Helmchen LA, Lehmann HP, Abramoff MD. Automated detection of retinal disease. Am J Manag Care 2014;11(17).

[12] Kocher R, Sahni N. Rethinking health care labor. N Engl J Med 2011;365:1370−2.

[13] Pugh JA, Jacobson JM, Van Heuven WA, Watters JA, Tuley MR, Lairson DR, et al. Screening for diabetic retinopathy. The wide-angle retinal camera. Diabetes Care 1993;16 (6):889−95.

[14] Lin DY, Blumenkranz MS, Brothers RJ, Grosvenor DM. The sensitivity and specificity of single-field nonmydriatic monochromatic digital fundus photography with remote image interpretation for diabetic retinopathy screening: a comparison with ophthalmoscopy and standardized mydriatic color photography. Am J Ophthalmol 2002;134(2):204−13.

[15] Shortliffe EH, Davis R, Axline SG, Buchanan BG, Green CC, Cohen SN. Computer-based consultations in clinical therapeutics: explanation and rule acquisition capabilities of the MYCIN system. Comput Biomed Res 1975;8(4):303−20.

[16] Fukushima K. Neocognitron: a self organizing neural network model for a mechanism of pattern recognition unaffected by shift in position. Biol Cybern 1980;36(4):193−202.

[17] Rumelhart DE, McClelland JL, University of California San Diego, PDP Research Group. Parallel distributed processing: explorations in the microstructure of cognition. Cambridge, MA: MIT Press; 1986.

[18] US Food and Drug Administration. FDA permits marketing of artificial intelligence-based device to detect certain diabetes-related eye problems. Washington, DC: US Food and Drug Administration; 2018.

[19] [No authors listed]. Fundus photographic risk factors for progression of diabetic retinopathy. ETDRS report number 12. Early Treatment Diabetic Retinopathy Study Research Group. Ophthalmology 1991;98:823−33.

[20] [No authors listed]. Progression of retinopathy with intensive versus conventional treatment in the Diabetes Control and Complications Trial. Diabetes Control and Complications Trial Research Group. Ophthalmology 1995;102(4):647−61.

[21] Browning DJ, Glassman AR, Aiello LP, Bressler NM, Bressler SB, Danis RP, et al. Optical coherence tomography measurements and analysis methods in optical coherence tomography studies of diabetic macular edema. Ophthalmology 2008;115(8):1366−71 1371.e1.

[22] Diabetic Retinopathy Clinical Research Network, Beck RW, Edwards AR, Aiello LP, Bressler NM, Ferris F, et al. Three-year follow-up of a randomized trial comparing focal/

grid photocoagulation and intravitreal triamcinolone for diabetic macular edema. Arch Ophthalmol 2009;127(3):245−51.

[23] [No authors listed]. Classification of diabetic retinopathy from fluorescein angiograms. ETDRS report number 11. Early Treatment Diabetic Retinopathy Study Research Group. Ophthalmology 1991;98(5 Suppl.):807−22.

[24] Gulshan V, Peng L, Coram M, Stumpe MC, Wu D, Narayanaswamy A, et al. Development and validation of a deep learning algorithm for detection of diabetic retinopathy in retinal fundus photographs. JAMA 2016;316(22):2402−10.

[25] Abramoff MD, Lou Y, Erginay A, Clarida W, Amelon R, Folk JC, et al. Improved automated detection of diabetic retinopathy on a publicly available dataset through integration of deep learning. Invest Ophthalmol Vis Sci 2016;57(13):5200−6.

[26] Abràmoff MD, Lavin PT, Birch M, Shah N, Folk JC. Pivotal trial of an autonomous AI-based diagnostic system for detection of diabetic retinopathy in primary care offices. NPJ Digit Med 2018;1(1):39.

[27] Hazin R, Barazi MK, Summerfield M. Challenges to establishing nationwide diabetic retinopathy screening programs. Curr Opin Ophthalmol 2011;22(3):174−9.

[28] Hazin R, Colyer M, Lum F, Barazi MK. Revisiting diabetes 2000: challenges in establishing nationwide diabetic retinopathy prevention programs. Am J Ophthalmol 2011;152 (5):723−9.

[29] Lee DJ, Kumar N, Feuer WJ, Chou CF, Rosa PR, Schiffman JC, et al. Dilated eye examination screening guideline compliance among patients with diabetes without a diabetic retinopathy diagnosis: the role of geographic access. BMJ Open Diabetes Res Care 2014;2 (1):e000031.

[30] McEwen LN, Herman WH. Health care utilization and costs of diabetes NIH Pub No. 17-1468 In: Cowie CC, Casagrande SS, Menke A, Cissell MA, Eberhardt MS, Meigs JB, Gregg EW, Knowler WC, et al., editors. Diabetes in America. 3rd ed. Bethesda, MD: National Institutes of Health; 2018. p. 1−78.

[31] Crossland L, Askew D, Ware R, Cranstoun P, Mitchell P, Bryett A, et al. Diabetic retinopathy screening and monitoring of early stage disease in Australian general practice: tackling preventable blindness within a chronic care model. J Diabetes Res 2016;2016: 8405395.

[32] Stevens GD, Shi L, Vane C, Peters AL. Do experiences consistent with a medical-home model improve diabetes care measures reported by adult Medicaid patients? Diabetes Care 2014;37(9):2565−71.

[33] Johansen ME. Comparing medical ecology, utilization, and expenditures between 1996-1997 and 2011-2012. Ann Fam Med 2017;15(4):313−21.

[34] Bae J, Encinosa WE. National estimates of the impact of electronic health records on the workload of primary care physicians. BMC Health Serv Res 2016;16:172.

[35] Bhargava HK, Mishra A. Electronic medical records and physician productivity: evidence from panel data analysis 2011. Available from: <http://ssrn.com/abstract = 1952287>.

[36] Chiang MF, Boland MV, Margolis JW, Lum F, Abramoff MD, Hildebrand PL. Adoption and perceptions of electronic health record systems by ophthalmologists: an American Academy of Ophthalmology survey. Ophthalmology 2008;115:1591−7.

[37] Haidar YM, Moshtaghi O, Mahboubi H, Ghavami Y, Ziai K, Hojjat H, et al. Association between electronic medical record implementation and otolaryngologist productivity in the ambulatory setting. JAMA Otolaryngol Head Neck Surg 2017;143(1):20−4.

[38] Lam JG, Lee BS, Chen PP. The effect of electronic health records adoption on patient visit volume at an academic ophthalmology department. BMC Health Serv Res 2016;16:7.

[39] Menachemi N, Collum TH. Benefits and drawbacks of electronic health record systems. Risk Manage Healthc Policy 2011;4:47—55.

[40] Redd TK, Read-Brown S, Choi D, Yackel TR, Tu DC, Chiang MF. Electronic health record impact on productivity and efficiency in an academic pediatric ophthalmology practice. J AAPOS 2014;18(6):584—9.

[41] Samaan ZM, Klein MD, Mansour ME, DeWitt TG. The impact of the electronic health record on an academic pediatric primary care center. J Ambul Care Manage 2009;32 (3):180—7.

[42] Stiroh KJ. Investing in information technology: productivity payoffs for U.S. Industries. Curr Issues Econ Finance 2001;7(6):1—7.

[43] Peng Y, Dharssi S, Chen Q, Keenan TD, Agron E, Wong WT, et al. DeepSeeNet: a deep learning model for automated classification of patient-based age-related macular degeneration severity from color fundus photographs. Ophthalmology 2019;126(4):565—75.

[44] Abramoff MD, Folk JC, Han DP, Walker JD, Williams DF, Russell SR, et al. Automated analysis of retinal images for detection of referable diabetic retinopathy. JAMA Ophthalmol 2013;131(3):351—7.

[45] Liu Y, Rajamanickam VP, Parikh RS, Loomis SJ, Kloek CE, Kim LA, et al. Diabetic retinopathy assessment variability among eye care providers in an urban teleophthalmology program. Telemed J E Health 2019;25(4):301—8.

[46] Lynch S, Folk J, Abramoff M. Autonomous artificial intelligence (AI) reliably detects diabetic retinopathy. Invest Ophthalmol Vis Sci 2019;59:1537-A0221.

[47] American Medical Association. Augmented intelligence in health care H-480.939 (Updated August 28, 2019). Available from: <https://policysearch.ama-assn.org/policyfinder/detail/augmented%20intelligence?uri = %2FAMADoc%2FHOD.xml-H-480.939.xml>.

[48] Fenton JJ, Taplin SH, Carney PA, Abraham L, Sickles EA, D'Orsi C, et al. Influence of computer-aided detection on performance of screening mammography. N Engl J Med 2007;356(14):1399—409.

[49] Klonoff DC, Schwartz DM. An economic analysis of interventions for diabetes. Diabetes Care 2000;23(3):390—404.

[50] Moyer VA. Force USPST. Screening for glaucoma: U.S. Preventive Services Task Force Recommendation Statement. Ann Intern Med 2013;159(7):484—9.

[51] Chou R, Dana T, Bougatsos C, Grusing S, Blazina I. Screening for impaired visual acuity in older adults: updated evidence report and systematic review for the US Preventive Services Task Force. JAMA 2016;315(9):915—33.

[52] McLaughlin CC, Wu XC, Jemal A, Martin HJ, Roche LM, Chen VW. Incidence of noncutaneous melanomas in the U.S. Cancer 2005;103(5):1000—7.

[53] McDonnell PJ. 'The Retinator': revenge of the machines. Ophthalmol Times 2010;35 (13):4.

[54] National Committee for Quality Assurance. HEDIS and performance measurement 2019 Available from: <https://www.ncqa.org/hedis/>, 2019.

[55] Finlayson SG, Chung HW, Kohane IS, Beam AL. Adversarial attacks against medical deep learning systems. arXiv:170809843. 2018.

[56] Lynch S, Abramoff MD. Catastrophic failure in image-based convolutional neural network algorithms for detecting diabetic retinopathy. IOVS 2017;58 (ARVO E-abstract 3776).

[57] Shah A, Lynch S, Niemeijer M, Amelon R, Clarida W, Folk J, et al., editors. Susceptibility to misdiagnosis of adversarial images by deep learning based retinal image analysis algorithms. In: Proceedings — International Symposium on Biomedical Imaging; 2018.

[58] Friedenwald JS. Diabetic retinopathy. Am J Ophthalmol 1950;33(8):1187—99.

[59] MacKenzie S. A case of glycosuric retinitis, with comments. (Microscopical examination of the eyes by Mr. Nettleship). Roy Lond Ophthal Hosp Rep 1879;9(134).

[60] Aldington SJ, Kohner EM, Meuer S, Klein R, Sjolie AK. Methodology for retinal photography and assessment of diabetic retinopathy: the EURODIAB IDDM complications study. Diabetologia 1995;38(4):437—44.

[61] Harding S, Greenwood R, Aldington S, Gibson J, Owens D, Taylor R, et al. Grading and disease management in national screening for diabetic retinopathy in England and Wales. Diabet Med 2003;20(12):965—71.

[62] US Center for Medicare and Medicaid Services. 2019 ICD-10-CM (updated June 20, 2019). Available from: <https://www.cms.gov/Medicare/Coding/ICD10/2019-ICD-10-CM.html>.

[63] Abramoff MD, Fort PE, Han IC, Jayasundera KT, Sohn EH, Gardner TW. Approach for a clinically useful comprehensive classification of vascular and neural aspects of diabetic retinal disease. Invest Ophthalmol Vis Sci 2018;59(1):519—27.

[64] Glassman AR, Beck RW, Browning DJ, Danis RP, Kollman C, Diabetic Retinopathy Clinical Research Network Study Group. Comparison of optical coherence tomography in diabetic macular edema, with and without reading center manual grading from a clinical trials perspective. Invest Ophthalmol Vis Sci 2009;50(2):560—6.

[65] Diabetic Retinopathy Study Group. Factors Influencing the development of visual loss in advanced diabetic retinopathy: DRS report 9. Invest Ophthalmol Vis Sci 1985;26:983—91.

[66] Chen JH, Goldstein MK, Asch SM, Altman RB. Dynamically evolving clinical practices and implications for predicting medical decisions. Pac Symp Biocomput 2016;21:195—206.

[67] Arbel Y, Qiu F, Bennell MC, Austin PC, Roifman I, Rezai MR, et al. Association between publication of appropriate use criteria and the temporal trends in diagnostic angiography in stable coronary artery disease: a population-based study. Am Heart J 2016;175:153—9.

[68] US Food and Drug Administration. E6(R2) good clinical practice: integrated addendum to ICH E6(R1) (updated August 24, 2018). Available from: <https://www.fda.gov/regulatory-information/search-fda-guidance-documents/e6r2-good-clinical-practice-integrated-addendum-ich-e6r1>.

[69] Kaplan RM, Irvin VL. Likelihood of null effects of large NHLBI Clinical Trials has increased over time. PLoS One 2015;10(8):e0132382.

Chapter 13

Digital foot care—leveraging digital health to extend ulcer-free days in remission

Bijan Najafi[1], Mark Swerdlow[2], Grant A. Murphy[2] and David G. Armstrong[2]

[1]*Division of Vascular Surgery and Endovascular Therapy, Michael E. DeBakey Department of Surgery, Interdisciplinary Consortium for Advanced Motion Performance (iCAMP), Baylor College of Medicine, Houston, TX, United States,* [2]*Department of Surgery, Southwestern Academic Limb Salvage Alliance (SALSA), Keck School of Medicine of University of Southern California, Los Angeles, CA, United States*

Abbreviations

DFU	diabetic foot ulcer
DPN	diabetic peripheral neuropathy
EMR	electronic medical record
IoT	Internet of Things
mHealth	mobile health
PTS	plantar tissue stress

Key points

- The alarmingly high rates of recurrence of ulcerations in the diabetic foot require a change in our approach to care and to the vernacular in the medical literature so that we can promote achieving ulcer-free days without recurrence following a sentinel incident and remission of a foot ulcer.
- With its high rates of morbidity and recurrence, the clinical significance of the complex diabetic foot may be aptly comparable to that of many forms of cancer.
- While it is in the early stage of development, ultimately, we envisage a connected home that, using voice-controlled technology and Bluetooth-radio connected peripherals, may improve the patient's central role and responsibility in enabling an optimized health-care ecosystem to better manage the diabetic foot problem.

Diabetes Digital Health. DOI: https://doi.org/10.1016/B978-0-12-817485-2.00013-4

Background

Diabetes and other noncommunicable diseases of decay are now the leading cause of global mortality in the developed and developing world [1]. While not many people might realize it, if the diabetes were a country, then it would be the third largest in the world with a population exceeding 425 million. Up to one-third of people with diabetes will develop a diabetic foot ulcer (DFU) in their lifetime [2]. Globally, it is estimated that 20 million people currently have an active DFU; an additional 130 million have a history of DFU or the precursor risk factor diabetic peripheral neuropathy (DPN) and are expected to develop a DFU without intervention [2]. Ulcers requiring acute care can result in treatment costs of up to US $28,000 per event, varying with wound severity. Unfortunately, even after the resolution of a foot ulcer, recurrence is common and estimated to be 40% within 1 year, approximately 60% within 3 years, and 65% within 5 years [2]. It is estimated that in the United States one-third of all diabetes-related costs are due to diabetic foot care, with two-thirds of these costs incurred in the inpatient settings, constituting a substantial cost to society. A study on the economic burden of DFUs and amputations showed that DFU patients on the average were seen in outpatient facilities 14 times/year and hospitalized approximately 1.5 times/year, for a total of $33,000 in annual Medicare costs [3].

Perhaps no subsequent complication of DFU is more significant than its associated 10%−20% rate of lower limb amputation per event, at least 70% of which are potentially preventable [4]. The consequences of DFU are not limited to amputation; DFUs may put people at risk for other adverse events such as falls, fractures, reduced mobility, frailty, and mortality. Mortality after DFU-related amputation is estimated to be 70% at 5 years, which exceeds that of many common malignancies such as breast cancer and prostate cancer.

In light of the impending diabetes epidemic and high prevalence of DFU and its recurrence, the need for enhanced prevention of DFUs and/or keeping patients with ulcers in "remission" [2] is clear. DFU rates can be reduced, but effective management is multifaceted and requires constant monitoring from patients, caregivers, and health-care providers [2]. Thanks to new "smart" sensors that communicate with a handheld device or the cloud, and communication technologies such as smartphones and smart connected home infrastructure, new opportunities exist to manage DFUs, as well as prevent their initial occurrence [5]. With the help of automation, patients can be prompted to check their feet, glucose levels, or weight, and enter results into mobile patient portals. Even better: they can transmit the results to their physicians in real time. These fast-growing, low-cost, and widely available resources can help predict one's risk for foot ulcers, infections, peripheral arterial disease, frailty, and other diabetes-associated complications, ultimately saving limbs and lives.

To better understand potential opportunities and challenges associated with implementing digital technologies for the management of DFU, this chapter reviews recent relevant literature and includes expert opinions from a multidisciplinary point of view, including podiatry, engineering, and digital health.

Digital health for effective prescription of offloading to prevent and manage diabetic foot ulcers

The most common pathway to develop a DFU is unchecked repetitive elevated plantar mechanical stress over time on insensate plantar foot tissue. Plantar tissue stress (PTS) is a concept that attempts to integrate several well-known mechanical factors into one measure, including plantar pressure, shear stress, daily weight-bearing activity, and time spent in prescribed offloading interventions (adherence) [6]. If PTS remains elevated, then it results in subdermal inflammation and eventually a DFU. In a sensate foot, patients relieve (offload) the inflamed regions aided by feedback from their intact sensory pathways. Unfortunately, loss of plantar sensation, or "the gift of pain," from DPN not only results in the inability to perceive elevated levels of PTS but can also cause gait abnormalities and foot deformities that potentially exacerbate PTS [7].

Management of PTS is essential to mitigating DFU incidence and severity while prompting safe mobility in people with high DFU risk. Currently, providers frequently reschedule patients for follow-up appointments and guide offloading treatments using their clinical intuition of the patient's average buildup of their preulcerative callus from activity and footwear. Over the last 20 years, these clinical judgments have been augmented by knowledge from objective measurements, that have demonstrated the capacity of various footwear and offloading devices to reduce PTS in controlled research settings. More recently, high-quality studies have gone further and demonstrated that objective measurements of plantar pressure can be used to successfully guide clinical treatment decisions and prolong ulcer-free days for the patient in diabetic foot remission [6]. This has led to international guidelines recommending that clinicians objectively measure plantar pressure to guide the prescription of their footwear-related offloading treatments [6].

Although measuring plantar pressure at one moment in time has proven clinically beneficial, it is not representative of a person's entire PTS. A key limitation of the current PTS assessment modalities is that they only measure PTS over a short period of time, which does not factor in daily weight-bearing physical activities such as walking, standing, and sitting while shifting weight to the feet. Currently, a major gap in managing DFUs is a lack of understanding about the association between volume of weight-bearing activity and increased DFU risk. Unless a person steps on a foreign body such as a sharp stone, the plantar pressure encountered in a single step is generally not of sufficient magnitude to develop a DFU or delay wound healing. Incorporating a time dimension (such as measuring pressure time integral as a surrogate of cumulative plantar stress) enables improved detection of those with a history of DFU. However, such measurements still lack specificity for predicting DFU formation [7]. Even prediction of DFU location using plantar pressure assessment is uncertain. For example, Veves et al. [8] reported that only 38% of ulcer locations matched the peak pressure location. They also found that the peak pressure location actually changed in 59% of patients over a mean follow-up time of 30 months.

To improve the specificity of DFU prediction, a person's weight-bearing activity should be considered when measuring PTS [6]. Early studies investigating weight-bearing activity in patients with neuropathy were dependent on a participant's self-reporting outcome. Such self-reporting suffers from both intentional (e.g., being afraid for potential consequence of carelessness) and unintentional (e.g., forgetting) errors. With advances in signal processing and multisensor devices, it is now possible to comprehensively monitor activity beyond counting steps. This includes measurements of total weight-bearing activity, bouts of weight-bearing activity, and activity intensity [9–11]. Najafi et al. [12] found that neuropathic patients spent approximately threefold as much time weight-bearing per day as walking, and that daily standing time may be predictive of worse DFU healing outcomes [13]. In a recent exploratory study [14], they noted that walking more than 3000 steps/day lowers the rate of wound healing irrespective of type of offloading (i.e., removable and irremovable). These recent studies suggest the importance of managing the dosage of weight-bearing activity for both the prevention and healing of DFU.

Thanks to advances in smart phones, mobile applications, and smart wearable sensors, the ability to continuously and simultaneously measure multiple mechanical factors comprising PTS has become more achievable. Smart flexible sensors implanted in insoles or socks combined with digital health apps have paved the way for monitoring PTS during activities of daily living. For people at risk of a DFU, in 2017 Raviglione et al. [15] proposed the concept of daily monitoring of plantar pressure using a smart textile (Sensoria socks, Sensoria Inc., Redmond, WA, United States; Fig. 13.1A). Their system contained 1) a textile pressure sensor attached to a stretchable band, 2) hardware that collects data and transmits them via Bluetooth to a smartphone, 3) an app that gathers the data and stores them in the cloud, and 4) a web dashboard that displays the data to the clinician. They concluded that this technology could determine optimal offloading in the community setting and assist with DFU prevention. However, their study was limited to a proof-of-concept design and no clinical study was conducted to support the conclusion. Recently, Sensoria and an Italian offloading company, Optima (Optima Molliter, Civitanova, Italy, Fig. 13.1B), collaborated to design the MOTUS Smart Boot that facilitates real-time assessment of offloading

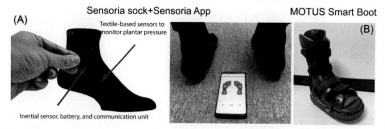

FIGURE 13.1 (A) Sensoria socks (Sensoria Fitness Inc., Redmond, WA, United States) monitor plantar pressure under three plantar regions of interest, including the heel, first metatarsal head, and fifth metatarsal head. They include an anklet that snaps to socks' sensors for transmitting data. (B) Recently Optima and Sensoria teamed up to design a smart offloading boot named MOTUS Smart Boot that facilitates real-time assessment of offloading efficacy and monitoring daily dosage of weight-bearing activities. *Images provided from Sensoria with permission to publish.*

efficacy and management of weight-bearing physical activity dosage. However, clinical validity of this offloading is unclear at the time of drafting this chapter.

Recently, there have been promising efforts to design smart footwear to better monitor PTS during activities of daily living. In 2017 Najafi et al. [16] introduced the concept of SmartSox (Fig. 13.2) using a highly flexible fiber optic to simultaneously measure plantar pressure, plantar thermal stress response (change in plantar temperature as a function of repetitive stress), and toe range of motion during walking. They validated the technology in 33 people at high risk of DFU and demonstrated a significant agreement between measured metrics of interest derived from SmartSox and gold standards, including computerized insole pressure measurement (F-Scan, Tekscan, Inc, Boston, MA, United States) and a thermal camera (Fluke Ti25, Fluke Corporation, WA, United States).

The recent revolution of wearable technologies and digital health has led to an exponential number of publications of studies claiming to measure plantar pressure and assists in DFU prevention [17]. They often include a combination of highly flexible pressure sensors to measure pressure and/or horizontal force (shear), a microstrip patch antenna to stream data to a smartphone or smartwatch, and a biofeedback device (e.g., text message, visual, audio, or vibratory feedback via smartphone and smartwatch), which notifies the wearer during excessive, insufficient, or incorrect foot offloading [17]. However, most of these studies were conducted in vitro or using healthy subjects. Hence, their ability to predict or prevent DFU still needs to be examined.

A recent study by Najafi et al. [18] suggests that real-time notification of harmful plantar pressure can be effective to extend ulcer-free days in remission in people with diabetes. In their study, 17 patients in diabetic foot

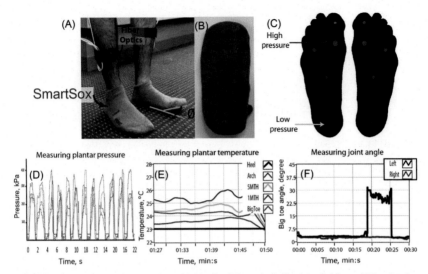

FIGURE 13.2 SmartSox is based on highly flexible optical fibers optic that enable simultaneous measurement of plantar pressure, plantar thermal stress response, and toe range of motion during walking irrespective of the type of footwear. *Taken from Najafi B, Mohseni H, Grewal GS, Talal TK, Menzies RA, Armstrong DG. An optical-fiber-based smart textile (Smart Socks) to manage biomechanical risk factors associated with diabetic foot amputation. J Diabetes Sci Technol 2017;11(4):668–77. https://doi.org/10.1177/1932296817709022. PubMed PMID: 28513212; PMCID: PMC5588846.*

remission (history of neuropathic ulceration) were instructed to wear a smart insole system (the SurroSense Rx, Orpyx Medical Technologies Inc., Calgary, Canada; Fig. 13.3) over a 3-month period. This device cues offloading by providing simple instructions via smartwatch (e.g., walk a few steps after prolonged sitting or standing, check the inside of shoes for a foreign object causing high pressure, and check formation of callus) to manage unprotected sustained plantar pressures in an effort to prevent foot ulceration. A successful response to an alert was defined as pressure offloading, which occurred within 20 minutes of the alert onset. Patient adherence, defined as daily hours of device wear, was determined using sensor data and patient questionnaires. While no ulcer reoccurrence was observed in their study, the results need to be confirmed with a larger sample size. However, an interesting observation in this study is the benefit of real-time notification to improve patient engagement and adherence to prescribed footwear. Specifically, these investigators found that alerting patients at least once every 2 hours improved adherence to prescribed footwear over time.

Other digital health products are available in the market exist to facilitate home monitoring of plantar pressure and gait. For example, FeetMe (FeetMe, Paris, France; Fig. 13.4) uses a smartphone to monitor high plantar

SurroSense Rx device (Orpyx Medical Technologies Inc.)

Illustration of high pressure
alert via smartwatch

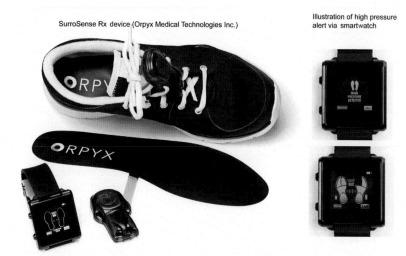

FIGURE 13.3 Recent advances in wearables enable providing timely and real-time feedback to patients to protect their feet against conditions that may increase the risk of a diabetic foot ulcer. The SurroSense Rx (Orpyx Medical Technologies Inc., Calgary, Canada) is an example of technologies that enable continuous screening plantar pressure through smart insoles and notify the patient via the smartwatch in the form of visual, vibratory, and audio feedback in case of a sustained plantar pressure beyond a predefined threshold [18]. This technology could be used to educate patients to avoid conditions leading to sustained plantar pressure (e.g., unbroken and prolonged standing), which, in turn, could assist with the prevention of diabetic foot ulcers. A recent study has also demonstrated the benefit of real-time feedback to improve adherence to footwear. *Taken from Najafi B, Ron E, Enriquez A, Marin I, Razjouyan J, Armstrong DG. Smarter sole survival: will neuropathic patients at high risk for ulceration use a smart insole-based foot protection system?. J Diabetes Sci Technol 2017;11(4):702−13. https://doi.org/10.1177/1932296816689105. PubMed PMID: 28627227; PMCID: PMC5588829.*

The system for
recharging insoles

FeetMe app

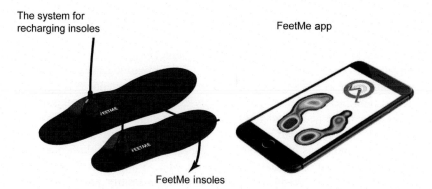

FeetMe insoles

FIGURE 13.4 FeetMe devices combine embedded and miniaturized sensors with smart algorithms to assess mobility and plantar pressure during activities of daily living. *Images provided by FeetMe with permission to publish.*

pressure. However, the clinical validation of these products and their ability to prevent DFU via daily plantar pressure screening are still unclear.

Digital health to improve triaging those at high risk of foot ulcers

Ideally, an at-risk diabetic foot should undergo regular podiatry evaluation. However, regular visits could easily overload an already overburdened health-care system. Even in specialty diabetes centers with dedicated staff and top-shelf resources, the current model of regular visits still is associated with a very high ulcer recurrence rate [19]. Thus a better referral model is needed. Because inflammation is one of the earliest signs of foot ulceration, technologies that capture markers of inflammation may assist in predicting DFU with sufficient lead time for effective intervention [19]. Inflammation has five symptoms: dolor (pain), calor (heat), rubor (redness), tumor (swelling), and functio laesa (loss of function). The most reliable measurement of inflammation, however, is based on thermography to measure heat, which has been shown to be promising for both the prediction and prevention of DFU [19].

Isolated plantar regions with increased temperature are indicative of inflammation due to damaged or near-damaged tissue. In 1997 Armstrong et al. [20] proposed the use of a portable hand-held infrared skin temperature probe as an effective technique to predict both foot injury and foot complications such as Charcot's arthropathy. Later on, in 2007, Lavery et al. [21] suggested that using thermography as a self-assessment tool is effective to prevent recurrence of DFU. Despite this evidence and the simplification of thermography using new devices such as the FLIR thermal camera (FLIR Systems, Inc., Wilsonville, OR, United States), daily plantar temperature monitoring is still not part of preventive care for managing the diabetic foot. This could be because of compliance issues such as adherence to daily use of thermography by the patient or his/her caregivers, the ease of use by non-tech savvy patients and caregivers (i.e., some may not be able to follow the instruction to accurately assess foot plantar temperature using either an app or a handheld thermography devices), or their ability to interpret the temperature difference (i.e., only the difference between two identical spots from left and right feet beyond of approximately 2°C is clinically meaningful).

To address the need to identify a temperature gap between feet, Frykberg et al. [22] proposed a smart mat based on the telehealth concept, which could address the limitations of previous thermography tools. They studied a novel in-home connected foot mat (Podimetrics Mat, Somerville, MA, United States; Fig. 13.5) to predict DFU risk and better stratify those who need urgent foot care. This simple-to-use system was designed to require no configuration or setup by the users who simply had to step on the mat with both feet for 20 seconds. Using an embedded cellular component, the collected

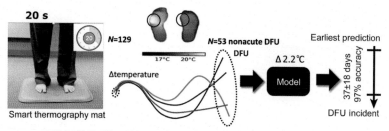

Everyday monitoring up to 34 weeks

FIGURE 13.5   In a prospective cohort observational study of patients in foot ulcer remission, Frykberg et al. [22] demonstrated that 20 seconds of daily monitoring plantar temperature using a smart mat (Podimetrics LLC, MA, United States) and an asymmetry temperature of greater than 2.22°C enables predicting the incidence of ulcer recurrence with 97% accuracy and an average lead time of 37 ± 18 days (mean ± standard deviation). In this study, 129 eligible subjects were recruited and followed for up to 34 weeks leading to 53 incidents of DFU. Then using a machine learning model, an optimum threshold of 2.22°C was identified to yield a trade-off between longest lead time and detection with the highest accuracy. *DFU*, Diabetic foot ulcer. *Based on Frykberg RG, Gordon IL, Reyzelman AM, Cazzell SM, Fitzgerald RH, Rothenberg GM, et al. Feasibility and efficacy of a smart mat technology to predict development of diabetic plantar ulcers. Diabetes Care 2017;40(7):973–80. https://doi.org/10.2337/dc16-2294. PubMed PMID: 28465454.*

data are streamed to a cloud. Thus, there is no need to use WiFi or smart-phones that might not be available at the patient's home. Using an image-processing tool, an integrated program compares the temperature profile between feet. In their study, they demonstrated that a threshold difference of ≥2.22°C between corresponding sites on opposite feet correctly predicts 97% of DFU with an average lead time of 37 days. Adherence to the mat was high with 86% of participants using the mat at least three times per week, and an average use of five times per week. While this accuracy and lead time could be sufficient to better target those who need urgent care, the technology suffers from an important limitation: while the 2.22°C threshold provided 97% sensitivity in Frykberg's study, it yielded only 43% specificity [22]. Increasing the threshold value increases specificity but decreases sensitivity. However, the observed high sensitivity and sufficient lead time (37 days) seem to be promising for effective triaging and coaching the individual and their caregiver to alter behavior to reduce DFU risk.

There are other wearables and digital health developments for improving daily monitoring of plantar temperature and potentially higher sensitivity and specificity to predict DFU and extend ulcer-free days in remission. Siren Care (Siren Diabetic Socks, Neurofabric, Siren Care Inc., San Francisco, CA; Fig. 13.6) [23] is an example of such recent developments. It uses smart textiles that allow continuous monitoring of plantar temperature and thus may improve specificity for DFU prediction and engage patients to reduce risk. But the validity and acceptability of these technologies and their advantage compared to a daily single point assessment like that offered by the

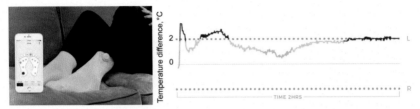

FIGURE 13.6 Siren socks enable continuous home temperature monitoring, which may be used as an early warning system, to provide people with objective feedback so they can modify their activity and protect their feet before ulcers develop. *Based on Reyzelman AM, Koelewyn K, Murphy M, Shen X, Yu E, Pillai R, et al. Continuous temperature-monitoring socks for home use in patients with diabetes: observational study. J Med Internet Res 2018;20(12):e12460. https://doi.org/10.2196/12460. PubMed PMID: 30559091; PMCID: PMC6315272.*

Podimetrics Mat remain to be studied. Similarly, new technologies enable temperature measurements between insole and shoe and simultaneous assessment of plantar pressure, temperature, and lower extremities joint angles [16]. These technologies may assist in the improvement of triaging those at a high risk of DFU and eventually assist with personalized prevention strategies by indirect measurement of shear stress and sweating during daily physical activities. However, such developments are in their infancy and remain to be examined in prospective and clinical trials.

Smartphones to improve management of diabetic foot ulcers

Smartphones and other consumer digital technologies have emerged as powerful tools to empower patients to take care of their own chronic conditions. In 2015 Parmanto et al. [24] proposed a smartphone app to support self-skincare tasks, skin condition monitoring, adherence to self-care regimens, skincare consultation, and secure two-way communications between patients and clinicians. Their app may help in supporting self-care and adherence to care management, while facilitating communication between patients and clinicians. Wang et al. [25] developed an app for analyzing wound images with the assistance of a physical image capture box. The software detects wound boundaries and determines healing status. Mammas et al. [26] evaluated the feasibility and reliability of a smartphone as a mobile-telemedicine platform by asking 10 specialists to remotely examine a diabetic foot based on simulating experimentation. The reference classification was determined from grades assigned by these specialists. They demonstrated that this platform allows remote classification of the wound with an average accuracy of 89%. In addition, the acceptability of the platform was 89%−100% among specialists. An app proposed by Foltynski et al. measures wound area, sends the data to a clinical database, and creates a graph of the wound area over time [27].

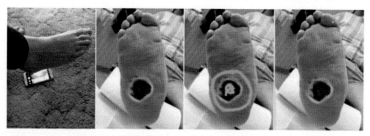

FIGURE 13.7 MyfootCare application developed by van Netten et al. to facilitate capturing high-quality photos from plantar wounds using a voice-assistant application. *Taken from Ploderer B, Brown R, Seng LSD, Lazzarini PA, van Netten JJ. Promoting self-care of diabetic foot ulcers through a mobile phone app: user-centered design and evaluation. JMIR Diabetes 2018;3 (4):e10105. https://doi.org/10.2196/10105. PubMed PMID: 30305266; PMCID: PMC6238831.*

A novel application of mobile health (mHealth) was proposed by Quinn et al. [28] to improve patient referral strategy from tertiary centers. They utilized smartphone technology to decentralize care from tertiary centers to the community, which improved efficiency and patient satisfaction and maintained patient safety. Their app enables remote collection and transmission of foot wound images. They demonstrated that images could be transmitted securely and that their platform is safe and reliable. Furthermore, their method could be used for remote wound bed assessment and determining skin integrity/color. They concluded that with minor adjustments, this application could be used across the clinical-community focusing on wound care to reduce patient attendances at vascular outpatient clinics while maintaining active tertiary specialist input to care. To facilitate capturing a high-quality picture from plantar wounds, Ploderer et al. [29] developed and evaluated the usability and usefulness of a smartphone application with voice-assistance called "MyFootCare" (Fig. 13.7). Their results suggest that using a voice assistant is beneficial to engage in tracking their plantar wound size and that wound size data measurements are useful to both monitor progress and engage patients with DFUs.

Smart home devices and voice-driven technologies better engage patients at diabetic foot ulcer risk

DFU management largely entails a home approach, including regular self-inspection (e.g., inspecting sighs of redness, callus, and blister) or self-measurement-based tips (e.g., assessing foot temperature), for the prevention of DFUs. One of the fast-developing infrastructures promising to revolutionize the diabetic foot-care industry is the Internet of Things (IoT) [5]. It is expected that up to 50% of health care over the next few years will be delivered through virtual platforms. This trend has accelerated the development of a new "digital wellness" market, which combines digital technology and health care [5]. Digital technology—based health care is regarded as a natural and cost-effective choice for remote, home-based, and long-term care of patients with chronic conditions because of its low cost, scalability, high accuracy, and continuous monitoring and tracking capabilities.

Thanks to recent advances in voice-driven technologies, voice-activated commands are evolving into an integral component of the IoT. Voice-controlled IoT technology is already ubiquitous and constantly improving from intelligent personal assistants (e.g., Apple's Siri, Amazon's Alexa, Google's Google Now, and Microsoft's Cortana) to devices that learn each individual person's unique voice and create an interface where that voice can reliably interact with a variety of applications (e.g., electronic medical record [EMR]) and medical devices (e.g., "wake" a device from "sleep" mode to "recognition" mode). Speech-recognition tools and voice-driven technologies are increasingly helping health-care providers to enhance patient electronic health records (EMR). For example, a physician can now speak directly to the EMR and hear it back. Voice-to-text enabled medical transcription allows doctors and nurses to record what they say as text, rather than having to type or handwrite forms. Some medical devices are also now using voice commands to "wake" the device from the low power detection mode ("sleep" mode) and switch to the "recognition" mode, by applying algorithms to spoken words and phrases. This is ideal for many wearable devices as well as other battery-operated devices.

Although much of the focus on voice recognition in the health-care industry is on developing technologies to aid providers directly, some efforts have focused to develop voice-driven technologies, which could be used for patient engagement and self-care applications. It is estimated that 40%—60% of American adults already use voice search and that 50% of all queries will be voice searches by 2020 [5]. This figure will grow as voice-enabled assistant devices such as the Amazon Alexa and Google Home become more commonplace. There are efforts taking place to utilize these systems for better health-care delivery and outcomes ranging from drug delivery to voice-activated technology for home-based exercise and caregiver engagement [5]. Some of these efforts have been for diabetes care; however, these efforts are still in their infancy and we could not identify any clinical trials yet to demonstrate the feasibility, acceptability, and/or effectiveness of such technology for the purpose of diabetic foot management. Recently, industrial supported initiatives have encouraged researchers to explore solutions for the use of voice-enabled technology for managing diabetes. In 2017 Amazon paired with Merck and Luminary Labs to launch the "Alexa Diabetes Challenge," calling on innovators to create Alexa voice-enabled solutions to improve the lives of those with type 2 diabetes. The challenge received 96 submissions from a variety of innovators; in October 2017, Sugarpod by Wellpepper was awarded [5]. They suggested building a voice-enabled IoT scale and foot scanner integrated with a voice-powered interactive care plan. Their system

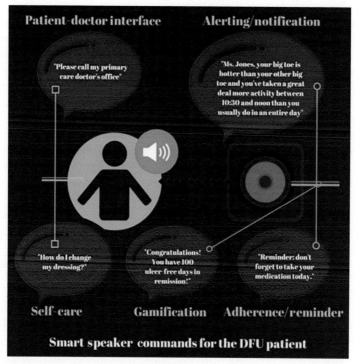

FIGURE 13.8   The model suggested by Basatneh et al. to integrate voice-enabled technologies and Internet of Things to improve management of DFU at home. *DFU*, Diabetic foot ulcer. *Taken from Basatneh R, Najafi B, Armstrong DG. Health sensors, smart home devices, and the Internet of medical things: an opportunity for dramatic improvement in care for the lower extremity complications of diabetes. J Diabetes Sci Technol 2018;12(3):577–86. https://doi.org/ 10.1177/1932296818768618. PubMed PMID: 29635931; PMCID: PMC6154231.*

delivers patient experiences via SMS, email, web, and a mobile application—and 1 day, through voice interfaces. In 2017 Basatneh et al. [5] published an expert opinion and review paper discussing different scenarios, in which voice-enabled technologies could be used for DFU home-management. This includes five different feature categories (Fig. 13.8): (1) patient—doctor interface, (2) patient—caregiver interface, (3) general alerting/notification, (4) time-effective alerting, and (5) optimum dosage recommendation of daily activities without risk.

Conclusion

In summary, lower extremity complications of diabetes remain too common. Next-generation technologies should be geared to the long-term monitoring of people both with the presence of DFU and after healing in remission. The integration of smart wearables and interactive communication systems will provide patients and clinicians with easily accessible, objective data that can be used to personalize treatment. These technologies will promote prevention of DFUs by (1) offloading to avoid excessive PTS, (2) timely scheduling of patients to allow effective preventive treatments, and (3) allowing self-care strategies to extend the number of ulcer-free days in remission. This personalized care approach will likely consist of epidermal, wearable, and implantable sensors combined with interactive user interfaces via smartwatches and smartphone and potentially with embedded voice-driven technologies. Physicians no longer will need to rely on the subjective history given by neuropathic patients who lack the ability to sense the deterioration of their own bodies. Creating unified methods of communication and interoperability that transcend the proprietary nature of individual devices will be critical to long-term success in helping people move through the world with greater ease. Although in an early stage of development, ultimately, we envisage the benefits of IoT and connected smart homes extending beyond the realm of consumer health care, assisting clinicians to continuously and remotely monitor patients. IoT technology will also empower patients and their families in the care of diabetic foot problems. While IoT is being celebrated as the future of medicine, there are still concerns that need to be addressed on patient engagement, battery-life issues, security, and privacy. Nonetheless, we find ourselves in the early stages of a dramatic change in health care: where the merger of consumer electronics, digital health, and medical devices has made the home the clinic of the future.

References

[1] Bloom DE, Cafiero E, Jané-Llopis E, Abrahams-Gessel S, Bloom LR, Fathima S, et al. The global economic burden of noncommunicable diseases. Program on the Global Demography of Aging; 2012.

[2] Armstrong DG, Boulton AJM, Bus SA. Diabetic foot ulcers and their recurrence. N Engl J Med 2017;376(24):2367−75. Available from: https://doi.org/10.1056/NEJMra1615439. PubMed PMID: 28614678.

[3] Margolis DJ, Malay DS, Hoffstad OJ, Leonard CE, MaCurdy T, Tan Y, et al. Economic burden of diabetic foot ulcers and amputations: data points #3. Data Points Publication Series. Rockville, MD; 2011.

[4] Rogers LC, Andros G, Caporusso J, Harkless LB, Mills Sr. JL, Armstrong DG. Toe and flow: essential components and structure of the amputation prevention team. J Vasc Surg 2010;52(3 Suppl.):23S−27SS. Available from: https://doi.org/10.1016/j.jvs.2010.06.004. PubMed PMID: 20804929.

[5] Basatneh R, Najafi B, Armstrong DG. Health sensors, smart home devices, and the internet of medical things: an opportunity for dramatic improvement in care for the lower extremity complications of diabetes. J Diabetes Sci Technol 2018;12(3):577−86. Available from: https://doi.org/10.1177/1932296818768618 PubMed PMID: 29635931; PMCID: PMC6154231.

[6] Lazzarini PA, Crews RT, van Netten JJ, Bus SA, Fernando ME, Chadwick PJ, et al. Measuring plantar tissue stress in people with diabetic peripheral neuropathy: a critical concept in diabetic foot management. J Diabetes Sci Technol 2019;. Available from: https://doi.org/10.1177/1932296819849092. PubMed PMID: 31030546.

[7] Wrobel JS, Najafi B. Diabetic foot biomechanics and gait dysfunction. J Diabetes Sci Technol 2010;4(4):833–45. Available from: https://doi.org/10.1177/193229681000400411. PubMed PMID: 20663446; PMCID: PMC2909514.

[8] Veves A, Murray HJ, Young MJ, Boulton AJ. The risk of foot ulceration in diabetic patients with high foot pressure: a prospective study. Diabetologia 1992;35(7):660–3 PubMed PMID: 1644245.

[9] Crews RT, Yalla SV, Dhatt N, Burdi D, Hwang S. Monitoring location-specific physical activity via integration of accelerometry and geotechnology within patients with or at risk of diabetic foot ulcers: a technological report. J Diabetes Sci Technol 2017;11 (5):899–903. Available from: https://doi.org/10.1177/1932296816651631. PubMed PMID: 27246669.

[10] Lemaster JW, Reiber GE, Smith DG, Heagerty PJ, Wallace C. Daily weight-bearing activity does not increase the risk of diabetic foot ulcers. Med Sci Sports Exerc 2003;35 (7):1093–9. Available from: https://doi.org/10.1249/01.MSS.0000074459.41029.75. PubMed PMID: 12840628.

[11] Sheahan H, Canning K, Refausse N, Kinnear EM, Jorgensen G, Walsh JR, et al. Differences in the daily activity of patients with diabetic foot ulcers compared to controls in their free-living environments. Int Wound J 2017;14(6):1175–82. Available from: https://doi.org/10.1111/iwj.12782.

[12] Najafi B, Crews RT, Wrobel JS. Importance of time spent standing for those at risk of diabetic foot ulceration. Diabetes Care 2010;33(11):2448–50. Available from: https://doi. org/10.2337/dc10-1224. PubMed PMID: 20682681; PMCID: PMC2963510.

[13] Najafi B, Grewal GS, Bharara M, Menzies R, Talal TK, Armstrong DG. Can't stand the pressure: the association between unprotected standing, walking, and wound healing in people with diabetes. J Diabetes Sci Technol 2017;11(4):657–67. Available from: https:// doi.org/10.1177/1932296816662959. PubMed PMID: 27510440; PMCID: PMC5588814.

[14] Najafi B, Armstrong DG, editors. Gait inefficiency induced by offloading – critically unintended consequences for the diabetic foot in remission. In: Eighth international symposium on the diabetic foot. The Hague, The Netherlands; 2019.

[15] Raviglione A, Reif R, Macagno M, Vigano D, Schram J, Armstrong D. Real-time smart textile-based system to monitor pressure offloading of diabetic foot ulcers. J Diabetes Sci Technol 2017;11(5):894–8. Available from: https://doi.org/10.1177/1932296817695339. PubMed PMID: 28627224.

[16] Najafi B, Mohseni H, Grewal GS, Talal TK, Menzies RA, Armstrong DG. An optical-fiber-based smart textile (Smart Socks) to manage biomechanical risk factors associated with diabetic foot amputation. J Diabetes Sci Technol 2017;11(4):668–77. Available from: https://doi.org/10.1177/1932296817709022. PubMed PMID: 28513212; PMCID: PMC5588846.

[17] Piaggesi A, Lauchli S, Bassetto F, Biedermann T, Marques A, Najafi B, et al. Advanced therapies in wound management: cell and tissue based therapies, physical and bio-physical therapies smart and IT based technologies. J Wound Care 2018;27(Sup6a):S1–137. Available from: https://doi.org/10.12968/jowc.2018.27.Sup6a.S1. PubMed PMID: 29902114.

[18] Najafi B, Ron E, Enriquez A, Marin I, Razjouyan J, Armstrong DG. Smarter sole survival: will neuropathic patients at high risk for ulceration use a smart insole-based foot protection system? J Diabetes Sci Technol 2017;11(4):702−13. Available from: https://doi.org/10.1177/1932296816689105. PubMed PMID: 28627227; PMCID: PMC5588829.

[19] Lavery LA, Armstrong DG. Temperature monitoring to assess, predict, and prevent diabetic foot complications. Curr Diab Rep 2007;7(6):416−19 PubMed PMID: 18255002.

[20] Armstrong DG, Lavery LA, Liswood PJ, Todd WF, Tredwell JA. Infrared dermal thermometry for the high-risk diabetic foot. Phys Ther 1997;77(2):169−75 discussion 76-7. PubMed PMID: 9037217.

[21] Lavery LA, Higgins KR, Lanctot DR, Constantinides GP, Zamorano RG, Athanasiou KA, et al. Preventing diabetic foot ulcer recurrence in high-risk patients: use of temperature monitoring as a self-assessment tool. Diabetes Care 2007;30(1):14−20. Available from: https://doi.org/10.2337/dc06-1600. PubMed PMID: 17192326.

[22] Frykberg RG, Gordon IL, Reyzelman AM, Cazzell SM, Fitzgerald RH, Rothenberg GM, et al. Feasibility and efficacy of a smart mat technology to predict development of diabetic plantar ulcers. Diabetes Care 2017;40(7):973−80. Available from: https://doi.org/10.2337/dc16-2294 PubMed PMID: 28465454.

[23] Reyzelman AM, Koelewyn K, Murphy M, Shen X, Yu E, Pillai R, et al. Continuous temperature-monitoring socks for home use in patients with diabetes: observational study. J Med Internet Res 2018;20(12):e12460. Available from: https://doi.org/10.2196/12460. PubMed PMID: 30559091; PMCID: PMC6315272.

[24] Parmanto B, Pramana G, Yu DX, Fairman AD, Dicianno BE. Development of mHealth system for supporting self-management and remote consultation of skincare. BMC Med Inform Decis Mak 2015;15:114. Available from: https://doi.org/10.1186/s12911-015-0237-4. PubMed PMID: 26714452; PMCID: PMC4696204.

[25] Wang L, Pedersen PC, Strong DM, Tulu B, Agu E, Ignotz R. Smartphone-based wound assessment system for patients with diabetes. IEEE Trans Biomed Eng 2015;62 (2):477−88. Available from: https://doi.org/10.1109/TBME.2014.2358632. PubMed PMID: 25248175.

[26] Mammas CS, Geropoulos S, Markou G, Saatsakis G, Lemonidou C, Tentolouris N. Mobile telemedicine systems in the multidisciplinary approach of diabetes management: the remote prevention of diabetes complications. Stud Health Technol Inform 2014;202:307−10. PubMed PMID: 25000078.

[27] Foltynski P, Ladyzynski P, Wojcicki JM. A new smartphone-based method for wound area measurement. Artif Organs 2014;38(4):346−52. Available from: https://doi.org/10.1111/aor.12169. PubMed PMID: 24102380.

[28] Quinn EM, Corrigan MA, O'Mullane J, Murphy D, Lehane EA, Leahy-Warren P, et al. Clinical unity and community empowerment: the use of smartphone technology to empower community management of chronic venous ulcers through the support of a tertiary unit. PLoS One 2013;8(11):e78786. Available from: https://doi.org/10.1371/journal.pone.0078786. PubMed PMID: 24265716; PMCID: PMC3827111.

[29] Ploderer B, Brown R, Seng LSD, Lazzarini PA, van Netten JJ. Promoting self-care of diabetic foot ulcers through a mobile phone app: user-centered design and evaluation. JMIR Diabetes 2018;3(4):e10105. Available from: https://doi.org/10.2196/10105. PubMed PMID: 30305266; PMCID: PMC6238831.

Chapter 14

Smart insulin pens and devices to track insulin doses

David C. Klonoff[1], Victoria Hsiao[2], Hope Warshaw[3] and David Kerr[4]

[1]*Diabetes Research Institute, Mills-Peninsula Medical Center, San Mateo, CA, United States,*
[2]*University of California, San Francisco, CA, United States,* [3]*Hope Warshaw Associates, LLC,*
Asheville, NC, United States, [4]*Sansum Diabetes Research Institute, Santa Barbara, CA,*
United States

Abbreviations

CGM	continuous glucose monitoring
CSII	continuous subcutaneous insulin infusion
IoT	Internet of Things
MDI	multiple daily insulin injections
PWDs	people with diabetes
SIP	smart insulin pens
T1D	type 1 diabetes
T2D	type 2 diabetes

Key points

- The majority of people with diabetes (PWDs) take insulin via injections (syringes or legacy pens). A current limitation of insulin delivered in this manner is a lack of automated systems that accurately and consistently record the dose and time of insulin administration as well as recognition of the amount of insulin on board.
- The use of new smart insulin pens, with automatic wireless transmission capabilities to send data by way of a mobile phone to the Cloud, can integrate insulin dosing data with other diabetes management data within an electronic logbook (such as glucose, carbohydrate consumption, and insulin on board) that can potentially reduce the personal day-to-day self-management burden for PWDs.
- Smart insulin pens are a digital health tool that will provide information to patients and caregivers about insulin dosing and adherence to treatment that is currently not available.

Diabetes Digital Health. DOI: https://doi.org/10.1016/B978-0-12-817485-2.00014-6

Introduction

Insulin has been available as a therapy in the management of diabetes for almost 100 years and remains a life-sustaining medication for type 1 diabetes (T1D) as well as an important part of the therapeutic armamentarium for type 2 diabetes (T2D). However, despite a long history of experience with insulin and an ever-increasing availability of modified insulin preparations and combinations, people with diabetes (PWDs) who use insulin still report challenges related to hypoglycemia, excess weight gain, and persistant sub-optimal glycemic control [1].

Furthermore, for certain subgroups (e.g., US minority populations with diabetes), there are also important cultural and socioeconomic barriers to insulin initiation [2]. For clinicians who prescribe insulin, there are a number of practical "rules" that can help one to maximize benefit and reduce therapeutic inertia [3], but in reality, two key and continuing limitations are (1) an inability for the person who takes insulin to accurately and consistently record the dose and time of insulin administration and (2) lack of a reliable method for measuring circulating insulin levels. Although the ability to have continuous real-time insulin measurements is not likely to be available in the near future, having access to reliable and accurate measurements of the dose and timing of insulin injections in a device other than an insulin pump or patch is now a clinical reality in the form of smart insulin pens (SIPs) and other tracking insulin dosing devices.

Challenges for people who take insulin and clinicians

For PWD, taking insulin is complex and challenging. Clinicians also face challenges in helping insulin users who use syringes or traditional "legacy" pens to maximize their potential benefits from a prescribed regimen due to the lack of objective data on the dose and timing of insulin administration. To date, for individuals using multiple daily injections of insulin (MDI), this assessment must be done through self-reports, logbooks, and other recording tools shared by the PWD. Extracting, reviewing, and analyzing these data for clinical decision-making are time-consuming and fraught with inaccuracies. Yet, over time these have been the data with which clinicians have had to make clinical decisions on insulin use and dosing.

Despite the considerable need, there are no national or international clinical practice guidelines that explicitly recommend that insulin users log information about their insulin doses and timing. Unlike insulin pump users, people who use legacy insulin dosing devices, such as syringes or durable/disposable pens, must make important daily decisions to administer insulin without access to reliable information on previous doses given, the residual insulin still active (insulin-on-board), and other confounding variables (e.g., exercise, travel across time zones, and changes in insulin sensitivity). Specifically, there is also the daily burden of remembering to take insulin.

Recent data from individuals using MDI and continuous glucose monitoring (CGM) devices suggest that one in four meals is associated with either a late or missed insulin bolus [4]. In a study using a Bluetooth-enabled insulin pen cap [5], insulin omission occurred in 100% of participants over a 1-month period. The impact of a missed insulin dose can be significant. For example, forgetting two meal-related doses each week is associated with a 0.3%−0.4% increase in HbA_{1c} levels and missing basal injections can lead to a 0.2%−0.3% change [6]. Improving adherence to a prescribed treatment regimen is associated with improved clinical outcomes [7] as well as lower disease-related medical costs [8].

Insulin omission and incorrect dosing can occur for a number of reasons, including simple forgetfulness, embarrassment, dose complexity, eating disorders, and/or financial cost. Another factor affecting the complexity of dosing insulin is numeracy skills. Calculating a safe and effective dose of insulin requires numeracy skills. Limited numeracy skills have been shown to influence achieved HbA_{1c} levels [9].

Choosing an insulin delivery device

For current insulin users and for individuals starting insulin, personal objectives and circumstances, clinician practice, and health plan coverage contribute to the choice of insulin(s) and delivery device. Traditionally, insulin has been given as an injection using a syringe or pen (legacy devices), or as a continuous subcutaneous insulin infusion (CSII) with a pump, via a pod or patch or more recently, as a fast-acting inhaled insulin currently used by a relatively small number of individuals. Overall, PWD and clinicians appear to prefer pens over vials and syringes [10]. This is not surprising given that pens (compared to vials and syringes) have been shown to be more accurate, more discreet, less painful, and associated with greater adherence [11,12]. Legacy insulin pens also have several potential advantages in the hospital setting [13]. Finally, there is less potential for waste of insulin with pens due to the volume of insulin contained in each insulin pen (300 U) versus the volume in vials (1000 U) [14].

The majority of people who use insulin do not use CSII for various reasons, including lack of desire to wear a device continuously, the burdensome requirement to master potentially complex technology, device insertion and changes, and maintaining an inventory of related supplies [15]. Although CSII can provide clinical and lifestyle benefits, this form of insulin delivery may be less cost-effective than MDI [16]. Also, CSII is used less often in minority populations with T1D [17,18]. In T2D, uptake of CSII continues to be very low across all populations.

Impact of the Internet of Things on smart insulin delivery

The Internet of Things (IoT) is a system of interrelated objects, sensors, and computing devices that each have unique identifiers and are able to transfer data over a network automatically without any human-to-human or human-to-computer interaction. The IoT allows the integration of medical monitoring devices to provide a complete picture in real time of a person's physiology and health. IoT uses smart sensors that are monitoring devices that make and process measurements and then send information to a smartphone or to the cloud. For open loop control, whereby a person who uses information to make a decision, smart sensors provide important real-time information as opposed to automatic closed loop control, whereby intelligent sensors are needed to make decisions and control an actuator or affect a process.

Increasingly, people are seeking methods that can automatically monitor their health in real time and also provide timely insights regarding various health parameters to themselves as well as to their clinicians. Clinicians are also seeking better methods to monitor numerous aspects of diabetes care to gain an understanding of outcomes between visits and the impact of treatment plans. Sensors are now available to monitor both various physiologic parameters and the presence of phenomena that can influence health outcomes. For PWD the first category of sensors includes commercially available blood glucose monitors for self-monitoring of blood glucose, CGM, blood pressure monitors, and exercise trackers. In the second category, monitors are becoming available to assess food intake, insulin dosing from a pump or a closed loop system, pillbox management, and pill ingestion.

Phenomena that can influence personal health outcomes include food preferences, how many pills are ingested, and how much insulin is given as well as glycemic control. This additional information is valuable as part of clinical decision-making processes. Currently, the administration and amount of an insulin dose can be detected by sensors contained in insulin pumps. Until 2017 there was no way to monitor the amount of insulin delivered by a syringe or a pen. The availability of information about the amount of insulin delivered by a pump is a major reason why the FDA cleared insulin dosing software in insulin pumps many years before they cleared any freestanding bolus or basal insulin dosing software. If a dose was associated with an adverse event, then by reviewing the amount of insulin delivered it would be possible to investigate what happened and possibly alter the software if necessary. This type of correction has not been possible with legacy self-administered insulin delivery systems such as pens and syringes.

Recording glucose, insulin dosing, and other diabetes-related data

The use of pen-and-paper logbooks appears to be declining [19]. This is unsurprising given that electronic logbooks are more accurate than traditional ones.

Data can be electronically linked to the sensor performing the measurement rather than stored in a book repository of manually entered sensor data. Furthermore, additional documentation features such as cameras or multiple physiological sensors can be added to these logbooks [20]. Although the use of paper and electronic logbooks is well established for recording glucose values and self-management information on food and exercise, the use of electronic logbooks for recording the time and dose of insulin injections has not been advocated [21]. However, it has been suggested that treatment may be enhanced with electronic recording of this type of data [22]. For people using MDI, Bluetooth-enabled SIPs that automatically collect information on the timing and dose of rapid-acting insulin doses and their timing, along with manual or Bluetooth-enabled entry of long-acting insulin doses, would transform currently available bolus dose advisors and allow MDI users and their clinicians to have the same access to clinical data, that is, currently available for people who use CSII [23].

Devices for tracking insulin doses

Over the last decade the major worldwide manufacturers of insulin, along with a number of small companies, have been working on a wide array and numerous iterations of SIPs and tracking dosing delivery devices. These include various types of devices, including pens and caps and clips, that go on or attach to a legacy insulin pen. An article by Sangave et al. offers several tables with detailed information about numerous SIPs and tracking dosing delivery devices [24]. The capabilities and key functions of SIPs vary. Kerr et al. identified nine critical functions that are integral to meet the criteria for SIPs. These are detailed in Table 14.1 [25].

A conceptual evolution from legacy insulin delivery systems to tracking insulin pens to SIPs can be expressed as progression over six stages. These include stage 0 that is vial and syringe or traditional insulin pens that provide no tracking or decisions support. Stage 1 is a tracking insulin pen with retrospective accurate dose data. Stage 2 is a real-time insulin tracking pen providing real-time dose data with insulin on board, reminders, and cloud connectivity. Stage 3 is an integrated tracking insulin pen that provides integrated diabetes management reports, including insulin doses, carbohydrate intake, and glucose concentrations. Stage 4 is a SIP with dose calculation, including autoprime detection and individualized settings, such as target glucose concentration, insulin to carbohydrate ratios, and insulin sensitivity ration. Stage 5 is a SIP with advanced decision support, including basal titration recommendations, educational modules, and coaching [25]. A significant benefit of SIPs that meet the criteria listed in Table 14.1 is that the intelligence and interface of the technology is located in the user's smart phone, an item most people carry as part of their everyday life. The SIP transmits the data to the user's mobile device and from there to the cloud where the

TABLE 14.1 Nine essential functions that meet the criteria for smart insulin pens [25].

1. No need to wear or carry an additional device beyond a smartphone
2. Provides continuous use for at least 1 year
3. Automatically responds to changes in a user's time zone
4. Automatically records and tracks the dose and timing of insulin administration with the option of sharing this information with a clinical team
5. Reminds if insulin dose not taken within a customized scheduled time frame
6. Ability to differentiate priming dose from a bolus dose. This is especially required to ensure accurate tracking of insulin-on-board estimations
7. Provides access to clinical decision support with personalized settings. These settings should include carbohydrate-to-insulin ratios, glucose level correction factors (also referred to as insulin sensitivity factor), and tracking insulin on-board information (also referred to as duration of insulin action) from prior bolus insulin doses for more precise insulin dosing and reducing the risk for hypoglycemia
8. Ability to integrate with other diabetes technologies (e.g., continuous glucose monitoring), wearables (e.g., activity monitors), and digital therapeutic platforms
9. Allows a person with diabetes and team to communicate virtually, which allows remote monitoring as a service

information can be analyzed and made available to the user, a designated significant other, and/or to their clinicians.

Regulatory review for smart insulin pens and tracking dosing delivery devices

As with other diabetes-specific devices, the regulatory review processes for approval vary from country to country. The level of regulatory review and process followed by entities and regulatory agencies for SIPs and other tracking dosing devices depends on the functionalities of the device. For example, SIPs that have the capability of calculating insulin doses and providing dosing recommendations and clinical decision support will require a higher level of review than smart dosing devices that serve as tracking tools. Dose-tracking devices will track the time and amount of insulin administered and can differentiate bolus doses from basal doses.

Other potential benefits of smart insulin pens

An indirect benefit of SIPs will also be the ability to use currently available and new insulins, including biosimilar and human insulin products. This will allow underserved populations of PWD to access intensive insulin therapy technologies more easily than at present. As with all technology-dependent devices, there are several challenges worth noting for SIPs coming to the market. These include cost and creating a user interface and user experience that will be "sticky" for subpopulations of PWD (e.g., young vs older, new onset vs established diabetes, and taking into consideration the specific needs of racial and ethnic groups).

The use of insulin dosing information to promote better treatment adherence that has been automatically sensed, analyzed, and presented to a PWD in the form of an app and to their clinician in a secure website is, potentially, a new paradigm for improving adherence to treatment. It must be noted, however, that the literature suggests that nonadherence to medication regimens in diabetes is multifactorial and can be related to beliefs, mood disorders, the burden of diabetes, and the intensity of the prescribed treatment regimen as well as the costs of treatment [26−28]. Thus the use of any new technology will have to be incorporated into a holistic diabetes care plan that addresses psychosocial barriers and the individual needs and lifestyle of the person to achieve an agreed treatment plan. A SIP could provide immediate benefits from recommending, confirming, and alerting insulin users about insulin dosing, but it will still be necessary for clinicians to engage with PWD to explain the benefits of insulin optimization, provide less costly therapies when possible, and provide a sense of caring.

Special situations

While SIPs are currently being developed for outpatient use, they also hold promise for inpatient and skilled nursing facility use, where the accurate recording of insulin doses is both essential and challenging. The use of SIPs could reduce dosing errors as well as provide clearer information about the administration of previous doses in the event that a pen user is unable to communicate.

Pregnancy is another stage of life in which SIP technology would be beneficial. The risks of uncontrolled diabetes in pregnancy are well documented for both mother and fetus. Insulin is the main glucose-lowering medication used in women who are pregnant with T2D [29], and approximately 30% of pregnant women who develop gestational diabetes will also require insulin [30]. By fine-tuning dosing and collecting data into one, easy-to-read location, SIPs will enable PWD and clinicians access to the data they need to achieve the tight glycemic control needed for a successful pregnancy.

Conclusion

For PWD and clinicians, there are many barriers to the initiation and continuation of insulin therapy. These burdens include remembering to take injections, determining the correct doses, and limiting hypoglycemia. In addition during time-limited appointments, clinicians may be concerned about the time involved in initiating, monitoring, and titrating insulin doses.

These factors can lead to delayed initiation of insulin, exposing PWD to a higher risk of complications at a younger age.

A positive result will be the replacement of legacy insulin dosing devices with SIPs and other tracking insulin dosing devices plus a combination of sensors, transmitters, and the capability to integrate with other diabetes data collecting systems. Overall, mobile/smartphone applications capable of integrating with Bluetooth-enabled diabetes devices will continue to improve and simplify diabetes management for all who are able to take advantage of their use. These technologies will enable expanded use of telemedicine and artificial intelligence. By harnessing the potential of technology to identify patterns from insulin dose data for the purpose of insulin decision support, we are at last on the verge of reducing the tremendous day-to-day burden faced by millions of PWD who use insulin.

References

[1] Saydah SH. Medication use and self-care practices in persons with diabetes. 3rd ed. Diabetes in America, 39. The National Institute of Diabetes and Digestive and Kidney Diseases, Health Information Center; 2014. p. 1–14.

[2] Gary TL, Narayan KM, Gregg EW, Beckles GL, Saaddine JB. Racial/ethnic differences in the healthcare experience (coverage, utilization, and satisfaction) of US adults with diabetes. Ethn Dis 2003;13(1):47–54.

[3] Kerr D, Cavan D. Treating obese patients with poorly controlled diabetes: confessions of an insulin therapist. Diabetes Metab Res Rev 1999;15(3):219–25.

[4] Norlander LM, Anderson S, Levy CJ, Ekhlaspour L, Lam DW, Hsu L, et al. Late and missed meal boluses with multiple daily insulin injections. Diabetes. 2018;67(Suppl. 1):992-P.

[5] Munshi MN, Slyne C, Greenberg JM, Greaves T, Lee A, Carl S, et al. Nonadherence to insulin therapy detected by bluetooth-enabled pen cap is associated with poor glycemic control. Diabetes Care 2019;42(6):1129–31.

[6] Randlov J, Poulsen JU. How much do forgotten insulin injections matter to hemoglobin a1c in people with diabetes? A simulation study. J Diabetes Sci Technol 2008;2(2):229–35.

[7] Huber CA, Rapold R, Brungger B, Reich O, Rosemann T. One-year adherence to oral antihyperglycemic medication and risk prediction of patient outcomes for adults with diabetes mellitus: an observational study. Med (Baltim) 2016;95(26):e3994.

[8] Sokol MC, McGuigan KA, Verbrugge RR, Epstein RS. Impact of medication adherence on hospitalization risk and healthcare cost. Med Care 2005;43(6):521–30.

[9] Marden S, Thomas PW, Sheppard ZA, Knott J, Lueddeke J, Kerr D. Poor numeracy skills are associated with glycaemic control in Type 1 diabetes. Diabet Med 2012;29(5):662–9.

[10] Meneghini LF, McNulty JN. Role of devices in insulin delivery. Diabetes Technol Ther 2017;19(2):76–8.

[11] Spollett G, Edelman SV, Mehner P, Walter C, Penfornis A. Improvement of insulin injection technique: examination of current issues and recommendations. Diabetes Educ 2016;42(4):379–94.

[12] Lasalvia P, Barahona-Correa JE, Romero-Alvernia DM, Gil-Tamayo S, Castaneda-Cardona C, Bayona JG, et al. Pen devices for insulin self-administration compared with needle and vial: systematic review of the literature and meta-analysis. J Diabetes Sci Technol 2016;10(4):959−66.

[13] Haines ST, Miklich MA, Rochester-Eyeguokan C. Best practices for safe use of insulin pen devices in hospitals: recommendations from an expert panel Delphi consensus process. Am J Health Syst Pharm 2016;73(19 Suppl. 5):S4−16.

[14] Page MR. Insulin pens: improving adherence and reducing costs, Available from: <https://www.pharmacytimes.com/publications/directions-in-pharmacy/2015/may2015/insulin-pens-improving-adherence-and-reducing-costs>; 2015 [updated 19.05.15].

[15] Blair JC, McKay A, Ridyard C, Thornborough K, Bedson E, Peak M, et al. Continuous subcutaneous insulin infusion versus multiple daily injection regimens in children and young people at diagnosis of type 1 diabetes: pragmatic randomised controlled trial and economic evaluation. BMJ. 2019;365:l1226.

[16] Pollard DJ, Brennan A, Dixon S, Waugh N, Elliott J, Heller S, et al. Cost-effectiveness of insulin pumps compared with multiple daily injections both provided with structured education for adults with type 1 diabetes: a health economic analysis of the relative effectiveness of pumps over structured education (REPOSE) randomised controlled trial. BMJ Open 2018;8(4):e016766.

[17] Foster NC, Beck RW, Miller KM, Clements MA, Rickels MR, DiMeglio LA, et al. State of type 1 diabetes management and outcomes from the T1D exchange in 2016-2018. Diabetes Technol Ther 2019;21(2):66−72.

[18] Willi SM, Miller KM, DiMeglio LA, Klingensmith GJ, Simmons JH, Tamborlane WV, et al. Racial-ethnic disparities in management and outcomes among children with type 1 diabetes. Pediatrics. 2015;135(3):424−34.

[19] Gibbons CJ. Turning the page on pen-and-paper questionnaires: combining ecological momentary assessment and computer adaptive testing to transform psychological assessment in the 21st century. Front Psychol 2016;7:1933.

[20] Gates RS, McLean MJ, Osborn WA. Smart electronic laboratory notebooks for the NIST research environment. J Res Natl Inst Stand Technol 2015;120:293−303.

[21] Scaramuzza A, Cherubini V, Tumini S, Bonfanti R, Buono P, Cardella F, et al. Recommendations for self-monitoring in pediatric diabetes: a consensus statement by the ISPED. Acta Diabetol 2014;51(2):173−84.

[22] Weissmann J, Mueller A, Messinger D, Parkin CG, Amann-Zalan I. Improving the quality of outpatient diabetes care using an information management system: results from the observational VISION study. J Diabetes Sci Technol 2015;10(1):76−84.

[23] Walsh J, Roberts R, Bailey TS, Heinemann L. Bolus advisors: sources of error, targets for improvement. J Diabetes Sci Technol 2018;12(1):190−8.

[24] Sangave NA, Aungst TD, Patel DK. Smart connected insulin pens, caps, and attachments: a review of the future of diabetes technology. Diabetes Spectr 2019;32 (4):378−84.

[25] Kerr D, Warshaw H, and Choi N. Smart insulin pens will address critical unmet needs for people with diabetes using insulin. Endocrine today. 2019, May.

[26] Krass I, Schieback P, Dhippayom T. Adherence to diabetes medication: a systematic review. Diabet Med 2015;32(6):725−37.

[27] Polonsky WH. Poor medication adherence in diabetes: what's the problem? J Diabetes 2015;7(6):777−8.

[28] Wu P, Liu N. Association between patients' beliefs and oral antidiabetic medication adherence in a Chinese type 2 diabetic population. Patient Prefer Adherence 2016;10:1161−7.

[29] Berry DC, Boggess K, Johnson QB. Management of pregnant women with Type 2 diabetes mellitus and the consequences of fetal programming in their offspring. Curr Diab Rep 2016;16(5):36.

[30] UCSF Health. Diabetes in pregnancy. University of California. Available from: <https://www.ucsfhealth.org/education/diabetes_in_pregnancy/>. Accessed on 13.03.2020.

Section 3

Technical aspects of digital health for diabetes

Chapter 15

Research end points for diabetes digital health

Kathryn L. Fantasia, Mary-Catherine Stockman and Katherine L. Modzelewski

Section of Endocrinology, Diabetes, and Nutrition, Boston University School of Medicine and Boston Medical Center, Boston, MA, United States

Abbreviations

CEEBIT	Continuous Evaluation of Evolving Behavioral Intervention Technologies
CGM	continuous glucose monitor
FDA	Food and Drug Administration
FGM	flash glucose monitoring
HbA1c	hemoglobin A1c
MOST	multiphase optimization strategy
RCT	randomized controlled trial
SMART	sequential, multiple assignment, randomized trials
UX	user experience
WHO	World Health Organization

Key points

- Diabetes digital health does not easily fit traditional models of research because of its rapid pace of change and the components that must be evaluated: technology, clinical efficacy, and behavioral change.
- Although randomized controlled trials are considered the gold standard for clinical trial design, alternative methodologies may better evaluate digital health technologies.
- Patient-reported outcomes should be considered alongside clinical end points such as glycemic control when evaluating digital health.

Diabetes technology has evolved dramatically since the first description of an insulin pump prototype by Kadish in 1963 [1]. Historically, diabetes technology meant using an instrument to directly affect blood glucose control, but more recently it has expanded to also include the broader topic of digital health. Digital health is defined as the use of digital technology to

Diabetes Digital Health. DOI: https://doi.org/10.1016/B978-0-12-817485-2.00015-8

impact health and health-care delivery; it can be divided into many subcategories, including eHealth, mHealth, wearables, and telehealth, among others [2]. While the field of digital health has been rapidly expanding and adopted by both providers and patients, two questions arise: why do we need to study these technologies, and if so, what research end points allow us to best accomplish this?

Why we need to study digital health for diabetes

The World Health Organization (WHO) first recognized the potential impact of digital technologies on health in 1998, and in 2005 it identified eHealth, which is the use of information and communication technologies for health, as a potential way to improve health-care delivery [3]. If eHealth is going to be recognized as an adjunct to traditional care models, then it seems fitting that it must also be studied and regulated in a similar manner.

As with any medication or medical device, patient safety is of the utmost importance when considering utilization of digital health. The Food and Drug Administration (FDA) is responsible for approving new medications and clearing new medical devices, which are instruments intended for use in disease diagnosis, treatment, or prevention. Digital health poses a challenge because available technologies do not necessarily fit the traditional definition of medical devices [2,4]. An example of this is the concept of Software as a Medical Device, which is using software for medical purposes without direct integration into medical device hardware [5]. Further adding to this challenge is the rapidity with which technology evolves and increasing communication among different devices. A continuous glucose monitor (CGM) can sync directly with a smartphone to send data to the cloud to be downloaded by a medical practitioner. Current controversies include whether each level of this interaction should be subject to the same regulations as blood glucose meters, insulin pumps and CGMs, or whether a different set of standards applies to each device. Pharmacologic and technological advancements in medicine have been subject to highly rigorous clinical trials and FDA oversight with the expectation that medications and devices result in clinical efficacy for our patients, but this same rigor has thus far not been applied to the burgeoning digital health market [6].

The interoperability of devices, often seen through the interaction between a smartphone, tablet, or computer with a medical device or patient portal, not only increases the utility of digital health, but also increases the potential risks. These risks occur on several levels, from the technology itself to increased access to protected health information. Using technology as an adjunct in health care adds an additional step for the patient. This leads to the risk of user error, as well as potential consequences related to failure of the technology to function as expected, be it from power failure or inability to connect to the internet or other devices.

Medical devices are evaluated for safety prior to approval, and if risks outweigh the benefits, then they are not approved. They may also be removed from the market if deemed problematic in postmarket surveillance, though this oversight is currently limited and primarily consumer-driven. This becomes more complicated when the idea of cybersecurity is introduced because medical devices are at risk for being hacked, but so are personal devices being used for portals or with mobile applications for health-care delivery. Concerns have previously been brought up about the potential ability to hack implantable cardiac devices, and presumably the same concerns are relevant to blood glucose monitors, smart pens, insulin pumps, and CGMs [7]. Altering a reported blood sugar or shutting off access to the report of a blood sugar level that must be accessed automatically for decision-making in a closed-loop insulin delivery system could lead to disastrous outcomes, so we must understand vulnerabilities of our technology to ensure that new risks are identified and adaptations can be made to mitigate these potential vulnerabilities as much as possible.

While much of the current focus on digital health research and oversight has been surrounding safety, the importance of establishing efficacy and effectiveness of digital technologies for diabetes management must not be diminished. Medications that are not clinically efficacious, even if safe, are not approved for clinical use, and the same standard should be held for digital health. Effectiveness, which is different from efficacy, must also be considered to know if a product is worthwhile. Effectiveness can be best assessed with real-world data collected in real-world evidence trials. If an intervention is not applicable in a "real-world" setting, the lack of effectiveness should preclude its use. Research into efficacy and effectiveness of digital health should be concurrent with safety research, and rapid approval of technologies should not occur at the expense of quality patient care.

While safety, efficacy, and effectiveness are the most important aspects of studying digital health for diabetes, there are countless other reasons why it should be studied. These include usability of technology, selection of ideal candidates for use of digital health, and tailoring treatment to individuals. Digital health expands access to health care to individuals to whom it may traditionally have been limited or unavailable, be it from lack of physical access to care, language barriers, or socioeconomic status. With an estimated 77% of Americans having access to smartphones and more than 5 billion unique mobile subscribers worldwide, the potential reach of digital health is nearly universal [8,9]. Given the spread of such technology and the increased capacity to reach underserved populations, digital health platforms are poised to significantly change health-care delivery. However, the capacity for mHealth, which uses mobile wireless technologies to impact health, to have meaningful impact in health-care delivery is directly linked to the quality of a technology; not all mHealth may be beneficial for all individuals simply because they have access to it. A patient may be able to upload data from a device to the cloud for review, but their health-care provider needs to be able to access the data and provide recommendations for there to be a benefit. For other patients, the vast amount of data available, such as CGM glucose trend data, may become overwhelming. And despite the increased patient reach using mobile technologies, disparities still exist surrounding technology use in different segments of the population, although these could potentially be reduced by tailoring mobile technologies to specific groups.

As the definition of digital health continues to evolve, certainly there will be countless more research questions that arise. The outcomes of interest may change with time, and we will need to continuously examine how we can best address these for ourselves, as a medical community, and for our patients. In thinking about the current state of digital health for diabetes management, and how best to assess efficacy of interventions, we must consider research end points from the perspectives of both study design and outcomes.

Research study design

The randomized controlled trial (RCT) is the current gold standard for assessment of efficacy of an intervention in research studies [10]. Just as digital health interventions do not necessarily fit within the traditional model for medical device regulation, the RCT may also no longer be the best fit for studying digital health interventions and alternative trial designs for research should be considered. It is no longer enough to demonstrate efficacy for a new product; we must also consider effectiveness, especially for products such as digital health tools, where part of the benefit seen, when studied in an RCT, comes from a health-care professional regularly reminding a subject to adhere to using the product.

Randomized controlled trials

The many advantages of RCTs are well established, particularly the reduction of unfounded causality and bias through random assignment to groups. Randomization allows for attribution of causality to an intervention by balancing confounding variables among different groups [11].

As no other trial design can establish causal relationships, RCTs have been widely accepted as the ideal for efficacy studies in medicine, which are designed to determine the effect of an intervention under idealized conditions [12]. While the rigor of the study design warrants this designation, the practicality of RCTs is frequently limited by their high cost, length of time to complete, and issues with generalizability as study populations are often highly selective. In order to provide a representative sample, RCTs tend to be large, multisite, and multiyear trials, which comes at a great cost. Much time is demanded of both participants and researchers, as RCTs have frequent participant follow-up visits and require a team with medical, clinical, and regulatory expertise. These demands are not always practical for diabetes digital health studies because RCTs are generally performed in academic or clinical settings that are not easily accessible to all patients, and increasing health-care access is a large part of the allure of digital health. The long-term follow-up needed for RCTs can prove challenging in the assessment of digital health technologies. Because of the rapid pace of technological development, these tools may be outdated, or even obsolete, once efficacy is established.

In an attempt to adapt RCTs to the rapidly advancing pace of digital health technologies, such as mHealth, effectiveness studies, in the form of pragmatic clinical trials, are increasingly being used. Real-world data is information gathered from clinical practice that can be organized into patterns. This concept has been expanded to clinical trials that closely approximate "real-world" clinical settings, which are called pragmatic trials, and real-world evidence is the conclusions that can be reached from these pragmatic trials [13]. Although efficacy is sometimes used as a surrogate for effectiveness, the ideal clinical settings in which RCTs are performed with intensive clinician support may not be practically applicable in "real-world" clinical settings. To bridge this gap, pragmatic trials measure benefit in broader patient groups in "real-world" clinical settings. These trials are performed in clinical practice settings and are tailored to achieve clinically relevant outcomes. In contrast to efficacy trials, pragmatic trials provide evidence of effectiveness and are often used to determine if interventions should be adopted into routine practice [12].

Using real-world data patterns collected from clinician and patient interactions in clinical practice and real-world evidence obtained from pragmatic studies developed to closely resemble routine clinical practice, data from traditional RCTs can be augmented to help to inform policy, practice, and future development of study hypotheses [13]. In line with the increasing use of pragmatic trials, the FDA is launching a real-world evidence program for drug and biologic review, although this has not yet been expanded to devices, a category into which diabetes digital health technologies often fall [14]. While pragmatic clinical trials have aimed to assess health-care innovations in the "real world," when utilized to determine effectiveness of digital health technologies, these studies may use small sample sizes and short-term follow-up to ensure that the technological innovation being evaluated is not outdated by the time benefits are demonstrated. Although this may be an improvement over traditional RCTs, the small sample sizes, which are frequently studied in digital health research, limit generalizability and power. Likewise, the short-term follow-up, which is a common characteristic of digital health research, increases the risk of bias, particularly the favorable impact of a novelty effect, which can be seen early after adoption of a new technology, but which can fade after a few months.

Alternative study design

While RCTs have been considered the gold standard in determining the efficacy of an intervention, given their above strengths and limitations, identification of methodologies more appropriately suited to the assessment of the rapidly changing field of digital health technology is necessary, particularly where effectiveness is concerned [15]. Furthermore, the potential impact of mHealth interventions is grounded in the quality of their design, both for usability and effectiveness. Evaluation to guide design of these platforms and determine their effectiveness is imperative and requires selection of methodology tailored to the intervention and the outcome being assessed. While some data about usability and effectiveness can be gleaned from cohort observational studies, alternative methodologies that may lend themselves better to the study of digital health include sequential, multiple assignment, randomized trials (SMART), multiphase optimization strategy (MOST), and continuous evaluation of evolving behavioral intervention technologies (CEEBIT).

Digital health applications are becoming increasingly complex. Interventions often involve multiple components that can adapt to real-time contextual data collected by digital devices and sensors, such as just-in-time adaptive interventions [16]. In these adaptive intervention settings, variables impact both the delivery of intervention components and the order in which these components appear. SMART design provides a way to assess the sequential intervention components of digital technologies through multiple serial randomizations for each enrolled individual [17,18]. By assessing sequential intervention components, decision rules are developed that allow for adaptation of the delivered treatment. These components can include inputs from sensors within digital devices or through patient provided inputs. SMART design can be used when evaluating interventions such as utilization of push notifications from a mHealth application. The optimal content, timing, and frequency of messaging would be determined through sequentially randomizing individuals to different interventions or variations over time to optimize the intervention.

For less complex devices and interventions, MOST trial design offers an alternative to build, optimize, and evaluate digital interventions that may contain multiple components. MOST methodology is a three-phase process consisting of (1) screening, (2) refining the individual components, and (3) confirming the efficacy of the completed intervention through an RCT. Randomized experimentation occurs in each step of the study to inform design and assess efficacy of an optimized intervention [18]. This process allows for prospective, thoughtful engineering of mHealth technologies, such as multiple iterations of a mobile application. It can also help to ensure that a technology is still relevant once a completed product is determined to be effective and is released to market as these trials emphasize efficiency.

Finally, for those digital health devices and applications that primarily utilize behavioral interventions to effect changes to patient health and well-being, application of CEEBIT may prove to be a useful methodologic framework to rapidly and iteratively assess various behavioral interventions supplied by these devices [19]. The CEEBIT methodology allows for real-time and "real-world" concurrent evaluation of multiple models of an intervention through direct deployment to consumers. CEEBIT methodology continually improves upon an intervention by promoting promising models for further use and evaluation, while discontinuing models that are inferior or ineffective from either a usability or clinical outcome perspective, until the "best" model is identified [19]. Such a framework proves advantageous in a rapidly evolving market. Unlike in RCTs, where the end points are set at the time of trial initiation, these strategies adapt and can be updated to include new evidence, technological advances, patient behaviors, or data trends.

While the RCT still dominates diabetes digital health clinical trials at present, with alternative study designs that better fit with the goals of digital health, this landscape is likely to continue to evolve. At present, we are seeing this in the increasing number of n-of-1 studies that are being used to determine effectiveness of digital health technologies. In n-of-1 studies, multiple crossover events within a single patient occur that can then be combined with other patients and extrapolated to population-level analyses [20]. As emphasis shifts more toward effectiveness and patient-related outcomes, use of study designs that better align with these outcomes will continue to expand.

Research outcomes

The study design selected for research into diabetes digital health is largely shaped by the outcomes of interest, which can be divided into technology-related or patient-related outcomes, including clinical and patient-reported outcomes.

Technology-related outcomes

In studying a new technology for diabetes digital health, user experience (UX) is an important consideration. A comprehensive outcome, UX indicates the usability, accessibility, usefulness, desirability, navigability, and credibility of the technology [21].

The International Organization for Standardization defines usability as the "extent to which a product can be used by specified users to achieve specified goals with effectiveness, efficiency and satisfaction in a specified context of use" [22]. Usability is frequently overlooked, though it is critical to the success of any digital health technology. Usability consists of at least three of the following components: learnability, memorability, low usability error rate, efficiency, and end-user satisfaction [23]. These components can be evaluated in a research setting using validated questionnaires to measure test level satisfaction, including the 10 item system usability scale [24]. If a technology is found to have poor usability for the patient, the provider, or the larger health system, other outcomes are irrelevant. With the high rates of technology abandonment, usability is crucial for an intervention to be sustainable.

Once a technology is determined usable, it is critical to consider who has access to such technology, which defines accessibility. While most interventions are performed in a traditional research setting, with one of the main goals of digital health being to increase access to care, the ability of technology to be accessible to different groups is an important research focus. Penetration is the integration of an intervention into a setting, while the reach indicates the number of people willing to participate in the intervention [25,26]. Both penetration and reach are important when studying digital health for diabetes, particularly when it comes to potentially closing gaps in health-care access.

After usability and accessibility are determined, researchers should evaluate the other components of the UX, such as desirability and navigability [21]. These components may be evaluated through user surveys, interactive interviews, or focus groups. It is important for both patients and providers to have positive UX to assure that digital health use is characterized by positive interactions that can potentially impact care without compromising patient safety. This concept is important for both the patient and provider, particularly since patients are more likely to continue using the digital health and its potential benefits with provider support. Patients may have a positive experience with a technology that is not considered to have any glycemic benefit by a provider, and in contrast, a provider may endorse a technology that improves glycemic control but may be challenging for a patient to use correctly. This creates a complex interaction that must be evaluated on both sides.

Clinical outcomes

Finger-stick blood glucose and the hemoglobin A1c (HbA1c) have long been the standard for measuring glycemic control as patient-related clinical diabetes outcomes. Self-monitoring of blood glucose can be used to evaluate glycemic trend patterns, including fasting, preprandial, and postprandial sugars. However, checking blood sugars can be labor-intensive and, depending on when the blood glucose concentration is checked, provides only a small piece of the bigger picture. Studies often use fasting blood glucose for medication titration, but this does not account for variability throughout the rest of the day, potentially targeting fasting blood sugar for treatment when the real issue is postprandial hyperglycemia.

The HbA1c also provides discrete data through a measurement of average blood glucose over a 3-month period. While this is a reasonable time period to measure for clinical trials that span years, it only reflects an average blood glucose and provides no information about variability to help better understand patterns of glycemic control. In addition, HbA1c is not reliable in all populations, such as those with end-stage renal disease or anemia who glycate hemoglobin at different rates; thus, large populations may be excluded from research studies [27].

Just as the RCT may no longer be the best option to study mobile or digital health, the HbA1c may be becoming an obsolete end point when studying digital health efficacy. Technology changes rapidly and if shifts in study design lead to more rapid pace of research, the outcome measures will need to be able to keep pace.

With the advent of CGM and flash glucose monitoring (FGM) technology, a new set of clinical outcomes has arisen that not only keeps up with changes in mobile health but also can provide more granular data. Rather than studying long-term glycemic control or using seven-point glucose profiles to gain a sense of glycemic trends and using different strategies for measuring glycemic variability, the capability now exists to follow glucose trends at 5-minute intervals [28]. Use of target ranges can allow studies to be tailored to different populations, and the time in range, hypoglycemia, and hyperglycemia, as well as composite metrics [29], can be measured to have a more detailed understanding of glycemic trends [30]. Targeting an HbA1c of 7% gives only a small piece of a larger picture—half of the time can be spent in hypoglycemia and half in hyperglycemia, but overall blood sugars appear to be in range; in contrast, CGM and FGM technology allow for focused interventions and better definition of blood glucose trends. While the use of such technology as an end point within clinical trials is nascent, it marks an exciting shift in clinical trial design and development.

Patient-reported outcomes

Glycemic control and glycemic variability have been favored as clinically relevant study outcomes from their data demonstrating associations with reducing microvascular complications of diabetes [31,32]. However, frequently missing from clinical trials in diabetes care are patient-reported outcomes [33]. Important to those living with diabetes, quality of life and burden of treatment have emerged as outcomes worthy of routine inclusion into clinical trials [33,34]. These patient-reported outcomes are of particular importance for diabetes-related digital technologies, as these interventions have evolved out of a movement to transition toward highly accessible, minimally disruptive, and patient-centered care delivery. The importance of patient-reported outcome measures has been increasingly recognized by the FDA and is now being integrated into evaluation and labeling of medical devices [35]. One of the goals of digital health is to improve health and well-being through frequent interaction with technology. As interoperability between technologies increases, the capacity for seamless diabetes care will be enhanced and digital diabetes technologies may have the potential to reduce the time and energy required by patients for self-care and chronic disease management. In this setting, quality of life and burden become increasingly important end points in the assessment of digital health. Any added burden or decrease of quality of life from digital health must be carefully weighed.

Conclusion

The expansion of digital health in diabetes over the last decade is just the beginning of an exciting new direction for diabetes care that is expected to expand health-care access. While digital health is already being adopted, there is little consensus about how best to study these rapidly evolving technologies that do not necessarily fit the current gold standards for research. To best understand digital health and the implications for our patients with diabetes, from safety, clinical efficacy, and quality of life perspectives, we must be willing to adapt our research to fit new technologies appropriately, even if this means straying from traditional research modalities.

As the way we study digital health technologies changes, so too must regulatory oversight adapt to the evolving digital health-care landscape to ensure patient safety and promote the scientific rigor necessary to determine effectiveness of digital health technologies. These are factors we have come to expect from, and should demand of, health-care interventions.

References

[1] Kadish AH. Automation control of blood sugar a servomechanism for glucose monitoring and control. Trans Am Soc Artif Int Organs 1963;IX:363−7.

[2] U.S. Food and Drug Administration. Digital Health [Internet]. [cited 2019 May 13]. Available from: <https://www.fda.gov/medical-devices/digital-health>.

[3] World Health Organization. eHealth at WHO [Internet]. [cited 2019 May 13]. Available from: <https://www.who.int/ehealth/about/en/>.

[4] U.S. Food and Drug Administration. Is the product a medical device? [Internet]. [cited 2019 May 28]. Available from: <https://www.fda.gov/medical-devices/classify-your-medi-cal-device/product-medical-device>.

[5] U.S. Food and Drug Administration. Software as a medical device (SaMD) [Internet]. [cited 2019 May 28]. Available from: <https://www.fda.gov/medical-devices/digital-health/software-medical-device-samd>.

[6] Bates DW, Landman A, Levine DM. Health apps and health policy: what is needed? JAMA-J Am Med Assoc 2018;320(19):1975−6.

[7] U.S. Food and Drug Administration. Cybersecurity vulnerabilities affecting Medtronic implantable cardiac devices, programmers, and home monitors: FDA safety communication

[Internet]. 2019 [cited 2019 May 13]. Available from: <https://www.fda.gov/medical-devices/safety-communications/cybersecurity-vulnerabilities-affecting-medtronic-implantable-cardiac-devices-programmers-and-home>.

[8] Pew Research Center. Mobile fact sheet [Internet]. Pew Research Center. 2018 [cited 2019 May 13]. Available from: <https://www.pewinternet.org/fact-sheet/mobile/>.

[9] GSMA Intelligence. The Mobile Economy 2018 [Internet]. 2018. [cited 2019 May 13]. Available from: <https://www.gsma.com/mobileeconomy/wp-content/uploads/2018/02/The-Mobile-Economy-Global-2018.pdf>.

[10] Bothwell LE, Greene JA, Podolsky SH, Jones DS. Assessing the gold standard—Lessons from the history of RCTs. N Engl J Med 2016;374(22):2175−81.

[11] Feinstein AR, Horwitz RI. Double standards, scientific methods, and epidemiologic research. N Engl J Med 1982;307(26):1611−17.

[12] G. Gartlehner, R.A. Hansen, D. Nissman, K.N. Lohr, T.S. Carey, Criteria for Distinguishing Effectiveness From Efficacy Trials in Systematic Reviews. *Technical Review 12* (Prepared by the RTI-International-University of North Carolina Evidence-based Practice Center under Contract No. 290-02-0016.) AHRQ Publication No. 06-0046. Agency for Healthcare Research and Quality, 2006.

[13] Klonoff DC. The expanding role of real-world evidence trials in health care decision making. J Diabetes Sci Technol 2020;14(1):174−9.

[14] ElZarrad MK. Framework for FDA's real-world evidence program [Internet]. 2019. [cited 2019 May 13]. Available from: <https://www.actiac.org/system/files/ElZarrad%20MK%20PPT%20to%20ACT-IAC%20-FIN.pdf > .

[15] Modzelewski KL, Stockman MC, Steenkamp DW. Rethinking the endpoints of mhealth intervention research in diabetes care. J Diabetes Sci Technol 2018;12 (2):389−92.

[16] Nahum-Shani I, Smith SN, Spring BJ, Collins LM, Witkiewitz K, Tewari A, et al. Just-in-time adaptive interventions (JITAIs) in mobile health: key components and design principles for ongoing health behavior support. Ann Behav Med 2018;52(6):446−62.

[17] Murphy SA. An experimental design for the development of adaptive treatment strategies. Stat Med 2005;24(10):1455−81.

[18] Collins LM, Murphy SA, Strecher V. The multiphase optimization strategy (MOST) and the sequential multiple assignment randomized trial (SMART): New methods for more potent eHealth interventions. Am J Prev Med 2007;32(5 Suppl.):112−18.

[19] Mohr DC, Cheung K, Schueller SM, Brown CH, Duan N. Continuous evaluation of evolving behavioral intervention technologies. Am J Prev Med 2013;45(4):517−23.

[20] Duan N, Kravitz RL, Schmid CH. Single-patient (*n*-of-1) trials: a pragmatic clinical decision methodology for patient-centered comparative effectiveness research. J Clin Epidemiol 2013;66(8 Suppl. 8):1−12.

[21] U.S. Department of Health and Human Services. User experience basics [Internet]. U.S. Department of Health and Human Services. [cited 2019 May 13]. Available from: <https://www.usability.gov/what-and-why/user-experience.html>.

[22] National Institute of Standards and Technology. Health IT usability [Internet]. 2017 [cited 2019 May 13]. Available from: <https://www.nist.gov/programs-projects/health-it-usability>.

[23] Staggers N, Xiao Y, Chapman L. Debunking health IT usability myths. Appl Clin Inf 2013;4(2):241−50.

[24] Sauro J. Measuring usability with the system usability scale (SUS) [Internet]. 2011 [cited 2019 May 13]. Available from: <https://measuringu.com/sus/>.

[25] Lewis CC, Fischer S, Weiner BJ, Stanick C, Kim M, Martinez RG. Outcomes for implementation science: an enhanced systematic review of instruments using evidence-based rating criteria. Implement Sci 2015;10(1):1−17.

[26] Gaglio B, Shoup JA, Glasgow RE. The RE-AIM framework: a systematic review of use over time. Am J Public Health 2013;103(6):e38−46.

[27] Sacks DB. Hemoglobin A1c in diabetes: panacea or pointless? Diabetes 2013;62(1):41−3.

[28] Rodbard D. The challenges of measuring glycemic variability. J Diabetes Sci Technol 2012;6(3):21−2.

[29] Nguyen M, Han J, Spanakis EK, Kovatchev BP, Klonoff DC. A review of continuous glucose monitoring-based composite metrics for glycemic control. Diabetes Technol Ther. 2020 Mar 4. Available from: https://doi.org/10.1089/dia.2019.0434. [Epub ahead of print].

[30] Wright LA-C, Hirsch IB. Metrics beyond hemoglobin A1C in diabetes management: time in range, hypoglycemia, and other parameters. Diabetes Technol Ther 2017;19(S2):S-16−26.

[31] Diabetes Control and Complications Trial Research Group. The effect of intensive treatment of diabetes on the development and progression of long-term complications in insulin-dependent diabetes mellitus. N Engl J Med 1993;329(14):977−86.

[32] UK Prospective Diabetes Study (UKPDS) Group. Intensive blood-glucose control with sulphonylureas or insulin compared with conventional treatment and risk of complications in patients with type 2 diabetes. Lancet 1998;352(9131):837−53.

[33] Rodriguez-Gutierrez R, McCoy RG. Measuring what matters in diabetes. JAMA-J Am Med Assoc 2019;321(19):1865−6.

[34] Spencer-Bonilla G, Quiñones AR, Montori VM. Assessing the burden of treatment. J Gen Intern Med 2017;32(10):1141−5.

[35] U.S. Food and Drug Administration. Patient-reported outcomes (PROs) in medical device decision making [Internet]. [cited 2019 May 28]. Available from: <https://www.fda.gov/about-fda/cdrh-patient-engagement/patient-reported-outcomes-pros-medical-device-decision-making>.

Chapter 16

Digital health technologies, diabetes, and driving (meet your new backseat driver)

Andjela Drincic[1], Matthew Rizzo[2], Cyrus Desouza[1] and Jennifer Merickel[2]

[1]*Division of Diabetes, Endocrinology & Metabolism, Department of Internal Medicine, University of Nebraska Medical Center, Omaha, NE, United States,* [2]*Mind & Brain Health Labs, Department of Neurological Sciences, University of Nebraska Medical Center, Omaha, NE, United States*

Abbreviations

CGM continuous glucose monitor
EU European Union
T1D type 1 diabetes

Key points

- Drivers with diabetes are at a greater risk for driver errors and vehicle crashes compared to the general population.
- The main factors contributing to this increased risk are hypoglycemia-associated cognitive impairment and comorbidities, including retinopathy, neuropathy, and sleep disorders.
- Advances in technology have transformed the vehicle into a "medical diagnostic tool" capable of analyzing real-time health data from wearable sensors (such as glucose and heart monitoring) to determine and respond to driving risk, preventing vehicle crashes.

A framework for assessing driver safety in medical disorders

Driving is a key activity of daily living that supports mobility, health, and quality of life. However, vehicle crashes are associated with over 1 million deaths and 50 million injuries worldwide each year, resulting in significant suffering, disability, and societal cost [1]. The risk and burden of vehicle

Diabetes Digital Health. DOI: https://doi.org/10.1016/B978-0-12-817485-2.00016-X
219

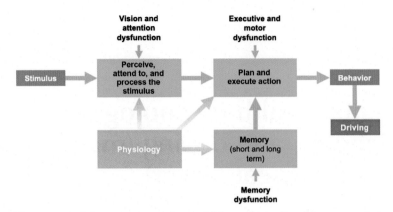

FIGURE 16.1 **An Information-processing model for understanding driver errors that may lead to vehicle crashes.** Driver behavior can be safe or unsafe because of impairments at one or more stages in the driving task. For people living with diabetes, changes in their glucose levels can affect processing at several stages.

crashes disproportionately affects drivers with medical disorders and may result in injury, death, driving curtailment, or loss of agency [2]—underscoring the need for innovative tools and strategies to detect, monitor, predict, and prevent unsafe driving in people with medical conditions such as diabetes.

Safe driving requires key functional abilities (perceptual, cognitive, and motor) that may be affected by a wide-range of medical disorders (e.g., endocrine, neurologic, sleep, cardiac, psychiatric, and visual) [2]. Impairments in these domains can increase the risk for driver errors that may lead to crashes (Fig. 16.1). Medical diagnoses or more static, driver-level demographic factors (e.g., age and gender) alone are often insufficient for predicting driver safety [2]. Critically, drivers with medical disorders may be safe at some times and in some settings, yet not in others, because of fluctuating disease processes over time and complex factors that mediate driver impairment.

To assess the contribution of driver behavior to unsafe driving, one must consider the driver's clinical status, their driving strategy, and surrounding driving environment:

- Driver's clinical status—including sleepiness, physiologic impairment, and stress—can have both acute and chronic effects.
- Driver strategies—including reducing exposure to higher-risk driving environments (e.g., snow, dense traffic, and low light), curtailing unnecessary driving, and avoiding driving while impaired—may all improve driver safety, yet can result in reduced personal mobility, quality of life, and independence.

- Driving environment factors—including roadway characteristics, weather/ lighting, and speed limit— can challenge impaired drivers and increase their risk of a crash.

Interventions aimed at preserving driver safety, mobility, and quality of life can focus on driver capacity, vehicle and roadway design, clinical practice, and public policy. Promising tools to improve driver safety include evidence-based assessments of driver safety, in-vehicle medical monitoring, and automated driving systems which can assist impaired drivers.

Driving risk in diabetes

Vehicle crash risk in diabetes

Drivers with diabetes are at significantly greater risk of vehicle crashes compared to those without diabetes [2−5]. Approximately 1.3% of vehicle crashes are due to driver-related medical emergencies and diabetes has been implicated in up to 20% of these crashes [6]. Based on a meta-analysis of 13 studies, drivers with diabetes have an estimated 1.19 times greater crash risk than drivers without diabetes [3]. While crash records are often incomplete and unable to characterize key factors that may have contributed to the crash (e.g., medication usage and glucose levels) [2], retrospective reviews of publicly available prescription data and crash records have linked crash risk to insulin usage and hypoglycemia [3−5]. Elevated crash risk in diabetes is also related to demographic factors, including older age [4,5]. These findings underscore the need to ascertain links between diabetes driver physiology, particularly glucose control, and real-time driver behavior with safety.

Solutions to minimizing driving-related risk in diabetes have primarily included driving restrictions [7,8]. These restrictions are typically general, with limited ability to screen and identify high-risk drivers. In the United States, licensure restrictions and regulations for drivers with diabetes are state-specific and vary widely [7]. Some states impose few if any restrictions, while others require detailed information about medications and a history of diabetes-related problems (e.g., hypoglycemia and vision loss) that could impact safe vehicle operation. Restrictions may not account for confounders (e.g., poor sleep, visual impairment, or neuropathy). A number of states provide waivers in specific situations (e.g., a single hypoglycemic episode after a recent change in medication). State-specific laws also vary in requirements for medical evaluation and physician-reporting requirements to state licensing authorities. To address the inconsistencies and pitfalls in current state licensing laws, the American Diabetes Association developed general guidelines for diabetes driver fitness assessments and licensure recommendations that are based on individual evaluations [7].

Laws also vary across countries. In the United Kingdom, physicians must report hypoglycemia occurring during waking hours to licensing authorities.

European Union (EU) regulations require licensure withdrawal after two or more severe hypoglycemic episodes within 12 months. Restrictive regulations have far-reaching impact on patient care and medical decision-making. In the EU, reports to medical providers of severe hypoglycemia among individuals with type 1 diabetes (T1D) dropped 55% after introduction of regulations requiring hypoglycemia reporting to licensing authorities. These findings serve as a call to action to create evidence-based criteria for driver safety evaluation and identification of high-risk drivers while preserving quality of life, mobility, and patient-physician relationships for the drivers with diabetes.

Hypoglycemia and driving in diabetes

Hypoglycemia is a key risk factor for crash risk in diabetes [3−5], particularly in T1D where hypoglycemia is common. Several laboratory-based studies have linked acute hypoglycemia to impaired driving performance in simulated driving tasks [9,10]. Acute hypoglycemia produces cognitive impairment in domains critical to driving (e.g., attention, visual perception, psychomotor speed, and executive function). Hypoglycemia-related cognitive impairment can persist for over an hour after an acute episode resolves, and the effects of hypoglycemia can vary widely across individuals [11]. Simulated driving experiments have shown that drivers with diabetes who have a history of driving mishaps show larger driving performance decrements during acute hypoglycemia than those without such a history [12]. Judgment and awareness are also affected in hypoglycemia, which may result in a patient failing to appropriately self-restrict driving while impaired [3].

Comorbid factors and driving risk in diabetes

Diabetes-related comorbidities are also recognized as contributory factors to driving risk. Retinopathy diminishes visual function. Neuropathy can affect tactile sensation, proprioception, and muscle strength that are critical for safe vehicle control. Obstructive sleep apnea is common in diabetes and may increase driver risk by increasing cognitive impairment because of poor sleep. Some data suggest that severe hyperglycemia can impact driver safety [13].

Linking diabetes to driver behavior using real-time monitoring technology

Driver safety data in diabetes derive primarily from controlled studies of simulated driving under hypoglycemic clamp conditions. Studies show decrements in driving performance, particularly in vehicle control, during mild−moderate hypoglycemia. Acute mild−moderate hypoglycemia is also linked to the loss of vehicle control (i.e., spinning out), driving into the opposing lane of traffic, or driving off the roadway [9]. Hypoglycemia has been linked to driver speed choice errors. Drivers with diabetes typically choose slower speeds than drivers without diabetes [9]. This may reflect a compensatory mechanism to improve driver safety while impaired by hypoglycemia, but it is unclear if it mitigates on-road risk. Most drivers with diabetes show driving performance decrements during hypoglycemia, and the magnitude of these decrements are likely associated with the extent of hypoglycemia-related cognitive, psychomotor, and neurological impairment.

Prior literature on driving and diabetes is limited by studying drivers in controlled, laboratory settings under artificial conditions (e.g., simulated driving and using a glucose clamp to induce hypoglycemia). While laboratory-based studies can provide insight into driver behavior, they are conducted in a controlled environment that ultimately reduces the predictive utility of laboratory-based data to real-world safety outcomes. Laboratory-based studies do not capture the complexity or context of a driver's typical driving environment, usual on-road behavior, changing physiology, and risk exposure over time (Fig. 16.2). For drivers with diabetes, risk exposure may include the driver's choice to drive while impaired from abnormal glycemia. Some drivers with greater awareness of hypoglycemia may choose not to drive during hypoglycemia, marginalizing their on-road risk and reducing the validity of simulator-based data where they are required to drive during hypoglycemia. Drivers may also behave differently in a simulator, engaging in riskier behaviors than they would when faced with their real-world scenario. Simulator-based studies, which often rely on a single driver assessment, cannot capture the myriad of complex, comorbid factors that mediate real-world risk.

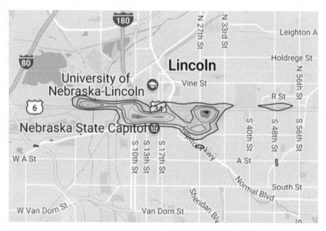

FIGURE 16.2 A driver's life space. GPS data collected over time during a naturalistic driving experiment show a driver's typical exposure and "life space." GPS "hotspots" (*red nodes*) correspond to the driver's home, gym, friend's house, and preferred grocery store.

Naturalistic driving studies can address these limitations by employing systematic, repeated observation of drivers in their own vehicle and typical driving environment across their typical physiology, sleep patterns, strategies, safety countermeasures, and adaptive behaviors [14–16]. Naturalistic driving studies use passive, in-vehicle sensor devices that can collect GPS, speed, accelerometer, video, and vehicle sensor data (Fig. 16.3). They record, unobtrusively, driver behavior, permitting objective assessment of real-world driver safety across the range of individual variation. While instrumentation can be built specifically for driving, these implementations can also take advantage of mobile and wearable devices.

These types of instrumentation can capture driver performance, errors (e.g., running a red light), and events such as near-crashes and crashes. Videos can provide information to discern driver states (e.g., distraction or sleepiness) and visible signs of hypoglycemia (e.g., sweating). Information on the driver, driving frequency, and environmental factors (e.g., traffic density and lighting) can be merged with databases that further contextualize the driving environment (e.g., weather and roadway databases). Such richly contextualized data (Fig. 16.4) can enhance laboratory-based data and add to the current often incomplete state-driving records that quantify driver risk from citations and vehicle crashes.

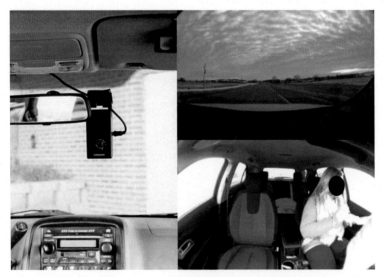

FIGURE 16.3 An example instrumentation package and video outputs for a naturalistic driving instrumentation system. The instrumentation is unobtrusively mounted on the forward, vehicle windshield, permitting collection of sensor (e.g., GPS, accelerometer, and speed) and video data. Video data capture the forward roadway and vehicle cabin. In this example, hyperglycemic drivers with T1D operate the steering wheel with their legs while eating and driving. *T1D*, Type 1 diabetes.

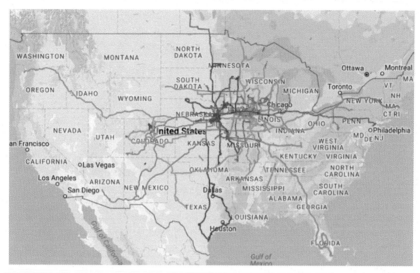

FIGURE 16.4 Data collection from a naturalistic driving study. Naturalistic driving studies permit collection of comprehensive, nuanced data on driver behavior and strategies. This figure shows GPS driving paths for a study of 77 drivers who were each observed for a 3-month period. Total data collection was >180,000 miles of driving across almost the entire United States. This dataset contains far more detailed information on driver behavior across wide-spread geographic environments than is possible with laboratory-based or retrospective studies.

Driving observations can also be combined with laboratory-based data (e.g., driver diagnosis and demographics), state records of crashes and citations, and contemporaneous data from wearable sensors monitoring driver mobility, sleep, and heart rate. For drivers with diabetes, real-world driving data can be combined with continuous glucose monitor (CGM) data to objectively link current and historical glucose control to contemporaneous driver safety [17]. CGM data can be used to derive metrics of glucose control (e.g., average glycemia, number/severity/duration of hypo- and hyperglycemic episodes) over time, which can then be mapped to a driver's behavior (e.g., frequency of driving during hypoglycemia), vehicle control, and errors.

Combining wearable sensors with naturalistic driving observation

To assess the feasibility and utility of combining wearable sensor and naturalistic driving technologies (Fig. 16.5), our group conducted a pilot study of 36 subjects (20 with T1D and 16 comparison drivers without diabetes) over 4 weeks of naturalistic observation [14]. Our primary hypothesis was that driver safety behavior would be impaired overall and related to poor glucose control in drivers with T1D relative to comparison drivers. Driver glucose control was assessed using CGMs. We investigated global metrics of driver

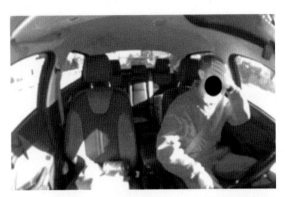

FIGURE 16.5 A hypoglycemic driver with T1D. In-vehicle video captures visible signs of hypoglycemia in a driver with T1D, observed to appear uncomfortable while wiping the sweat from his brow. The driver's CGM confirms a severely hypoglycemic episode (<40 mg/dL) that occurred during the drive and was linked to a concurrent lapse in vehicle control. *T1D*, Type 1 diabetes.

vehicle control related to braking/accelerating and steering behaviors across the T1D driver's contemporaneous glycemic state [hypoglycemia (<70 mg/dL), euglycemia-moderate hyperglycemia (70–299 mg/dL), and severe hyperglycemia (≥300 mg/dL)].

Vehicle control in the pilot study was measured with lateral (side–side/steering) and longitudinal (front–back/braking or accelerating) acceleration variability [18,19]. Increased acceleration variability indexes erratic steering and braking/accelerating that maps to swerving, variability in lane position, and variance in vehicle speed. Reduced acceleration variability can index driver inattention/attentional impairment and failure to adjust the vehicle appropriately to driving environment dynamics. All analyses are controlled for roadway speed limit to account for changes in vehicle acceleration due to speed.

Our results linked contemporaneous glucose levels to at-risk vehicle control behavior [14]. Drivers with T1D, who were hypo- or hyperglycemic, exhibited significantly different vehicle control behaviors than those who were euglycemic or moderately hyperglycemic. Hypoglycemic drivers showed increased acceleration variability rates manifested as erratic steering or swerving and harsh braking/accelerating. Severely hyperglycemic drivers showed decreased acceleration variability, manifested as reduced vehicle control adjustments. Observed changes in driving during hypo- and hyperglycemic conditions are to a degree similar to those observed during distracted driving. Distraction was associated with reduced steering control manifested as an increase in steering variability. In addition, elderly drivers, compared to middle-aged drivers, exhibited decreased speed variability during distraction [20].

These novel, preliminary data underscore the promise of combining advancements in technology to develop more accurate models of driver risk in diabetes with the goal of informing driver safety and health interventions.

The promise of technology in diabetes driver safety

Technology has the potential at multiple levels for improving driver safety in diabetes. At one level, applying wearable sensor and naturalistic monitoring technologies can assess relationships between driver health, physiology, and comorbid factors with the goal of developing methods for detecting, monitoring, and improving safety for drivers with diabetes. Naturalistic monitoring of real-world behavior shows special promise for addressing variations in driving performance by quantifying individual risk factors that mediate real-world safety, quality of life, and health outcomes.

Passive-monitoring technologies can also permit large-scale observations across a range of individuals, diseases, and comorbid factors. These data can be mined and used to develop predictive algorithms for health and safety outcomes. Naturalistic studies of real-world behavior and physiology provide evidence-based metrics for mapping clinical (e.g., cognitive and medical) test results to real-world behavior and outcomes to help clinicians. Furthermore, evidence-based models could inform the development of targeted, personalized treatment regimens or therapeutic approaches that mitigate real-world risk and adverse health outcomes in relation to driving.

With advances in data-analytic techniques, such as machine learning, vehicles can now be taught to process and interpret patterns of health data from a person's wearable devices, parse information to determine risk in-the-moment, and respond effectively. These data can be combined with other driver-monitoring data, including real-time data on driver attention and sleepiness from eye movements, stress and autonomic function from heart rate, and physiologic monitoring from wearable devices such as CGMs. Systems have the potential to learn—in real time—from incoming data to adjust predictions relative to individual behavior patterns. These systems may help one reduce on-road risks resulting from impaired driver decision-making, performance, and maladaptive driver strategies (e.g., reducing speed to compensate for impairment, which may increase the risk of a rear end crash). Several vehicle manufacturers are now developing sensor systems to alert drivers that can be combined with semiautomated vehicle systems that are capable of operating the vehicle. With technological advances, these systems may be trained to take over vehicle control when the driver is impaired, such as during hypoglycemia.

Industry efforts to develop driver-monitoring technology for diabetes

Multiple vehicle manufacturers are collaborating with health-focused technology companies, engineers, and researchers (clinical and behavioral). For example, Ford, in 2011, partnered with WellDoc's Diabetes Manager (a mobile phone–based diabetes management software) to integrate glucose and heart rate monitoring with its vehicle systems. This collaboration was further pursued with Medtronic to link CGMs with vehicle systems and provide driver feedback on glucose levels through the vehicle's sound systems and visual displays. Nightscout, a diabetes technology group, has worked to connect CGM devices to vehicles (e.g., Tesla, Honda CR-V) and permit drivers with diabetes to view CGM data in real time. Other vehicle manufacturers (e.g., Mercedes, VW, and Audi) have attempted real-time monitoring of driver fatigue through observations of at-risk behaviors (e.g., swerving, harsh acceleration) and alerts that warn the driver of potential risk.

Toyota's Collaborative Safety Research Center is working with clinicians, researchers, and engineers to integrate CGM data with in-vehicle safety systems. This effort is aimed at detecting real-time driver safety in diabetes and intervening during at-risk situations. Toyota is also investigating changes in heart rate to develop systems capable of detecting cardiac events so that the vehicle may take over or stop driving if the driver becomes incapacitated because of medical emergency. General Motors has worked to develop a system capable of monitoring driver attention through video and infrared light-based tracking of driver head position. This system is designed to stop the vehicle and engage its hazard lights if the driver becomes inattentive. Mercedes has implemented an in-vehicle system that stops the vehicle when it is determined that the driver is no longer controlling the vehicle. Honda and BMW are deploying biometrics and facial-recognition sensors to monitor driver health. Should an abnormality in driver health be detected, the vehicle is designed to take over driving and call 911.

Conclusion and new directions

Advancements in-vehicle technology now offers innovative possibilities to use the vehicle as a safety intervention tool to support at-risk drivers and as a diagnostic tool—capable of monitoring, classifying, and reporting real-world patient health and behavior over extended time frames (the backseat driver you actually want in your car). However, new technology brings new challenges. Real-world implementations of in-vehicle safety systems raise concerns over increased driving complexity, driver workload, and distracted driving. Further research is needed on how to integrate in-vehicle driver monitoring in an effective and safe manner and determine which parameters of driver demographics, disease, behavior, cognitive, and physiologic status should be classified to index risk. There are also legal and cybersecurity concerns. Standards are being developed for wireless diabetes device security and will need further integration with advances in vehicle technologies as automotive, medical, research, and engineering communities collaborate to improve and support safety and health in patients with diabetes.

References

[1] World Health Organization. Road traffic injuries. World Health Organization; 2018. Available from: <http://www.who.int/mediacentre/factsheets/fs358/en/>.

[2] Rizzo M. Impaired driving from medical conditions: a 70-year-old man trying to decide if he should continue driving. J Am Med Assoc 2011;305(10):1018−26.

[3] Treager S, Rizzo M, Tiller M, Schoelles K, Hegmann KT, Greenberg MI, editors. Diabetes and motor vehicle crashes: a systematic evidence-based review and meta-analysis. In: Proceedings of the fourth international driving symposium on human factors in driving assessment, training, and vehicle design; 2007.

[4] Lorber D, Anderson J, Arent S, J D, Frier BM, Greene MA, et al.; American Diabetes Association. Diabetes and driving. Diabetes Care 2012;35(Suppl. 1):S81−6.

[5] Inkster B, Frier BM. Diabetes and driving. Diabetes Obes Metab 2013;15(9):775−83.

[6] National Highway Traffic Safety Administration. The contribution of medical conditions to passenger vehicle crashes. In: Report no.: DOT HS 811 219. Washington, DC: National Highway Traffic Safety Administration, Transportation USDo, Administration NHTS; 2009.

[7] Lorber D, Anderson J, Arent S, Cox DJ, Frier BM, Greene MA, et al. Diabetes and driving. Diabetes Care 2014;37(Suppl. 1):S97−103.

[8] Kohrman DB. Driving with diabetes: precaution, not prohibition, is the proper approach. J Diabetes Sci Technol 2013;7(2):350−5.

[9] Cox DJ, Gonder-Frederick L, Clarke W. Driving decrements in type I diabetes during moderate hypoglycemia. Diabetes 1993;42(2):239−43.

[10] Cox DJ, Gonder-Frederick LA, Kovatchev BP, Julian DM, Clarke WL. Progressive hypoglycemia's impact on driving simulation performance. Occurrence, awareness and correction. Diabetes Care 2000;23(2):163−70.

[11] Zammitt NN, Warren RE, Deary IJ, Frier BM. Delayed recovery of cognitive function following hypoglycemia in adults with type 1 diabetes: effect of impaired awareness of hypoglycemia. Diabetes 2008;57(3):732−6.

[12] Cox DJ, Gonder-Frederick LA, Singh H, Ingersoll KS, Banton T, Grabman JH, et al. Predicting and reducing driving mishaps among drivers with type 1 diabetes. Diabetes Care 2017;40(6):742−50.

[13] Disruptive effects of hyperglycemia on driving in adults with type 1 & 2 diabetes. In: Cox DJ, Ford D, Ritterband L, Singh H, Gonder-Frederick L, editors. Diabetes, 60. 2011. p. A223.

[14] Merickel J, High R, Smith L, Wichman C, Frankel E, Smits K, et al. Driving safety and real-time glucose monitoring in insulin-dependent diabetes. Int J Automot Eng 2019;10 (1):34−40.

[15] Feng F, Bao S, Sayer JR, Flannagan C, Manser M, Wunderlich R. Can vehicle longitudinal jerk be used to identify aggressive drivers? An examination using naturalistic driving data. Accid Anal Prev 2017;104:125−36.

[16] Seppelt BD, Seaman S, Lee J, Angell LS, Mehler B, Reimer B. Glass half-full: on-road glance metrics differentiate crashes from near-crashes in the 100-Car data. Accid Anal Prev 2017;107:48−62.

[17] Klonoff DC, Ahn D, Drincic A. Continuous glucose monitoring: a review of the technology and clinical use. Diabetes Res Clin Pract 2017;133:178−92.

[18] Fung NC, Wallace B, Chan A, Goubran R, Porter M, Marshall S, et al. Driver identification using vehicle acceleration and deceleration events from naturalistic driving of older

drivers. In: IEEE international symposium on medical measurements and applications (MeMeA). 2017;33−8.

[19] Kluger R, Smith B. Pattern matching longitudinal acceleration time series data to identify crashes in naturalistic driving data. In: 21st world congress on intelligent transport systems, ITSWC 2014: Reinventing Transportation in Our Connected World; 2014.

[20] Thompson KR, Johnson AM, Emerson JL, Dawson JD, Boer ER, Rizzo M. Distracted driving in elderly and middle-aged drivers. Accid Anal Prev 2012;45:711−17.

Chapter 17

Standards for digital health

Syed Umer Abdul Aziz, Mariam Askari and Shahid N. Shah
Netspective Media LLC, Silver Spring, MD, United States

Abbreviations

ADT	admissions, discharge, and transfer
API	application programming interface
CCOW	Clinical Context Object Workgroup
CDA	Clinical Document Architecture
CMD	consumer mobile device
CMS	Center for Medicare and Medicaid Services
CPT	Current Procedural Terminology
DTMoSt	Diabetes Technology Society Mobile Platform Controlling a Diabetes Device Security and Safety Standard
DTS	Diabetes Technology Society
DTSec	Standard for Wireless Diabetes Device Security
EHR	electronic health record
FHIR®	Fast Healthcare Interoperability Resources
HbA1c	hemoglobin A1c
HL7	Health Level 7
HTTP	HyperText Transfer Protocol
ICD	International Classification of Diseases
ICD-10-CM	International Classification of Diseases, 10th Revision, Clinical Modification
IEEE	Institute of Electrical and Electronics Engineers
IHE	Integrating the Healthcare Enterprise
JSON	JavaScript object notation
LOINC	Logical Observation Identifiers Names and Codes
OAuth	Open Authorization
OAuth2.0	Open Authorization version 2.0
REST	representational state transfer
SAML	Security Assertion Markup Language
SMART	Substitutable Medical Applications, Reusable Technologies
SNOMED-CT	Systematized Nomenclature of Medicine—Clinical Terms
SOAP	Simple Object Access Protocol

Diabetes Digital Health. DOI: https://doi.org/10.1016/B978-0-12-817485-2.00017-1

SSO	single sign on
UMLS	Unified Medical Language System
W3C	World Wide Web Consortium

Key points

- No diabetes technology can be successful in a standalone manner. Any tech that cannot integrate and interoperate widely with patient-facing devices, applications, and professional-facing solutions (e.g., electronic health records [EHRs]) will have significantly lower overall value to patients and their care providers.
- When building future devices or apps or upgrading existing ones, it may be hard to choose the best standards. For patient-facing tech, our advice is to target Fast Healthcare Interoperability Resources (FHIR®), 4.0 application programming interfaces (APIs), and Institute of Electrical and Electronics Engineers (IEEE) 11073 device taxonomies. There are many standards and taxonomies to choose from, but a "FHIR-first" strategy is a good one to start with for connectivity decisions. For professional-facing tech that needs to connect to EHRs or other institutional software, targeting Health Level 7 (HL7) v2.x (HL7 2.x) first and then FHIR 4 is a good approach.
- Understanding standards is not only beneficial for developers but also for patients and health-care providers. Patients will learn how their information travels and what security standards are recommended to protect their data, while physicians and other providers can ensure that their current systems are equipped with the most recent standards to optimize interoperability and as a result enhance diabetes management. Patients and clinicians need to demand that app and device developers make their offerings integration friendly by refusing to purchase solutions that only work stand-alone.

Interoperability is the ability for different information systems, devices, or applications to cooperatively use and exchange data within and across organizations to ultimately enhance patient care and improve health outcomes [1]. Interoperability can mean *business model interoperability*, which means that regulatory and commercial ecosystems encourage integration across institutions and their business units, as well as *technical* interoperability, which means that hardware and software solutions are built to exchange data with each other. This chapter focuses on technical interoperability; business model and ecosystem interoperability are beyond the scope of this chapter but are a very important prerequisite to successful interoperability between solutions across the ecosystem.

While interoperability may not be achievable on a global scale for all patient data across all systems, it is quite possible and sometimes quite easy for specific use cases and disease-specific data sets. For a patient who self-monitors blood glucose levels either intermittently or continuously, provider teams should be notified when glucose levels are outside a target range, but not enough devices support that level of integration with EHRs. If this same patient has an implantable or a wearable device with an accelerometer incorporated into the device, then the care team could gauge if the patient's physical activity levels may have contributed to an abnormal glucose reading. The integration of information from multiple devices can better inform the context of a reading, but reliable flow of information through multiple systems requires interface and data-exchange standards.

Standards that allow current and future hardware and software to communicate with each other exist and any solution developers looking to make a difference in their patients' lives can do so today.

This chapter covers interoperability concepts and standards, and describes how device manufacturers and innovators can develop products that can be easily adopted by clinicians and patients. Understanding these standards is not only imperative for innovators and solution developers, but also for patients and physicians. For patients, understanding standards can empower them to make better purchasing decisions or determine the security of their information for a particular device. It can also help with determining whether a particular care team is implementing more recent technologies when administering their care. For physicians, it can also be a matter of assisting with a buying decision, because physicians and care team members should never approve purchases of stand-alone solutions when "connected" offerings are available. If a physician group decides to deploy a diabetes-management solution in their practice and learns later on that this software does not integrate with their EHR, then this would lead to a greater burden on the practice staff and less satisfied patients. Without proper data integration, staff members would need to spend extra time adding patients into the platform, monitoring patients through the platform, and saving reports to attach to the patient's EHR. For innovators, it is important to understand the landscape of the various standards as they develop a new product or technology to ensure that the product they build can be used within existing clinical workflows. Similar to the previous example of the diabetes management software, if an innovator creates a diabetes-management platform that can be accessed through an EHR, does not require additional logins for clinic users, and automatically adds patients to the platform without needing manual entry, then a clinic practice would be much more likely to purchase the product because it does not add additional burden to their existing workflow.

Although many standards exist, this chapter primarily focuses on four specific classes: device standards, medical standards, integration standards, and other IT standards.

Device standards

Device standards are standards used to integrate medical devices to an external system. Device standards matter in diabetes care because they allow patients to not only measure their glucose levels but also communicate those levels to another device, such as a mobile phone, and share this information with both family caregivers and providers. Medical standards are standards used in the medical industry to store or communicate information to other systems. Medical standards are useful because in the health-care industry, medical information passes through many hands. Medical information flows from physicians and nurses to labs, billing departments, and insurance companies to name just a few. As such, standards are needed to ensure that communication is clear and uniform between all parties involved. Similarly, we also have Integration standards that are used to communicate information between different systems. Integration standards can allow data from a device to be sent to a physician, allowing the care team to monitor their patients. Integration standards can also be used to improve communication from the care team to the patient. Lastly, we will talk about the other IT standards that are often used in the health-care space. Although these IT standards are not specifically oriented toward digital health, their applications can directly benefit users in the digital health space.

When working on interoperability, one of the primary guiding tools is the IEEE 11073 standards, which enable communication between medical devices and external computer systems [2]. In the case of diabetes technology, this could be a glucose monitor interacting with a mobile device in order to upload glucose levels to a web platform. There are two specific standards of communication that are of importance to the diabetes community:

1. IEEE 11073-10417-2015
2. IEEE 11073-10425-2017

IEEE 11073-10417-2015 establishes the standards of communication for self-monitoring blood glucose tools, specifically between glucose meters and a computer engine that acts as a monitor [3]. IEEE 11073-10425-2017 narrows the focus to establishing the standards of communication for continuous glucose-monitoring devices [4]. The functionality of these two devices lend them to have disparate communication standards. While a blood glucose monitor used on a daily or weekly basis will capture highly accurate glucose levels with individual readings more easily studied, a continuous glucose monitor generates a magnitude of more data points that are currently slightly less accurate but enable predictive glucose level abilities and require less operational effort from the patient [5]. These standards leverage existing IEEE 11073 standards, including terminology, information models, application profile standards, and transport standards.

Diabetes Technology Society (DTS) has also developed applicable standards in the digital health space. The Standard for Wireless Diabetes Device Security (DTSec) was published with the goal of ensuring that electronic products provide the security protections claimed by their developers. DTSec specifies security requirements for wireless devices that are codified as "protection profiles and security targets" [6].

DTS has also developed a second standard called Diabetes Technology Society Mobile Platform Controlling a Diabetes Device Security and Safety Standard (DTMoSt) that goes with DTSec. DTMoSt expands on the guidance of DTSec but applies primarily to mobile devices that are used to control wearable or implantable devices used in diabetes care. DTMoSt provides the guidance on what innovators need to keep in consideration when designing around consumer mobile devices (CMDs) and the challenges associated with relying on a CMD [7].

Medical standards

There are a few terminology and vocabulary standards that are immediately applicable to interoperability for digital health.

Diagnosis codes

Diagnosis codes are used by hospitals and clinic practices to code the patient diagnoses for the primary purposes of reimbursement and claims processing. Diagnosis codes are also used for the purposes of research and outcomes measurement [8]. Diagnosis codes are critical to EHRs and are useful when EHRs need to communicate medical data to other systems if the technology is dependent on a diagnosis code to power a workflow. If a patient is admitted to an emergency room with a diabetes-related diagnosis code, then the primary care physician monitoring the patient through a diabetes management platform may find it beneficial to know about this emergency room visit. Alternatively, if a patient is diagnosed with diabetes for the first time, then the diagnosis code could initiate a workflow to add the patient into a diabetes management platform, invite them to download a diabetes management app, and educate them on their disease. Because cardiovascular risk factors impact clinical outcomes most meaningful to patients with diabetes, such as myocardial infarction or ischemic stroke, physician-coordinated teams can also be alerted when patients are discharged with a diagnosis code indicating the development or worsening of such a risk factor to reassess a disease-management plan.

International Classification of Diseases (ICD) Codes: ICD codes are published by the World Health Organization. Several US agencies, including the Center for Medicare and Medicaid Services (CMS) and the National Center for Health Statistics, are authorized to modify these codes for implementation in the United States [9]. The current and active version of these codes is called the International Classification of Diseases, 10th Revision, Clinical Modification (ICD-10-CM). ICD-10-CM codes are multifunctional and are used to process claims for health insurers, conduct quality of care and outcomes research, and track morbidity and mortality statistics as a result of being used to define a patient's primary and secondary diagnoses in EHRs [10]. The ICD-10-CM codes classifying a diabetes-related diagnoses range from E08 to E13 [11]. ICD-10-CM codes may also express abnormal glucose readings or an insulin pump malfunction. In addition to the ICD-10-CM codes, CMS developed a set of International Classification of Diseases, 10th Revision, Procedure Coding System codes to denote procedures performed on hospitalized inpatients and, similarly to ICD-10-CM codes, their use is limited to US health-care facilities [12].

Systematized Nomenclature of Medicine—Clinical Terms (SNOMED-CT): This is another standard that can be used for clinical diagnosis. SNOMED-CT is more comprehensive than ICD and other code standards with over 340,000 concepts. SNOMED-CT is a key terminology under the CMS Promoting Interoperability Program, which focuses on interoperability and information exchange, reducing clinician burden, and improving patient access to data [13]. SNOMED-CT allows clinicians to query codes using more intuitive language and it maps to other international standards, enabling interoperability between different classification systems.

Current Procedural Terminology (CPT) Codes: This code standard is maintained by the American Medical Association and aims to guide claims processing and enable accurate information exchange [14]. While ICD-10 codes record a diagnosis claim, CPT codes target services rendered, including evaluation and management, anesthesia, surgery, radiology, and laboratory services [13]. These codes are predominantly used to reflect services performed in an outpatient setting. For example, CPT code 82948 indicates a blood-glucose test performed using a reagent strip and code 82962 represents the dispensation of a glucose-monitoring device cleared by the Food and Drug Administration [15].

Laboratory measurements

It is important to know and understand how systems capture laboratory measurements in diabetes technology, because there are a number of important measurements used to monitor a patient's diabetes and signal possible hyper- or hypoglycemia. The most common measurement and direct marker of glycemic control is blood glucose levels. This measurement can be in mg/dL or mmol/L and a value can obviously reveal different levels of glycemic control based on the unit for interpretation. Thus it is important to know what the units are for each laboratory measurement. The basic standard that defines the units for measurement is LOINC.

LOINC stands for *Logical Observation Identifiers Names and Codes* and is a universal standard for identifying laboratory observations and measurements. For instance, LOINC 2345-7 defines the standard measurement for "Glucose [Mass/Volume] in Serum or Plasma" [16]. This standard includes the units of measurement as well as reference ranges. LOINC codes vary in specificity as well and associated code descriptors can indicate patient status at the time of a test. LOINC 1558-6 builds on 2345-7 by detailing a test as "Fasting glucose [Mass/volume] in Serum or Plasma." LOINC can also specify the method used to obtain a laboratory value. Hemoglobin A1c (HbA1c) is a frequently used surrogate marker of glycemic control and, similar to blood glucose levels, has a range of LOINC codes associated with it. LOINC code 4548-4 simply denotes "Hemoglobin A1c/Hemoglobin total in Blood," while other codes describe the method used to ascertain the value, including electrophoresis (4549-2) and high performance liquid chromatography (17856-6) [17].

Medication/drugs

If the technology is used to communicate drug or medication changes, then it is important to utilize a standard such as RxNorm. RxNorm provides normalized names for clinical drugs and links those names to drug vocabularies used in pharmacy management software [18]. An example of this would be a diabetes management platform, which a physician uses to communicate with their patient, and to communicate a change of insulin prescription or dosage based on the glucose readings a patient has been uploading.

National Institutes of Health Unified Medical Language System (UMLS): It integrates and distributes key terminology, classification and coding standards, and associated resources to promote creation of more effective and interoperable biomedical information systems and services, including EHRs [19]. UMLS allows users to link health information across multiple systems that use different diagnosis codes, drug names, and billing codes. The UMLS consists of three tools called knowledge sources: the Metathesaurus, the semantic network, and the SPECIALIST Lexicon and Lexical tools [18]. The UMLS integrates many terminologies mentioned in this chapter, including ICD-9, ICD-10, CPT, SNOMED-CT, LOINC, and RxNORM. UMLS is a great resource for interoperability because it allows users to work across the many different standards used in healthcare.

An example of the potential utility of the UMLS is in research. If a researcher wanted to identify all patients in a health system who have diabetes, then it may be necessary to deal with nearly 2600 different diabetic diagnoses. With the UMLS, they simply have to search for all descendants of Diabetes Mellitus (UMLS CUI: C0011847) [20].

Determining which standard to use for diagnosis codes depends on a number of factors, including which diagnosis codes are used in the EHR and which diagnosis codes are most relevant to the user in question. A payer may find ICD codes more valuable because they receive diagnosis codes during billing and can use those to power specific workflows for their patients. However, the clinician may find that documenting the SNOMED code is more useful to capture the medical diagnosis. The National Library of Medicine published a tool called I-MAGIC that can help one to map SNOMED-CT to ICD-10 Codes. In either case, knowing the user's needs can help determine which type of diagnosis codes a digital health tool should integrate with.

Interoperability standards

There are many communication standards that can be used to implement interoperability between diabetes devices. Health-care-specific interoperability standards include the following:

HL7 2.x is the most widely implemented standard in the health-care industry. HL7 has extensive methods of integrating, and many chapters could be written on the types of HL7 integration methods. Some important types of HL7 Messages in diabetes digital health would be ADT (admissions, discharge, and transfer), which could be used to communicate demographics information from an EHR to a digital health platform.

HL7 Fast Healthcare Interoperability Resources (FHIR®) is the latest standard for exchanging health-care information electronically. FHIR has strong foundations in Web Standards such as JavaScript object notation (JSON), HyperText Transfer Protocol (HTTP), and Open Authorization (OAuth) [21]. FHIR solutions utilize resources to build interfaces in a modular fashion. In the case of diabetes digital health, the Diagnostic Medicine Module in FHIR has an observation resource that would be highly useful. This resource can be used to upload blood glucose levels from a blood glucose monitor to an EHR. Another example is the communication of a diabetes care plan, which would be found under the Clinical Module in the Resource CarePlan.

SMART (Substitutable Medical Applications, Reusable Technologies) on FHIR is a set of open specifications to integrate digital health apps within EHRs and other Health IT systems. SMART on FHIR enables clinicians in accessing third-party apps directly from an EHR, allowing for a more seamless workflow [22]. Through SMART on FHIR, a clinician could be logged into their EHR, and from the EHR access a third-party patient management system to create a care plan for the patient based on their needs.

HL7 Version 3 Clinical Document Architecture (CDA) is a standard that specifies the structure and semantics of clinical documents for the purposes of interoperability. CDAs have six characteristics: persistence, stewardship, potential for authentication, context, wholeness, and human readability [23].

HL7 Clinical Context Object Workgroup (CCOW) developed the CCOW Context Management Specification to ensure secure and consistent access to patient information from multiple sources [24]. CCOW is beneficial for large health systems that use multiple independent applications to manage their patient population. CCOW enables single-sign on solutions as well as eliminates the need for duplicative input into applications [9]. Going forward, SMART on FHIR is meant to provide the same functionality with a more modern interface.

Integrating the Healthcare Enterprise (IHE) Profiles are meant to provide a common language for purchasers and vendors to discuss the integration needs of health-care sites and the integration capabilities of health-care IT products [25]. IHE Profiles provide definitions on how different integration standards can be implemented to meet specific clinical needs [10]. The IHE developed a white paper that provides an example of diabetes care management and how it can be represented through IHE Profiles [26].

Other IT standards

There are many communication standards outside of the health-care space that one might find useful. Here are a few examples of communication standards and how they can be used in this space.

Application programming interfaces

APIs allow users to enable data transfer and workflows in new and unique ways. Many web-based applications support APIs for data transfer and interoperability. FHIR is actually just an API for exchanging health-related information. There are a few different types of API styles that innovators can use to integrate digital health data.

Simple Object Access Protocol (SOAP) API is a protocol that relies heavily on XML and is explicitly defined. SOAP structures are simply an XML element with two child elements, the header and the body. SOAP messages are transported via other transport protocols such as HTTP and SMTP [27]. SOAP specifications are official standards built and maintained by the World Wide Web Consortium.

REST (representational state transfer) API is an architectural style for designing APIs. REST mostly uses JSON and is easier to use compared to SOAP [28]. REST most often uses HTTP but there is no standard for the description format in REST [16].

GraphQL is a query language for APIs and is similar to REST in many ways. GraphQL is typically served over HTTP and is also commonly used with JSON [29].

Single sign on

Single sign on (SSO) refers to enabling access to an ancillary application using credentials from a primary application. For example, allowing the clinician to access a diabetes management platform from the EHR from a button in the EHR that opens the diabetes management platform without requiring the clinician to sign in. This kind of workflow can be enabled through the use of SSO. Two major standards to accomplish SSO include *Security Assertion Markup Language (SAML)* and *Open Authorization v2.0 (OAuth2.0)*. SAML is a standard protocol for web browser SSO using secure tokens. OAuth2.0 is an open standard for token-based authentication.

There are some differences between the two standards but they both attempt to accomplish the same goal, allow users to access an application without having to enter credentials multiple times. It is important to point out here that SMART on FHIR utilizes OAuth2.0 that is the recommended method for digital health innovators to integrate their tools into clinical workflows.

Selecting the right standards

If you are a patient considering buying a diabetes digital health product, then you may want to investigate what kind of integration capabilities such a product has. What may be most important to you is, does the product you are purchasing integrate with your cellular phone and provide you a way to view your data? Also, does the product you are purchasing integrate with your doctor's EHR? As a physician, you may be interested in whether the digital health product you are purchasing integrates with your EHR system as well as whether the product can be integrated into your clinical workflow.

As a developer or innovator, you need to determine which integration methods will support clinical workflows of your users. There are many standards to integrate with. Determining the right standard that your users need is key to building a successful product.

For new ("greenfield") applications that are *not* being built on legacy infrastructure (or older stand-alone systems that are adding connectivity), solution developers should build FHIR 4.x + data integration and SMART on FHIR clinical user interfaces. HL7 2.x could be considered optional when the greenfield applications are being installed in modern EHRs, but smart innovators that can afford to do so would support FHIR and HL7 2.x simultaneously. While REST APIs are now common, innovators should add an optional GraphQL layer for easier querying and simpler access for mobile and web app developers.

For legacy applications or those solutions that are already connected using older standards and are being upgraded, they should maintain their HL7 data-integration capabilities and add first SMART on FHIR if they have clinical user bases or add FHIR 4.x if they have a patient user base.

Conclusion

Digital health and medical devices in the service of diabetes patients and their caregivers are now quite common. Even more will be entering the market over the coming years. In the early days, just having *any* tech was helpful but now the explosion of apps for patients and clinicians, clinician-facing devices for hospitals, and patient-facing devices appear to be an excess of riches. But that is not the case—most solutions being marketed and sold today are stand-alone offerings creating potentially harmful data silos.

Any modern offering that is not "connectable"—that is, transferring data from patient-facing devices and apps to clinician EHRs at the very least—should not be considered a valuable part of the diabetes technology ecosystem. There are many vendors of solutions that make excuses for why interoperability is difficult or why connectivity is not possible, and they often point to a lack of standards. However, not only the standards are available, but there are also many existing software libraries, hardware components, and integration partners that make diabetes technology connectivity both possible and profitable.

If you are a patient, then you should not purchase any solution that is not ready to connect to the digital health tech ecosystem. If you are a health system buyer or a clinician, then you should add language to your upcoming requests for proposals and procurement contracts that force vendors to share data through connection-ready solutions.

Vendors can make their products interoperable—but only if patients and their health systems demand this functionality.

References

[1] HIMSS. What is Interoperability? [Internet]. 2016 [cited 2019 May 13]. Available from: <https://www.himss.org/library/interoperability-standards/what-is-interoperability>.

[2] IEEE Std 11073-20601-2014. IEEE Health informatics—Personal health device communication − Part 20601: Application profile—Optimized exchange protocol. IEEE Std 11073-20601-2014 (Revision of ISO/IEEE 11073-20601:2010); 2014. p. 1−253.

[3] IEEE Std 11073-10417-2015. IEEE Health informatics − Personal health device communication Part 10417: Device Specialization − Glucose Meter. IEEE Std 11073-10417-2015 (Revision of IEEE Std 11073-10417-2011); 2015. p. 1−78.

[4] IEEE Std 11073-10425-2017. Health informatics − Personal health device communication − Part 10425: Device Specialization − Continuous Glucose Monitor (CGM). IEEE Std 11073-10425-2017 (Revision of IEEE Std 11073-10425-2014); 2018. p. 1−83.

[5] Klonoff DC. Continuous glucose monitoring: roadmap for 21st century diabetes therapy. Diabetes Care 2005;28(5):1231−9.

[6] Diabetes Technology Society. Standard for Wireless Diabetes Device Security (DTSec) [Internet]. 2017. Available from: <https://www.diabetestechnology.org/dtsec.shtml?ver = 5>.

[7] Diabetes Technology Society. Guidance for use of mobile devices in diabetes control contexts [Internet]. 2018. Available from: <https://www.diabetestechnology.org/dtmost.shtml>.

[8] Bowman SE. Why ICD-10 is worth the trouble. J AHIMA 2008;79(3):24−9.

[9] Sanders TB, Bowens FM, Pierce W, Stasher-Booker B, Thompson EQ, Jones WA. The road to ICD-10-CM/PCS implementation: forecasting the transition for providers, payers, and other healthcare organizations. Perspect Health Inf Manag [Internet]. 2012;9(Winter):1f [cited 2019 May 13]. Available from: <https://www.ncbi.nlm.nih.gov/pmc/articles/PMC3329203/>.

[10] ICD. ICD-10-CM – International Classification of Diseases, (ICD-10-CM/PCS Transition [Internet]. 2019 [cited 2019 May 13]. Available from: <https://www.cdc.gov/nchs/icd/icd10cm_pcs_faq.htm>.

[11] ICD-10-CM Official Guidelines for Coding and Reporting [Internet]. [cited 2019 May 13]. Available from: https://www.cdc.gov/nchs/icd/data/10cmguidelines-FY2019-final.pdf.

[12] ICD. ICD-10-CM, ICD-10-PCS, CPT, and HCPCS Code Sets; 2018. p. 6.

[13] U.S. National Library of Medicine. Overview of SNOMED CT [Internet]. [cited 2019 May 11]. Available from: https://www.nlm.nih.gov/healthit/snomedct/snomed_overview.html.

[14] American Medical Association. CPT® overview and code approval [Internet]. [cited 2019 May 13]. Available from: <https://www.ama-assn.org/practice-management/cpt/cpt-over-view-and-code-approval>.

[15] Fu Associates, Ltd. Medicare National Coverage Determinations (NCD) coding policy manual and change report (ICD-10-CM) [Internet]. 2017 [cited 2019 May 13] p. 1539–605. (190.20 – Blood Glucose Testing). Available from: <http://www.healthnet-worklabs.com/pdf/icd10/Blood%20Glucose%20Testing%20-%20190.20.pdf>.

[16] LOINC. LOINC 2345-7 - Glucose [Mass/volume] in Serum or Plasma [Internet]. [cited 2019 May 13]. Available from: https://loinc.org/2345-7/.

[17] Centers for Disease Control and Prevention. Public Health Information Network Vocabulary Access and Distribution System (PHIN VADS) [Internet]. [cited 2019 May 13]. Available from: https://phinvads.cdc.gov/vads/ViewValueSet.action?oid = 2.16.840.1.114222.4.11.4239.

[18] RxNorm [Internet]. [cited 2019 May 13]. Available from: <https://www.nlm.nih.gov/research/umls/rxnorm/>.

[19] U.S. National Library of Medicine. Unified Medical Language System (UMLS) [Internet]. [cited 2019 May 11]. Available from: https://www.nlm.nih.gov/research/umls/.

[20] Anderson D. Introduction to the Unified Medical Language System (UMLS) [Internet]; 2019. Available from: <https://www.nlm.nih.gov/bsd/disted/video/clin_info/umls.pptx>.

[21] HL7. Introducing HL7 FHIR [Internet]. [cited 2019 May 13]. Available from: http://www.hl7.org/FHIR/summary.html.

[22] SMART Health IT. What Is SMART? [Internet]. 2012 [cited 2019 May 13]. Available from: <https://smarthealthit.org/an-app-platform-for-healthcare/about/>.

[23] HL7. HL7 Standards Product Brief – CDA® Release 2 [Internet]. [cited 2019 May 11]. Available from: https://www.hl7.org/implement/standards/product_brief.cfm?product_id = 7.

[24] HL7 Standards Product Brief – HL7 Context Management Specification (CCOW), Version 1.6 | HL7 International [Internet]. [cited 2019 May 11]. Available from: <https://www.hl7.org/implement/standards/product_brief.cfm?product_id = 1>.

[25] IHE International. Profiles [Internet]. [cited 2019 May 11]. Available from: <https://www.ihe.net/resources/profiles/>.

[26] Orlova A, Reed-Fourquet L. Knowledge representation in chronic care management: example of diabetes care management [Internet]. Integrating the Healthcare Enterprise; 2010. Available from: <https://www.ihe.net/Technical_Framework/upload/IHE_QRPH_WP_Diabetes_Care_Mngt_PC_2010_06_04.pdf>.

[27] Curbera F, Duftler M, Khalaf R, Nagy W, Mukhi N, Weerawarana S. Unraveling the web services web: an introduction to SOAP, WSDL, and UDDI. IEEE Internet Comput 2002;6:86–93.

[28] SoapUI. SOAP vs REST 101: Understand The Differences [Internet]. [cited 2019 May 12]. Available from: https://www.soapui.org/learn/api/soap-vs-rest-api.html.

[29] The GraphQL Foundation. GraphQL: A query language for APIs. [Internet]. [cited 2019 May 12]. Available from: http://graphql.org/.

Chapter 18

Are digital therapeutics poised to become mainstream in diabetes care?

Pablo Salazar and Adam Somauroo

McKinsey & Company, New York, NY, United States

Abbreviations

AI	artificial intelligence
FDA	Food and Drug Administration
HbA1c	a measure of glycated hemoglobin, which allows clinicians to measure average blood sugar levels over a period of weeks/months
RCT	randomized clinical trial
RWE	real-world evidence
TA	therapeutic area

Key points

- Digital therapeutics, although nascent, have shown great promise in addressing the burden of chronic disease but are still struggling for widespread adoption.
- The level of robust clinical evidence generated to support these technologies is limited, with higher volumes and quality required to differentiate them from "health and wellness" apps.
- Current business models will need to evolve in line with changes in the health-care ecosystem, while other external enablers, such as regulatory clarity, demand from health systems, an improvement in underlying technologies, and sustained investment, will need to be addressed to support mainstream adoption.

For the pharmaceutical and digital therapeutics industries, the precise nature of digital therapeutics is still a matter of debate. One practical and useful definition describes them as "evidence-based therapeutic interventions to patients that are driven by high quality software programs to prevent,

Diabetes Digital Health. DOI: https://doi.org/10.1016/B978-0-12-817485-2.00018-3

manage, or treat a medical disorder or disease ... [and] are used independently or in concert with medications, devices, or other therapies to optimize patient care and health outcomes" [1].

Diabetes is well placed to become the poster child for digital interventions because of three factors: the prevalence and the high and growing cost burden it imposes on many countries' health systems; the chronic and progressive nature of the condition; and the potential for improving patient outcomes through lifestyle modification and better disease management. Perhaps as a result, digital health technologies focused on diabetes have attracted more venture capital funding over the past few years than technologies targeting other therapeutic areas (TAs). The body of published scientific research on digital therapeutics also features diabetes more prominently than other TAs, according to our research (Fig. 18.1).

Existing evidence shows that new digital therapies have the potential to improve outcomes for patients. These digital therapies have used a variety of different approaches and target populations, including a digital therapeutic platform for type 1 and type 2 diabetes with embedded algorithms to support insulin initiation and optimization, which is a technology aimed at reversing type 2 diabetes or reducing the need for insulin and other costly medications through a combination of technology and online coaching as well as the use of an implantable device for long-term continuous glucose monitoring [2,3,4].

Given results like these, it is perhaps surprising that digital therapies have yet to join the mainstream of diabetes treatments. Why don't more physicians prescribe them, and more patients use them?

We believe two factors are preventing these therapies from reaching their potential. First, without sufficient high-quality clinical evidence to validate their usage, they risk getting lost in the sea of digital health and well-being products that span everything from diet trackers to fitness apps. Second, the companies offering these treatments have not yet created a business model that aligns incentives for providers, payers, and patients to adopt their products. If digital diabetes therapeutics is to achieve wider uptake, stakeholders, including regulators, payers, investors, and innovators, will all have a part to play.

Bridging the clinical evidence gap

To promote adoption and differentiate themselves from the plethora of health and wellness apps on the market, leading digital therapeutics companies are beginning to generate clinical-grade evidence using established endpoints that can be directly compared to the current standard of care for therapeutics or medical interventions. As yet, though, the evidence gap between digital and traditional therapeutics persists, and there are differences in the type and strength of evidence available for different technologies. To understand these

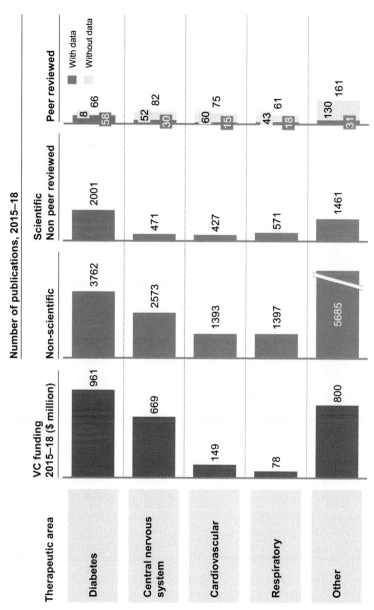

FIGURE 18.1 An overview of funding and publishing by therapeutic area.

variations, we conducted a retrospective analysis of published literature. This showed that despite intense activity in digital therapeutics (21,725 publications), only 384 appeared in peer-reviewed scientific journals, furthermore only 153 of those included hard data (Fig. 18.2).

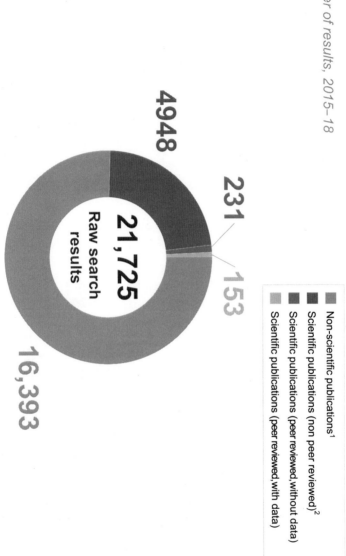

FIGURE 18.2   Digital therapeutics has been the focus of much research activity but few peer-reviewed publications.

Even so, the clinical evidence generated for digital therapeutics in diabetes is stronger than in other TAs. In October, 2018 McKinsey randomly selected a sample of 30 retrospective peer-reviewed studies from the set of the 153 above described data-containing studies. They found that two-thirds were based either on real-world evidence (RWE) or randomized clinical trials (RCTs). More than 70% of the studies showed statistically significant results, and more than 90% used well-defined traditional endpoints that would give confidence about comparability with existing therapies (Fig. 18.3).

However, the quantity and quality of data generated is not the only measure of a product's value. A 2019 study of 371 self-management apps for diabetes found that even though the majority of apps (58%) could alert users to hypoglycemic or hyperglycemic events, only a small proportion of them (less than 30%) went on to prompt those users to consume food or seek medical attention [5]. This suggests that the apps tend to focus on providing diagnostic insights to support self-management rather than recommending actions for users to take, even though the data generated could support such recommendations. This limitation may be due to the relative newness of the technologies concerned or from a conscious decision by developers not to subject their apps to the greater regulatory scrutiny and data requirements applicable to technologies that drive—rather than inform—clinical management [6]. In any case, it is clear that the apps still have some way to go before they can be regarded as fully mature, holistic offerings.

Moreover, some health-care stakeholders will want to take other factors into consideration. Payers, for instance, will likely want to see digital health technologies demonstrate tangible real-world impact in populations similar to their own members. If robust protocols are followed, RWE can provide insights into safety, effectiveness, and resource utilization for a specific intervention or enable it to be compared with multiple alternatives. RWE can also be used to supplement data on clinical validity to provide greater confidence in the effect of a digital therapeutic on a large population [7].

Payers may require such additional evidence in order to support digital therapeutics. If a digital therapeutics company has proved the clinical benefit of its technology *and* deployed it to large populations *and* demonstrated cost savings, better outcomes, or both, then the payer is likely to feel more confident that the technology is viable and that the company is able to deliver on its promise at scale. In addition, if the company has established itself in a particular area and formed relationships with local providers and other stakeholders, then the payer can be reassured that the conditions required to improve its members' health are in place.

To bridge the clinical evidence gap, digital therapeutics companies will need to balance their evidence-generation strategies to include both RCTs and RWE. They will also need to continue collecting data to support future growth and the long-term sustainability of their business. If they can demonstrate that their digital therapeutics increase treatment compliance, boost patient satisfaction, and improve health-care outcomes, then health-care stakeholders are likely to consider a different approach to disease management, and adoption could reach an inflection point.

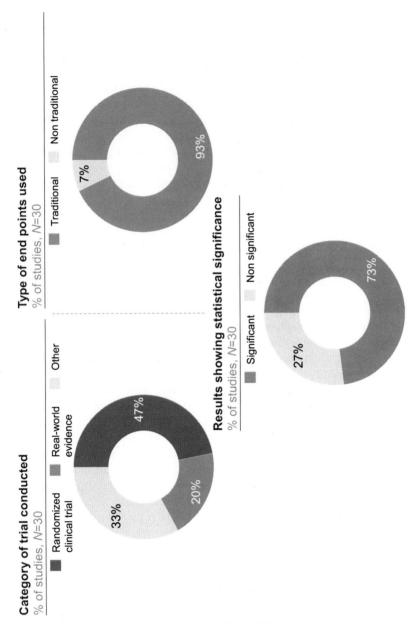

FIGURE 18.3   The majority of studies used traditional clinical endpoints and showed statistically significant results.

Developing the right business model

Even if digital therapeutics manage to bridge the evidence gap and be recognized as therapeutically equivalent to traditional medicines, they still face barriers in getting their products into the hands of end users. In many health systems the best way to secure widespread adoption from physicians and patients and improve affordability, is through reimbursement from payers.

To consider paying for a new therapy, payers want to know that it offers a clear improvement in outcomes in the form of better management of a condition and/or reduced costs for the health system. The challenge for digital health product developers lies in demonstrating measurable material outcomes that are clearly tied to their offerings and can be captured by the payer within a reasonably short timeframe. Most digital diabetes therapies target patients in the early onset of the disease before they represent a major cost to the health system. The real costs—of stroke, amputation, or dialysis, for instance—tend to come more than 10 years later. In the intervening decade a typical patient in the United States, for instance, might change their health plan more than once.

Our research suggests that most leading digital therapeutics companies use a subscription model to sell their products to payers and large employers-sponsored health plans and offer a value proposition based on saving costs across the population covered. There are a few success cases, where leading digital therapeutic companies started to generate real-world evidence of improved patient outcomes and cost savings. For instance, one study showed that one digital diabetes management program could reduce a member's medical spending by 22%, or $88 per month after the first year [8].

If the benefits of digital therapeutics are well established and user acceptability is no longer an issue, then we expect to see the emergence of either integrated technologies addressing multiple conditions or, more likely, a consolidated platform offering a harmonized approach across multiple digital therapeutics. As the shift toward standardization and interoperability continues, individual patients may eventually be able to assemble a personalized suite of technologies to support their unique blend of conditions and needs. How such a business model would work in practice and who would act as intermediaries remain to be seen. Such a future is some distance from today's business models with their focus on separate manageable conditions.

Until a harmonized platform is established, digital therapeutics companies have two viable strategies to broaden patient impact. One option is to widen their focus from preventing to managing disease. Many companies aim to prevent the onset of diabetes by encouraging people at risk of the disease to modify their behavior. Such companies may have opportunities to broaden the reach of their products to intervene more directly in diabetes after it is established. They could follow the example of businesses that uses artificial intelligence (AI) to analyze a diabetes patient's blood glucose levels, food consumption, physical activity, and so on, and then recommend an appropriate dose of insulin dose, as well as provide broader guidance to help the patient manage their condition more effectively.

The second viable strategy for digital therapeutics companies is to focus on customer segments that take a long-term perspective on health and disease prevention. As already mentioned, some commercial health plans in the United States tend to focus on near-term value because of the frequency with which customers move from one plan to another. However, well-established companies with employee health plans aim to retain their employees for a long time and have an interest in keeping them healthy and productive while minimizing health-care costs. To that extent, their objectives are perfectly aligned with those of digital therapeutics companies, and so they may offer opportunities for partnerships geared to maintaining workforce health.

Alternatively, digital therapeutics companies may wish to focus on the segment of health-conscious consumers who are willing to pay out of pocket for tools to help them maintain or improve their long-term health, including through diabetes prevention. One such tool uses AI-augmented health coaching in combination with human support and connected devices to help prevent and manage a number of chronic diseases.

Tackling other enablers of adoption

Bridging the evidence gap and deciding on the right business model are two of the key steps in establishing digital therapeutics in diabetes treatment. However, regulatory clarity, demand from health systems, an improvement in underlying technologies, and sustained public or private investment will also be needed to support widespread adoption.

Regulatory agencies

Regulators around the world are aware of this changing environment as well as the importance of guaranteeing patient safety while supporting innovation. Greater clarity will be important on how digital products are classified and assessed, along with the development of new pathways for products that do not fit within existing review mechanisms.

In the United States the Food and Drug Administration (FDA) is charting one such new pathway. This agency established a digital health program that led to a new pathway for these products and launched a precertification pilot program in 2017 [9]. The precert program aims to regulate company procedures rather than individual products and seeks to consider how clinical and real-world evidence can be balanced. Regulating products based on AI and machine-learning technologies is a difficult task because the underlying algorithms are constantly evolving and therefore the products themselves change over time. The FDA is taking a leading role in exploring possibilities and involving digital companies in the process.

Regulatory agencies also need to deal with wider issues surrounding digital products, such as cybersecurity. Health data is extremely sensitive, and regulators need to define ways to share and use data that will ensure privacy, trust, and accountability in health-care and society more broadly.

Payers/health systems

A key enabler for digital therapeutics products to be adopted into the mainstream is establishing platforms and standards to support the sharing of patient data and the interoperability with the electronic health record (EHR) systems of payers and providers. This would enable patients to access multiple digital therapeutics technologies or tools under one platform and to easily review which other tools are recommended/covered by providers and payers, respectively.

Innovators

To take digital diabetes therapeutics into the mainstream, companies should explore options for forming ecosystems with peers and allow cross-selling between partners to promote adoption and user acceptance. Some competing companies are already making their connected devices and apps interoperable across brands, enabling patients to select individual building blocks of a treatment platform—for example, insulin brand, digital app, connected device, sensors, exercise program, diet plan—to suit their lifestyle and help them achieve their treatment goals.

Investors

Venture capital investment in digital diabetes therapeutics continues to be strong and shows no sign of abating. Emerging markets may offer an opportunity to broaden the investor base through social-impact investment, public/private partnerships, or both. Given the health-care costs of the diabetes epidemic and the increasing ubiquity of mobile digital health tools, public health systems may start to pursue innovative approaches to control costs. If digital therapeutics companies are able to provide evidence of their effectiveness in tackling growing public health issues at the population level, then they may be able to attract long-term, large-scale government investment, as vaccination programs did in the past to combat infant mortality.

If digital therapeutics companies continue to innovate in their diabetes offerings and can demonstrate clinically validated value propositions to health-care stakeholders, then this market could experience exponential growth.

References

[1] Digital Therapeutics Alliance, 2019 <https://www.dtxalliance.org/>.

[2] Offringa R, Bose T, Greenfield MS. Diabetes management application improves self care behavior and glycemic control. Glooko. [no date]. 2019, Available from <https://get.glooko.com/rs/352-OEL-682/images/11-7-16_DTS%20Poster%20Final.pdf>.

[3] Hallberg SJ, McKenzie AL, Williams PT, Bhanpuri NH, Peters AL, Campbell WW, et al. Effectiveness and safety of a novel care model for the management of type 2 diabetes at 1 year: an open-label, non-randomized, controlled study. Diabetes Ther 2018;9(2):583−612.

[4] Christiansen MP, Klaff LJ, Brazg R, Chang AR, Levy CJ, Lam D, et al. A prospective multicenter evaluation of the accuracy of a novel implanted continuous glucose sensor: PRECISE II. Diabetes Technol Ther 2018;20(3):197−206.

[5] Lum W, Jimenez G, Huang Z, et al. Decision support and alerts of apps for self-management of blood glucose for type 2 diabetes. J Am Med Assoc 2019;321(15):1530−2.

[6] Food and Drug Administration. Software as a medical device (SAMD): clinical evaluation. December 8, 2017 at <https://www.fda.gov/media/100714/download>.

[7] Klonoff DC, Gutierrez A, Fleming A, Kerr D. Real-world evidence should be used in regulatory decisions about new pharmaceutical and medical device products for diabetes. J Diabetes Sci Technol 2019;.

[8] Whaley CM, Bollyky JB, Lu W, Painter S, Schneider J, et al. Reduced medical spending associated with increased use of a remote diabetes management program and lower mean blood glucose values. J Med Econ 2019.

[9] Food and Drug Administration. Digital health software precertification (pre-cert) program. December 8, 2017 at <https://www.fda.gov/medical-devices/digital-health/digital-health-software-precertification-pre-cert-program>.

Chapter 19

The US Food and Drug Administration regulation of digital health

Yarmela Pavlovic

Manatt, Phelps & Phillips, LLP, San Francisco, CA, United States

Abbreviations

AI	artificial intelligence
CDS	clinical decision support
FDA	US Food and Drug Administration
FD&C Act	Food, Drug, and Cosmetic Act
GMLP	good machine learning practices
ML	machine learning
MMA	Mobile Medical Applications: guidance for Industry and Food and Drug
Guidance	Administration Staff
NSE	not substantially equivalent
PreCert	Precertification
PDS software	patient decision support
PMA	premarket approval
SaMD	software as a medical device
SE	substantially equivalent

Key points

- Many digital health solutions are regulated by the US Food and Drug Administration (FDA). Determining whether an individual product is regulated requires review of the FDA's definitions for regulated products, as well as consideration of a set of policies designed to define the scope of products over which FDA exercises active regulatory authority.
- If a product is actively regulated by FDA, it may require clearance/approval by the Agency prior to commercialization, as well as compliance with a set of basic regulatory requirements applicable to all regulated products.

Diabetes Digital Health. DOI: https://doi.org/10.1016/B978-0-12-817485-2.00019-5

- FDA regulation is continuing to evolve in order to meet the demands of technological evolution. The Agency is developing additional regulatory programs aimed at addressing the unique issues presented by digital health technology.

Introduction

The rapid development and evolution of digital health products designed for use by persons with diabetes requires thoughtful and, in many cases, novel regulatory approaches and paradigms. Depending on the design, features, and intended use of digital health products, they may be regulated by the US Food and Drug Administration (FDA), the federal agency that oversees regulation of medical products and technologies, including medical devices, diagnostics, drugs, and biologics. New technologies wishing to enter the market may need to first comply with the Agency's regulatory requirements.

Determining whether a product is regulated by US Food and Drug Administration

Medical device definition

Most digital health products that are regulated by the FDA fall under the Agency's definition of a "medical device." Thus when considering whether a medical product, including a digital health solution, is regulated by the FDA, the first question to be asked is whether the product meets the statutory definition of a medical device. Per Section 201(h) of the federal Food, Drug, and Cosmetic Act (FD&C Act), a medical device is defined as

[A]n instrument, apparatus, implement, machine, contrivance, implant, in vitro reagent, or other similar or related article, including any component, part, or accessory, which is —

1. *recognized in the official National Formulary, or the United States Pharmacopeia, or any supplement to them,*
2. *intended for use in the diagnosis of disease or other conditions, or in the cure, mitigation, treatment, or prevention of disease, in man or other animals, or*
3. *intended to affect the structure or any function of the body of man or other animals, and*

   which does not achieve its primary intended purposes through chemical action within or on the body of man or other animals and which is not dependent upon being metabolized for the achievement of its primary intended purposes.

In addition, the FD&C Act was amended in 2016 to explicitly exclude certain types of medical software functions from the definition of a medical device, including

1. software intended for administrative support of a health-care facility, such as processing bills and claims, scheduling, inventory management, analysis of historical data to predict utilization, and determination of benefit eligibility;
2. software intended for maintaining or encouraging a healthy lifestyle where the use is unrelated to the diagnosis, cure, mitigation, prevention, or treatment of a disease or condition (i.e., general health and wellness);
3. software intended to serve as electronic patient records, if such records are created and used by health-care providers and constitute health information technology as certified under Public Health Service Act Section 3001(c)(5), and the software does not interpret or analyze patient records for the purpose of diagnosis, cure, mitigation, prevention, or treatment of a disease or condition;
4. software intended to transfer, store, convert formats, or display (but not analyze) laboratory and device data, results, associated findings by a health-care professional, and general background information about a test or device; and
5. clinical decision support (CDS) software that displays/analyzes medical information and makes recommendations for health-care professionals regarding prevention, diagnosis, or treatment of a disease/condition. However, such software
   a. cannot be processing or analyzing medical images (e.g., CT scans, MRIs, and X-rays), data from in vitro diagnostic devices, or "a pattern or signal from a signal acquisition system" and
   b. must be transparent and its recommendations reviewable, such that it does not serve as the sole basis for a health-care professional's determination regarding a particular patient.

Determining whether a product meets the definition of a medical device, and is not excluded by the subsequent statutory amendment, requires assessment of both design and intended use. Intended use of a product is determined by the intent of the manufacturer as evidenced by the design of the product and the product labeling. Importantly, the agency interprets the above definition broadly to assert jurisdiction over a variety of products. In addition, the statutory changes described above include a "catch-all" provision reserving FDA authority, under certain conditions, to regulate software functions that would otherwise be excluded from the definition of medical device, if it is "reasonably likely to have serious adverse health consequences" and identified as such in a final order after an opportunity for public comment. FDA has not yet taken advantage of this authority for any products.

Further, where a product has multiple functions, at least one of which does not meet the definition of a medical device, FDA focuses oversight on the regulated functions, though is permitted to consider the interaction between the multiple functions.

Enforcement discretion policies

If a product meets the definition of a medical device and is not excluded from FDA regulation by statute, the next question that must be considered is whether the Agency has announced a policy that would informally exclude the product from regulation. As an enforcement agency, FDA sometimes uses a policy of "enforcement discretion" and exercises discretion to refrain from enforcing some or all FDA requirements for certain types of products. Generally these policies focus on types of products that the Agency believes are very low risk and for which FDA regulation would not add significantly to the protection of public health. Examples of these policies are described next.

General wellness policy

In 2019 FDA issued a final guidance, entitled *General Wellness: Policy for Low Risk Devices* (General Wellness Guidance) [1]. The General Wellness Guidance explains that FDA does not intend to examine low risk general wellness products to determine whether they are devices under the FD&C Act, or, if they are devices, to determine whether they comply with the relevant regulatory requirements. Put another way, the Agency will not actively enforce the medical device regulatory requirements for products meeting the criteria in this guidance.

The General Wellness Guidance describes two categories of intended uses that are eligible for this treatment under the guidance:

- An intended use that relates to maintaining or encouraging a general state of health or a healthy activity without making reference to diseases or medical conditions (e.g., claims that focus on weight management, physical fitness, relaxation, and enhancing learning capacity).
- An intended use involving promoting, tracking and/or encouraging choices, which, as part of a healthy lifestyle, may help reduce the risk or impact of certain chronic diseases or conditions (e.g., coaching breathing techniques and relaxation skills for those with migraine headaches).

Notably, for software only products, the first of these categories was officially deregulated under the statutory changes made later in 2016 and described in the previous section. However, products that include hardware and fall within the first category, as well as the second category would continue to potentially fall within the medical device definition and, for that reason, the General Wellness Guidance remains relevant.

FDA's General Wellness Guidance further explains the Agency's perspective regarding the types of products that would no longer be considered medical devices and provides examples of products that are no longer considered medical devices, such as those with claims related to sustaining or offering general improvement of functions associated with a general state of health and that do not make any reference to diseases or conditions. Examples of such claims include weight management, physical fitness, relaxation or stress management, mental acuity, self-esteem, sleep management, or sexual function [2].

If the product does make medically oriented claims, the product may still fall under the existing General Wellness Guidance policy so long as the intended use relates the role of healthy lifestyle with helping to reduce the risk or impact of certain chronic diseases or conditions and where it is well understood and accepted that healthy lifestyle choices may play an important role in health outcomes of the disease or condition. To be considered a low risk product under this policy, the product should not be (1) invasive, (2) implanted, or (3) involved in an intervention or technology that may pose a risk to the safety of users and other persons if specific regulatory controls are not applied, such as risks from lasers or radiation exposure. In addition, the relationship between the lifestyle or behavioral recommendations and the reduced risk of disease or improved outcomes must be well established.

Mobile medical applications

Well before the FD&C Act was modified to exclude certain types of software, FDA had announced a policy related to "Mobile Medical Applications." The original guidance has been revised several times by the Agency and most recently issues as the final guidance Policy for Device Software Functions and Mobile Medical Applications [3]. In that guidance, the Agency defined mobile apps as software applications that can be run on a mobile platform or web-based software applications that are tailored to a mobile platform but run on a server. The guidance sets forth FDA policy regarding which mobile apps are not considered to be medical devices, which may be medical devices but are subject to enforcement discretion for purposes of compliance with FDA regulatory obligations, and which are considered medical devices subject to active FDA regulation. Notably, while the guidance originally focused on mobile applications, FDA has subsequently updated the guidance to clarify that the Agency regulates products based on intended use and functionality and not based on platform. Thus the concepts articulated in the guidance would also be relevant for products that use some platform other than a mobile app.

According to the MMA Guidance, FDA actively regulates only those mobile applications that meet the definition of a medical device and are intended to be used either as an accessory to a regulated medical device or to transform a mobile platform into a regulated medical device. This includes apps that

1. connect to a medical device to control that device or for use in active patient monitoring or analyzing medical device data;
2. use attachments, display screens, or sensors, or otherwise include functionalities similar to those of currently regulated medical devices; or
3. perform patient-specific analysis and provide patient-specific diagnosis or treatment recommendations.

Apps that fall into one of the above categories are subject to active FDA regulation because they have the same or similar intended use and technological characteristics as software or software-based devices that have been cleared or approved by FDA. Such apps present higher risk to users than products that simply record daily activities such as adherence to a medication regimen.

On the other hand, the guidance also includes an extensive list of examples of apps for which FDA plans to exercise enforcement action. However, unless a potential product fits within one of the examples in the guidance, the enforcement discretion policy in the guidance may be of limited help to a company.

Clinical and patient decision support tools

As noted above, certain types of CDS software are no longer considered medical devices, though they must be specific narrow criteria in order to be unregulated. To further explain the scope of their regulatory authority, the FDA has issued a draft guidance on CDS software [4].

As noted above, the FD&C Act now states that software functions meeting all of the following four criteria are no longer considered devices subject to FDA regulation:

1. *not* intended to acquire, process, or analyze a medical image or a signal from an in vitro diagnostic device or a pattern or signal from a signal acquisition system;
2. intended to display, analyze, or print medical information about a patient or other medical information (such as peer-reviewed clinical studies and clinical practice guidelines);
3. intended for the purpose of supporting or providing recommendations to a health-care professional about prevention, diagnosis, or treatment of a disease or condition; and
4. intended to enable such health-care professional to independently review the basis for such recommendations that such software presents so that it is not the intent that such health-care professional rely primarily on any of such recommendations to make a clinical diagnosis or treatment

decision regarding an individual patient (see Section 502(o)(1)(E) of the FD&C Act).

For purposes of the CDS Guidance, FDA interprets CDS to refer to tools that meet the first three criteria above. However, a CDS function is *only* excluded from the definition of a device (i.e., non-device CDS) when it also meets criterion 4 and enables independent review of the software's basis for clinical recommendations. The crux of this fourth criterion is that a health-care professional must be able to rely on his/her own judgment, rather than primarily on the software's recommendations, to make clinical decisions for individual patients. To that end, according to the draft guidance, the tool should clearly explain its purpose or intended use, the intended user, the inputs used to generate the recommendation (e.g., patient age), and the ratio-nale or support for the recommendation. The intended user should be able to reach the same recommendation on his/her own, so the sources supporting the recommendation or underlying the rationale for it should be identified, easily accessible, and understandable to the intended user.

If a CDS product does not meet all four of the Cures Act criteria, then it would be a device CDS and could be regulated by FDA. Notably, a CDS product intended for use by a patient or caregiver rather than a health care provider is a device CDS and could be regulated by FDA. However, the draft guidance explains that such products could be under enforcement dis-cretion if they meet certain additional criteria. Specifically, FDA intends to leverage factors developed in "Software as a Medical Device: Possible Framework for Risk Categorization and Corresponding Considerations" (IMDRF Framework) to apply a risk-based policy for determining whether CDS devices are subject to enforcement discretion. The IMDRF Framework, as explained in the draft guidance, deploys two major factors in a matrix to assign risk categorization of Software as a Medical Device (SaMD): (A) the significance of information provided by a SaMD to the health care decision, and (B) the state of the health care situation or condi-tion (i.e., critical, serious, or non-serious). The significance of the informa-tion to the health care decision is categorized as (in descending order of risk) "treat or diagnose," "drive clinical management," or "inform clinical management." FDA explains that it only considers software that is used to "inform clinical management" as CDS, because CDS functions − per the Cures Act criteria − are intended to provide information that supports or serves as a recommendation about prevention, diagnosis, or treatment of a disease/condition, but is not necessary to decision-making for a patient's care. Accordingly, SaMD functions which "drive clinical management" or "treat or diagnose" are not considered CDS and are more likely to be regu-lated. Building on the risk-based framework, the draft guidance indicates that FDA does not intend to enforce compliance for device CDS software functions under certain circumstances. Per the draft guidance, the following combinations of intended CDS audience, severity, and transparency would be subject to enforcement discretion:

- Device CDS intended for health care professional users for "non-serious situations or conditions" where the user cannot independently review the basis
- Device CDS intended for the patient or caregiver for "non-serious situations or conditions" and where the user can independently evaluate the basis for the recommendations.

Examples of CDS functions that are not devices because they meet all four criteria set forth above from the Cures Act include, among others,

- Software intended to aid in diagnosing suspected diabetes mellitus, where the health-care practitioner enters patient parameters and laboratory test results and the device suggests whether the patient's condition meets the definition of diabetes per established guidelines.
- Software that provides recommendations by matching patient-specific information (e.g., diagnosis, allergies, and symptoms) to reference information routinely used by the medical community in clinical practice (e.g., practice guidelines and FDA-approved drug labeling), to facilitate assessment or treatment of specific patients; and
- Software that provides recommendations on the use of a prescription drug that are consistent with the current FDA-required labeling.

US Food and Drug Administration regulatory framework for digital health

Where products are actively regulated by FDA as medical devices, the Agency's regulatory framework for medical devices is a risk-based approach where the risk posed by a device dictates the level of regulatory scrutiny to which it is subject. Accordingly, three device classes have been established, as described briefly next.

Class I devices present the lowest risk of harm to patients or users. Because of the low risk nature of these devices, most class I devices have been exempted by regulation from premarket clearance or approval requirements. Thus a manufacturer may begin marketing class I exempt devices without FDA authorization, so long as the company complies with FDA's General Controls for medical devices. Class I diabetes-related devices include tools such as lancets and mobile application used for retrospective display and review of continuous glucose monitor data.

Class II devices represent an intermediate level of risk. This class includes a wide range of products, some of which have also been exempted from the premarket notification requirements. Those that have not been exempted, however, must receive FDA clearance prior to marketing under Section 510(k) of the FD&C Act, which is based on a finding by FDA that a proposed device is "substantially equivalent" (SE) to a legally marketed "predicate device." Examples of class II diabetes-related digital health devices include blood glucose meters, insulin-dosing calculators, and standalone insulin pumps.

Finally, class III devices include high-risk products such as life-sustaining, life-supporting, or implantable devices or novel devices that are not SE (NSE) to any predicate and for which de novo reclassification (where a device with no suitable predicate is downclassified to class II based on its being sufficiently low-to-moderate risk) is not deemed appropriate. Manufacturers must obtain FDA authorization to market class III devices via a premarket approval (PMA) application, which requires reasonable assurances of the device's safety and effectiveness. In the context of diabetes-related digital health products, examples of class III devices include artificial pancreas systems, as well as some continuous glucose monitors.

The specifics of FDA's requirements for clearance/approval and general regulatory controls are provided in the following sections.

General controls

All medical devices, regardless of classification, are subject to FDA's "general controls." These are the basic regulatory requirements that must be adhered to regardless of final classification. General controls include statutory provisions that

- prohibit the commercial distribution of adulterated or misbranded devices (Sections 501 and 502 of the FDC Act; 21 U.S.C. Sections 351 and 352);
- require device manufacturers, importers, and distributors to register their establishments with FDA and submit device listing information (Section 510 of the FDC Act, 21 U.S.C. Section 360);
- grant FDA the authority to ban certain devices (Section 516 of the FDC Act, 21 U.S.C. Section 360f);
- provide for notification of risk and of repair, replacement, and refund (Section 518 of the FDC Act; 21 U.S.C. Section 360h);
- restrict the sale, distribution, or use of certain devices (Section 520(e) of the FDC Act; 21 U.S.C. Section 360j(e));
- establish good-manufacturing practices for medical devices (Section 520 (f) of the FDC Act, 21 U.S.C. Section 360j(f));
- require the submission of records and reports (Section 519 of the FDC Act, 21 U.S.C. Section 360i); and
- permit FDA inspection (Section 702 of the FDC Act; 21 U.S.C. Section 372).

These general controls apply to actively regulated medical devices regardless of classification and are discussed in further detail in the sections that follow.

510(k) pathway and substantial equivalence

If at all possible, where FDA marketing authorization is required, companies generally prefer to have their products fall within the 510(k) premarket notification process because that path is faster and typically less burdensome than the PMA or de novo review processes. The 510(k) process relies on a determination that a new device is "SE" to a legally marketed "predicate device" in terms of both intended use and technological characteristics. Only class I, class II, and pre-1976 class III products (so long as FDA has not required PMA applications) may serve as predicate devices.

In assessing whether a device is SE, the Agency first asks whether the device has the same general intended use as the predicate product(s). If the intended use differs, the analysis stops and the device is deemed "NSE" and, thus, ineligible for 510(k) clearance. While the new device must have the same general intended use as a predicate to be found "SE," the new device can have differences in terms of "indications for use." Per guidance issued by FDA in 2014, differences in the indications for use statements will not render a new device NSE, provided that the differences do not raise different questions of safety and effectiveness and, therefore, preclude a meaningful comparison with the predicate device [5]. Consequently, a new device with the same intended use as a predicate device may have a slightly different labeling and still be found SE and cleared via the 510(k) process.

When FDA evaluates the intended use and indications for use of potential predicate devices to determine whether the device that is the subject of a 510(k) notice is SE to those predicate devices, only the claims that have been cleared by FDA for the predicate devices are considered by the agency. Thus, although some predicate devices may be commonly used beyond the scope of their FDA-cleared indications, these uses will not be considered by FDA in determining the substantial equivalence of the new device.

Assuming the device is found to be SE in terms of intended use and indications for use, the Agency then asks whether the new device has the same technological characteristics as the predicate device (e.g., design, materials, and energy sources). If the characteristics are the same or very similar, the device may be found SE. However, if there are new or different characteristics, the FDA reviewer must further ask whether any differences raise "different questions of safety or efficacy" when compared to the cited predicate.

If the new or different technological characteristics raise different types of safety or effectiveness issues from the predicates, the device is deemed NSE. If the new or different characteristics do not raise any different types of questions of safety or effectiveness, the device may be found SE if accepted scientific methods exist to assess the effects of the different characteristics, and if data are available to demonstrate that the new or different characteristics do not impact safety or effectiveness.

In some instances, multiple predicate devices may be used to demonstrate substantial equivalence, although FDA prefers the use of only one predicate. For example, somewhat commonly, digital health products may combine the features of prior devices into a single new device. When multiple predicates are cited, FDA recommends that manufacturers identify the "primary predicate" that supports a substantial equivalence determination. In addition, each predicate must have the same intended use as the new device and, if the devices have different technological characteristics, then these must not raise different questions of safety or effectiveness.

The type and amount of data that must be included in a 510(k) notice varies depending on the type of product, the intended use, and the extent of new technological features. Although many 510(k) notices are cleared on the basis of human factors, bench testing and/or animal testing alone, an increasing proportion of 510(k) submissions also must include clinical data. If there are any serious safety or effectiveness concerns, the Agency may require 510 (k) data similar to those needed to support a PMA filing.

The timeframe for FDA review of 510(k) notifications ranges from a few months to a year or longer depending on the complexity and novel nature of the product. Specifically, FDA has 90 days by statute to perform its review of a 510(k) notice. In practice, it is common for FDA to issue an initial set of questions after approximately 45−60 days of review. Once the manufacturer responds to the Agency's questions, FDA aims to complete all substantive review within 90 total days of FDA review time (i.e., not including time taken by the manufacturer to respond to FDA questions). For a 510(k) with clinical data, it is not uncommon for the total process to take 9−12 months from submission to clearance. By comparison, 510(k) notices that do not involve clinical data are routinely cleared in 3−6 months, depending on whether FDA requires multiple rounds of review.

De novo pathway

If a product does not have a suitable predicate device and does not fit into a 510(k)-exempt classification, it automatically defaults to a class III classification. However, if the product is low-to-moderate risk, the de novo pathway may be used to reclassify the product type to class I or II and simultaneously authorize the individual device for marketing. Under that framework, a manufacturer submits a de novo request to FDA, requesting reclassification, and the Agency grants the request and simultaneously creates a new regulatory classification.

Historically, companies were only able to use the de novo pathway after submitting a 510(k) and receiving an NSE decision. In 2012 congress created the "direct de novo" process, allowing a company with a novel product to skip the 510(k) process and submit a de novo request. That process involves submission of an application to the agency requesting reclassification of the device under Section 513(f)(2) of the FD&C Act. The statutory timeframe for review of a de novo submission is 120 days from the date of the request. However, this timeframe has always been a challenge for the Agency to meet and the review process regularly exceeded this deadline. Recently enacted user fees for de novo submissions target a total FDA review time of 150 days, excluding the time required for a manufacturer to respond to any questions. The content and general requirements for a de novo request that follows a 510(k) and a direct de novo request are the same.

Regardless of whether a de novo request is direct or follows a 510(k), the submission is typically viewed as being more involved than a 510(k) submission, but less so than a PMA application. In addition to the device description and testing information typically included in a 510(k), a de novo request additionally includes reasons for the recommended classification, a discussion of the risks and benefits of the device, including how known risks can be effectively mitigated, as well as proposed general or special controls that the sponsor believes would provide reasonable assurance of safety and effectiveness for the device [6]. A de novo request must also contain data demonstrating that general and/or special controls support a classification of class I or class II; typically this involves submission of clinical data. Recently proposed changes to the de novo process would additionally allow FDA, at their option, to conduct premarket manufacturing and bioresearch monitoring inspections.

If FDA grants the request for de novo reclassification, the device is authorized for marketing as a class I or II device and may, in the future, serve as a legitimate predicate device for competitors.

PMA pathway

In the event that a device is found NSE to a predicate device and is not considered low to moderate risk, the product must be approved for marketing via the premarket approval (PMA) pathway.

PMA approval requires that the safety and effectiveness of the device be established with valid scientific evidence, a process that requires substantial supporting clinical data, generally from randomized, controlled multicenter studies. PMA submissions are typically more extensive than 510(k) notices, although 510(k) notices requiring clinical data in some cases may approach the complexity of a PMA. Approval of a PMA also requires detailed information on the sponsor's quality system in a dedicated manufacturing section and a preapproval inspection of the sponsor's manufacturing facilities by FDA, neither of which is required for the other regulatory pathways.

The timeframe for FDA review of PMA applications under the FD&C Act is considerably longer than comparable review times for a routine 510 (k) notice without clinical data. Specifically, FDA has 180 days to perform its review of a PMA submission, with a corresponding timeframe of 90 days for a 510(k) notice. However, FDA's initial PMA review typically results in a "major deficiency letter," which requests additional information from the sponsor and resets FDA's review clock. In our experience, multiple rounds of such agency questions are routine for PMA submissions. Assuming that the deficiencies raised by the agency can be successfully addressed, novel, first-in-class PMA devices are typically referred to as advisory panel. Advisory panels comprise experts (e.g., clinicians and statisticians), patient representative(s), and an industry representative. The panel is charged with evaluating the device and providing FDA a nonbinding advisory opinion on the safety and effectiveness profile of the device. From submission to ultimate approval of a PMA, the process generally requires a minimum of 18–24 months.

US Food and Drug Administration's Pre-Submission Program

For some types of products, the Agency's expectations regarding regulatory pathway and testing may already be well established. For more novel types of products, it is often advisable to discuss these issues with the Agency in advance of a marketing submission. The process used to facilitate such discussions is known as the Pre-Submission or Pre-Sub process.

FDA's guidance document, entitled *Requests for Feedback and Meetings for Medical Device Submissions: The Q-Submission Program—Guidance for Industry and Food and Drug Administration Staff*, outlines processes for obtaining feedback from FDA on specific questions necessary to guide product development and/or preparation of marketing applications [7]. Through this program, companies are able to obtain feedback on a variety of topics, including potential hurdles for approval/clearance or the agency's expectations as to the elements that must be included in a marketing application. Sponsors submit a written background package (referred to as a Pre-Sub) that includes specific questions for discussion. After submission of the background package, a face-to-face meeting or teleconference is scheduled typically within 60–75 days of submission. Under current procedures, 5 days prior to the scheduled meeting or teleconference, FDA provides written feedback in response to the sponsor's questions. That feedback is then used by the sponsor to further inform the discussion at the meeting. Following the meeting, the sponsor must provide written meeting minutes within 15 days and the Agency returns comments on those minutes 30 days after submission.

When submitting a Pre-Sub meeting request, the briefing document should include, among other things, a detailed description of the product and intended use, an overview of product development (including an outline of nonclinical and clinical testing either planned or already completed), and a discussion of the expected regulatory pathway. If feedback is sought on the planned testing, the sponsor should consider including complete draft protocols.

Regulation of combination products

Some digital health tools are meant to be used in conjunction with a prescription drug or biological product. When that is the case and both the digital health tool and the drug/biological product are essential to achieve the overall intended use, the FDA may regard the two products together as a combination product. Combination products are required to comply with the regulatory requirements applicable to the component with the primary mode of action, which is typically viewed as the drug product. When determining whether the two products should be regulated together, the agency looks to whether the products are copackaged. For example, prepackaged insulin pens are typically regulated as combinations products. By comparison, reusable insulin pens or pumps that are used with a variety of different insulin products, and not distributed along with the drug, are generally regulated as devices.

Regulation as a combination product requires that the system (drug/biologic and digital tool) obtain FDA approval via the Agency's process for a new drug application or biologics license application. Postmarket, manufacturers of combination products, must adhere to requirements applicable to drugs and biologic products. For example, any safety data collected by the digital health tool may need to be considered as part of the pharmacovigilance requirements for the drug/biological product.

Evolving regulatory paradigms

Given the constantly evolving nature of digital health technology, it is perhaps not surprising that the FDA's regulatory approach has also been evolving. Two initiatives, in particular, warrant the discussion.

US Food and Drug Administration precertification program

On July 27, 2017, FDA announced the pilot of a precertification (PreCert) program for companies developing software as a medical device (SaMD) [8]. The PreCert program, which is still in development, is a plan to "precertify" software companies that "demonstrate a culture of quality and organizational excellence based on objective criteria, for example, that they can and do excel in software design, development and validation (testing)." The PreCert by FDA would allow those developers to market low-risk devices and software without FDA review or through a more streamlined premarket review with reduced submission content and faster review. Precertified firms could also collect postmarket data to affirm the regulatory status of the product, as well as support new product functions. FDA has also indicated that certification may be accomplished through use of third parties.

The program has been in development since 2017 with a small group of companies initially accepted into the program, several of which are developing diabetes-related products. While FDA has not released any criteria for future entry into the program, FDA has stated that five excellence principles will drive the criteria: patient safety, product quality, clinical responsibility, cybersecurity responsibility, and proactive culture.

US food and drug administration artificial intelligence and machine-learning framework

It has become increasingly common for SaMD products to be based on machine learning (ML) and other artificial intelligence (AI) techniques. Historically, FDA has cleared or approved only "locked" algorithms, meaning that it has expected manufacturers to submit verification/validation performed on a device design that includes a frozen algorithm. Any subsequent algorithm updates are then assessed under the framework outlined in FDA's guidance, *Deciding When to Submit a 510(k) for a Software Change to an Existing Device* (Software Modifications Guidance) [9]. Under the current framework, a new 510(k) notice or PMA approval for an AI/ML-based SaMD would be required for essentially any software modification that significantly affects device performance, safety, or effectiveness, as well as any new intended use and any major change to the software algorithm.

Recently, FDA initiated development of a framework that would allow for greater change to algorithms without the need for new clearance or approval. To that end, the Agency released a discussion paper entitled *Proposed Regulatory Framework for Modifications to AI/ML-Based SaMD* [10]. In that discussion paper, the Agency proposes to allow for ongoing algorithm changes that are implemented according to prespecified performance objectives, follow defined algorithm change protocols, utilize a validation process that is committed to improving the software's performance, safety, and effectiveness, and include real-world performance monitoring. While the specific types of data required to ensure safety and effectiveness would continue to depend on the software's function, the risk it poses, and its intended use, FDA believes these pillars may allow for greater latitude for postmarket change without additional clearance or approval.

Key to the Agency's potential approach is the concept of "good ML practices" (GMLP) to capture AI/ML best practices (e.g., data management, feature extraction, training, and evaluation) that the Agency would expect of SaMD developers. GMLP considerations include

- relevance of available data to the clinical problem and current clinical practice;
- data acquired in a consistent, clinically relevant, and generalizable manner that aligns with the SaMD's intended use and modification plans;
- appropriate separation between training, tuning, and test datasets; and
- appropriate level of transparency (clarity) of the output.

This proposed approach will undoubtedly continue to evolve as FDA moves forward in discussions with the Agency.

References

[1] Food and Drug Administration. General wellness: policy for low risk devices—guidance for Industry and Food and Drug Administration Staff, <https://www.fda.gov/regulatory-information/search-fda-guidance-documents/general-wellness-policy-low-risk-devices>; 2019 [accessed 12.06.19].

[2] Food and Drug Administration. Changes to existing medical software policies resulting from section 3060 of the 21st century cures act: guidance for Industry and Food and Drug Administration Staff, <https://www.fda.gov/downloads/MedicalDevices/DeviceRegulation andGuidance/GuidanceDocuments/UCM587820.pdf>; 2019 [accessed 12.06.19].

[3] Food and Drug Administration. Policy for device software functions and mobile medical applications, <https://www.fda.gov/regulatory-information/search-fda-guidance-documents/policy-device-software-functions-and-mobile-medical-applications>; 2019 [accessed 12.06.19].

[4] Food and Drug Administration. Clinical support software: guidance for industry and Food and Drug Administration Staff, <https://www.fda.gov/regulatory-information/search-fda-guidance-documents/clinical-and-patient-decision-support-software>; 2019 [accessed 12.06.19].

[5] Food and Drug Administration. Guidance for Industry and Food and Drug Administration Staff: The 510(k) Program: evaluating substantial equivalence in premarket notifications [510(k)], <https://www.fda.gov/regulatory-information/search-fda-guidance-documents/510k-program-evaluating-substantial-equivalence-premarket-notifications-510k>; 2014 [accessed 12.06.19].

[6] Food and Drug Administration. De novo classification process (evaluation of automatic class III designation): guidance for Industry and Food and Drug Administration Staff, <https://www.fda.gov/regulatory-information/search-fda-guidance-documents/de-novo-classi fication-process-evaluation-automatic-class-iii-designation>; 2017 [accessed 12.06.19].

[7] Food and Drug Administration. Requests for feedback and meetings for medical device submissions: the Q-submission program – guidance for Industry and Food and Drug Administration Staff, <https://www.fda.gov/regulatory-information/search-fda-guidance-documents/requests-feedback-and-meetings-medical-device-submissions-q-submission-program>; 2019 [accessed 12.06.19].

[8] King F, Klonoff DC, Ahn D, Adi S, Berg EG, Bian J, et al. Diabetes technology society report on the FDA digital health software precertification program meeting. J Diabetes Sci Technol 2019;13(1):128–39. Available from: https://doi.org/10.1177/1932296818810436 Epub 2018 Nov 5 *See also* Food and Drug Administration. Digital Health Software Precertification (Pre-Cert) Program <https://www.fda.gov/medical-devices/digital-health/digital-health-software-precertification-pre-cert-program> [accessed 05.07.19].

[9] Food and Drug Administration. Deciding when to submit a 510(k) for a software change to an existing device: guidance for Industry and Food and Drug Administration Staff, <https://www.fda.gov/regulatory-information/search-fda-guidance-documents/deciding-when-submit-510k-software-change-existing-device>; 2017 [accessed 12.06.19].

[10] Food and Drug Administration. Proposed regulatory framework for modifications to artificial intelligence/machine learning (AI/ML)-based software as a medical device, <https://www.fda.gov/media/122535/download>; 2019 [accessed 12.06.19].

Chapter 20

Cybersecurity of digital diabetes devices

Christine Sublett[1] and William "Brad" Marsh[2]

[1]Sublett Consulting, San Mateo, CA, United States, [2]U.S. Army, Washington, DC, United States

Abbreviations

CDS	clinical decision support
CGM	continuous glucose monitor
CIA Triad	Confidentiality, Integrity, and Availability Triad
CISO	chief information security officer
DTMoSt	Diabetes Technology Society Mobile Platform Controlling a Diabetes Device Security and Safety Standard
DTS	Diabetes Technology Society
DTSec	Diabetes Technology Society Standard for Connected Diabetes Devices Security
EHR	electronic health record
FDA	Food and Drug Administration
HCIC	Health Care Industry Cybersecurity Task Force
HDO	healthcare delivery organization
HHS	Health and Human Services
HIPAA	Health Insurance Portability and Accountability Act
HSCC	Healthcare Sector Coordinating Council
IoMT	Internet of Medical Things
IT	information technology
JSP	Medical Device and Health IT Joint Security Plan
NIST	National Institute of Standards and Technology
OWASP	Open Web Application Security Project
PGHD	patient-generated healthcare data
SBOM	software bill of materials
SMBG	self-monitoring of blood glucose
TLS	transport layer security

Diabetes Digital Health. DOI: https://doi.org/10.1016/B978-0-12-817485-2.00020-1

Key points

- Security of medical devices is a shared responsibility between device manu-facturers, health information technology (IT) vendors, and health-care delivery organizations (HDOs).
- Standards, guidance, and security best practice publications are available for HDOs, clinicians, and security specialists to analyze and reduce medical device integration risk.
- Security of medical devices and health IT systems are no longer the singular responsibility of the chief information security officer (CISO). Rather, all stakeholders have a role from acquisition through implementation.

Burning platform

Recently, your hospital was victim of a successful ransomware attack. How did this happen? The chief information security officer (CISO) reports that this ransomware is common to a particular type of chip widely used in at-home medical devices. It becomes evident that an infected device with a known vulnerability became connected to your system to upload patient data for review by a clinician. The electronic health record (EHR) processed that data and ingested the ransomware. Now, your entire patient population is at risk and the fines for the breach are growing. How could this have been prevented?

It is vitally important to get the most complete picture of a patient's health status inside and outside the clinical setting. Getting this picture requires aggregation of multiple data points from a variety of sources. At certain points in the care continuum, your organization may have to share the data out to another entity to best take care of the patient. In this chapter, we discuss how to get and share this complete picture and how to balance this with the security of the entire healthcare sector. It is imperative to understand that these two requirements are not diametrically opposed, nor are they mutually exclusive. We outline key requirements and guardrails to put in place for the best patient care while maintaining system and data security.

Clinical requirements and evidence-based practice

In the outpatient setting, there are many different wearable/carriable medical devices for the management of diabetes, including blood glucose monitors, continuous glucose monitors (CGMs), insulin infusion pumps, smart insulin pens, and closed-loop artificial pancreas systems, used by these patients in their everyday lives. Children with Type 1 diabetes can apply a continuous monitoring device that connects wirelessly to a phone that will notify their parents should they fall out of a patient-specific glucose range. This technology provides much needed early warning. Blood glucose monitor systems are available for all ages to provide the patient and their families or caregivers quantifiable results to control blood glucose. Connected insulin pens can automatically calculate an appropriate dose for the current blood sugar level, decreasing the time to administration in some emergency situations. Insulin pumps and continuous glucose monitoring devices work in tandem to provide a closed-loop artificial pancreas system providing insulin as needed. This system measures glucose levels and automatically delivers the required insulin without needle injections and lancets. Other systems combine Bluetooth-enabled devices, sensors, and apps and upload data to the Cloud for analysis. Blood sugar management has entered the digital age and reflects a new paradigm of treatment.

Strict monitoring of an insulin-requiring diabetes patient's glucose level is the standard of practice in the inpatient setting. Upon admission, orders are often written for glucose checks before every meal and before bed. This allows for tight control of the patient's blood glucose, which reduces probability of infections and other complications [1]. The provider or care-team professional performs these tests, usually as a point of care test at the bedside and the data is entered into the medical record. In most cases the hospital or HDO has an interface to send the resulting data into the appropriate fields within the EHR, removing the human error element. Once in the EHR, two things can occur: first, the provider can see and identify trends with the patient's glucose level over time; second, the clinical decision support (CDS) software available in many commercial EHRs provides recommendations to ensure that the provider considers all pertinent treatment plans to improve the patient's outcome. These frequent tests, the incorporation of data, and the actions taken based on the data continue until the patient meets conditions for discharge.

Patients must be able to continue to treat themselves after they leave the walls of the hospital. Patients are instructed to obtain a blood glucose monitor system for home use in order to measure their glucose levels and to determine how much insulin they require. The nurse or educator provides the patient and/or their caregivers generic instruction on proper use of a commercial glucose monitor, insulin delivery system, and other pertinent medications. Often the patient is taught to keep a journal of all readings. The intent is that the patient will conduct self-monitoring of blood glucose (SMBG). Diabetes Technology Society (DTS) in 2010 published a consensus article that underscored the intrinsic benefits of SMBG in the outpatient diabetes population. They proposed that the data from SMBG provides the patient with insight into their personal care regimen to include medication impact on glucose levels, dietary intake, and activity habits in their natural setting. Without SMBG the hemoglobin A1c, which is a key indicator of long-term glucose control, fluctuates to a greater extent, which increases the risk of admission and readmission jeopardizes patient safety, increases expenditure for HDOs, and potentially decreases payer reimbursement [2].

In the out-of-hospital care setting of the average patient, the patient or their caregiver conducts the blood glucose check. Some blood glucose monitor systems provide a digital reading of the patient's glucose that the patient would have to handwrite in a journal. Others provide a cable or wireless connection to a computer and/or a network resource that uploads the resulting data to a vendor-specific data portal. Whether maintained in a handwritten journal, the device, a patient's computer, or the vendor's proprietary portal, the data is not available to the provider as readily as it was in the inpatient setting. The information is "silo-ed." The patient would need to provide documentation from either the journal or a printout to the provider, who can analyze the data and incorporate it into their care plan. This is a manual process, which is prone to human error and does not incorporate any CDS capability. Intentional misreporting of data to a handwritten logbook has been reported and can confound efforts to understand a patient's true glycemic pattern. For an experienced endocrinologist, interpreting data that is external to the EHR and making clinical decisions are commonplace. However, 80% of persons with diabetes are not under the care of an endocrinologist or diabetologist [3]. It is this population, which is usually followed by a general practice provider, that benefits most from the integration of SMBG data into the EHR.

The accumulated data from the patient's glucose monitoring devices provides essential information that can give a longitudinal picture of their overall health. Incorporation of this data into the EHR and making it available to the CDS capabilities is the optimal solution.

In January of 2018 the Office of the National Coordinator published "Conceptualizing a Data Infrastructure for the Capture, Use, and Sharing of Patient-Generated Health Data in Care Delivery and Research through 2024" [4]. This document outlined the importance of incorporating patient-generated healthcare data (PGHD) in the EHR. The inclusion of this data allows for the use of CDS capabilities to interpret and analyze PGHD, which can display a more complete picture of the patient and their condition. The CDS can apply the most current evidence-based diabetes management practices to improve the outcomes for the patient [4]. With this capability the general practice provider has access to advice and resources previously only held by endocrinologists, diabetologists, and other specialists. The ingestion and inclusion of this data not only comes with great rewards, but it also comes with increased cybersecurity risk.

To analyze and incorporate PGHD within the EHR, the data must be incorporated into the patient's record. Some medical practices instruct the patient to bring in their SMBG device and connect it to a computer on the clinical network (via USB or Bluetooth connection) for purposes of uploading data or device configuration. The data can then be transmitted via the internet to the manufacturer's portal and/or imported directly into the EHR as a data file. However, this process opens the entire EHR database to any viruses or malware contained on the SMBG device.

For the most part, medical devices in the hospital setting are controlled within the hospital. A patient-owned blood glucose monitor system or an insulin pump leaves the hospital and could then be exposed to any number of potential physical or electronic threats, including digital. Even in today's world of daily announcements of compromised data, people connect to public

Wi-Fi without a VPN or leave their phones discoverable to other Bluetooth devices. SMBG devices are no different. These devices are always seeking a connection. Should a nefarious actor connect to and manipulate an SMBG device, they could compromise it. A compromised blood glucose monitor system transmitting data to the clinical network exposes the HDO to a variety of threats, including malicious encrypting (ransomware) and viruses or other malware that create a backdoor through which patient-specific information can be stolen and sold, increasing liability on the HDO. In addition, a compromised device could put the patient at risk depending on the type of attack. For instance, an event that manipulates the configuration of the device or destroys data could harm the patient.

The Office for Civil Rights for Health and Human Services (HHS), the regulatory agency with Health Insurance Portability and Accountability Act (HIPAA) enforcement responsibility, issues penalties for noncompliance of the protection of health-care data based on the level of negligence and can range from $100 per violation (or per record) to a maximum penalty of $1.5 million per year dependent on the penalty tier [5]. However, this fine pales in comparison to the impact to the patient's safety and public's trust in that organization and in our health-care system as a whole, where a breach can have devastating effects.

Mitigation starts well before the patient has PGHD to incorporate into the record; it starts when these SMBG devices are designed and built. Through vendor product security and postimplementation support and HDO purchasing and supply chain management, HDOs can protect themselves more effectively.

Extending the security perimeter

Evidence-based practice clearly indicates the need to incorporate digital health data. This data plays an important role in diabetes treatment, given the constraints and limitations of budgets and staffing. In addition to the many different medical devices for the treatment of diabetes, including wearables/carriables, there are multiple apps available for mobile phone platforms that generate and compile PGHD. These applications include software for photographing foods, food calories trackers, diet software, and wearable exercise trackers.

Increasingly, both patient-owned and implanted medical devices such as glucose monitoring, pacemakers/defibrillators, and others within the hospital walls, including ultrasound systems, and MRI/CT machines, are gaining Internet, wireless, and Bluetooth connectivity. With this greater number of interfaces comes an increased capability of connecting and transferring, as well as an expanded attack surface. In digital terms, a compromise is any nefarious action resulting in loss of confidentiality, integrity, and/or availability of patient data. These three components form the Confidentiality, Integrity, and Availability Triad (CIA Triad) as shown in Table 20.1 [6]. A violation of any of the triad elements can lead to an adverse impact on security, privacy, and/or patient safety. All three are important and require a

TABLE 20.1 Definition of the CIA Triad elements.

CIA triad [6]
Confidentiality: limits information access to only those people who are authorized and prevent access by anyone else
Integrity: provides assurance that data quality remains whole, unaltered, and uncorrupted
Availability: provides uninterrupted system and data access

balance. Much effort is placed on confidentiality in regard to HIPAA and penalties. This chapter tries to bring integrity and availability into balance. And while there are no publicly reported incidents of patient harm due to hacked medical devices, vulnerabilities in these devices exist and have been identified by security researchers over the past several years. In 2016 flaws in the Animas OneTouch Ping insulin pump were reported that would allow an adversary within sufficient proximity to trigger unauthorized injections and harm the patient [7]. In 2009, the Food and Drug Administration (FDA) announced that Medtronic was recalling remote controllers for some of their insulin pumps for potential cybersecurity risks [8].

Most health-care organizations think about information security in the context of HIPAA or other regulatory requirements, but more importantly, compromised security also presents risks to patient safety. Safety can be jeopardized if a virus or other type of malware attack changes the configuration of a device, alters data values, or makes the device inaccessible. Those closest to both the devices and the patient, i.e., the technicians and clinicians, are the first and last line of defense for the patient. Compromised security could result in a loss of faith in medical devices, our health-care technology, and the health-care delivery infrastructure. This loss of faith presents a significant public health and national security threat [9] and is the foundation for the US Presidential Policy Declaration, which includes the health-care industry as one of the 16 critical infrastructure sectors in the United States. The 16 critical infrastructure sectors shown in Table 20.2 are those sectors whose virtual or physical systems, networks, and assets are considered so vital to the United States that their destruction or incapacitation would have a debilitating effect on national security, national economic security, and national public health or safety.

Securing health IT systems and medical devices is a combined responsibility. Healthcare stakeholders such as HDOs, health IT vendors, medical device manufacturers, clinicians, and patients all play pivotal roles securing Internet of Medical Things (IoMT). Clinicians and patients rely on medical device manufacturers and health IT system vendors to develop safe and secure products. They must address not only the CIA Triad but also consider

TABLE 20.2 16 Critical infrastructure sectors.

Critical infrastructure sectors [9]

- Chemical
- Commercial Facilities Sector
- Communications sector
- Critical Manufacturing Sector
- Dams Sector
- Defense Industrial Base Sector
- Emergency Services Sector
- Energy Sector
- Financial Services Sector
- Food and Agriculture Sector
- Government Facilities Sector
- Healthcare and Public Health Sector
- Information Technology Sector
- Nuclear Reactors, Materials and Waste Sector
- Transportation Systems Sector
- Water and Wastewater Systems Sector

patient safety and reliability to develop resilient devices and systems. In addition, the final balanced "equation" must include a consideration of cost. This is a collaborative effort that requires HDOs and clinicians to be aware of the security requirements they outline in order to purchase devices secure enough to be allowed to contribute to the EHR CDS data.

In 2009 the American Reinvestment & Recovery Act included a financial incentive for HDOs to implement and effectively use EHRs [10]. With the rapid deployment of EHRs, there was a subsequent marked increase in breaches and cybersecurity incidents. Seeing the implications, both to patient safety and financial penalties, focus in the Healthcare and Public Health industry shifted from adoption of EHRs and digital health-care information sharing to identification, management, and reduction of cybersecurity risk. Professional organizations such as DTS and the Open Web Application Security Project (OWASP), as well as regulatory and governmental bodies, including the FDA, the HHS Health Care Industry Cybersecurity (HCIC) Task Force, the National Institute of Standards and Technology (NIST), and the Healthcare Sector Coordinating Council (HSCC) issued cybersecurity recommendations, guidance, standards, and best practices. These recommendations help HDOs, health IT vendors, medical device manufacturers, clinicians, and patient organizations develop, deploy, and support medical devices, including those for the treatment and management of diabetes.

Product security

Building a secure product requires manufacturers and system vendors to build security into the design of their product. OWASP published a set of design principles called "security by design" to help companies minimize the risk of successful cyberattacks [11]. These comprehensive principles guide application developers to (1) consider the value of the data they are managing, (2) design controls that prevent misuse of the application and address the CIA Triad, and (3) build security measures to cover all types of risks from targeted attacks to accidental deletion of data. The principles also call for developers to think like an attacker. How would a cyberattacker or other malicious individual seek to attack their product? This approach assists developers in identifying and rating threats posed by their product.

The FDA provides manufacturers with pre- and postmarket guidance regarding cybersecurity device design, labeling, and documentation. The premarket recommendations outline those security elements that are optimally included prior to FDA approval to use as a medical device and make available on the open market. The postmarket guidance addresses the management and mitigation of risks once the medical devices are available to HDOs and are actively used in a health-care setting. This postmarket guidance is vital because cyber-threats are continually growing and changing, while medical devices and their embedded software (including firmware) historically are static, providing a tempting target for nefarious actors [12].

In 2018 the FDA issued a new draft premarket cybersecurity guidance, an update to the cybersecurity guidance first issued in 2014 [13] which updated medical device cybersecurity requirements in premarket submissions. The new draft guidance includes a two-tier cybersecurity risk categorization system for devices, risk management recommendations, requirements for inclusion in premarket submissions, including premarket approval, 510(k), and a software bill of materials (SBOM), for devices posing cybersecurity risk.

Table 20.3 outlines the criteria to categorize a medical device as either Tier 1 (Higher Cybersecurity Risk) or Tier 2 (Standard Cybersecurity Risk). Tier 1 devices include connected insulin and infusion pumps, the connected systems that interact with them (including home monitors), and devices with command and control functionality such as programming hardware. The connected nature of these devices and the fact that they provide life sustaining

TABLE 20.3 FDA security risk tiers explained.

Tier 1—Higher cybersecurity risk

- Capable of connecting to another product (medical/nonmedical), network, and/or the Internet
- Compromised of security can directly result in patient harm

Tier 2—Standard cybersecurity risk

- All other devices

services that, if compromised, jeopardize patient safety, require their categorization as a Tier 1 device. Tier 2 devices, on the other hand, include standalone devices, such as defibrillators and other devices without Wi-Fi and/or Bluetooth connectivity [13].

The FDA recommend that Tier 1 manufacturers include design documentation to show that the device is trustworthy and secure using the NIST Framework for improving critical infrastructure cybersecurity, and implementing security controls that demonstrate that medical devices provide a reasonable level of reliability and availability, perform its intended functions, is reasonably secure from cybersecurity misuse and intrusion, and adheres to generally accepted security procedures. On the contrary, the FDA expects that Tier 2 device premarket submissions include documentation that all Tier 1 security controls have been incorporated or else the manufacturers must provide a risk-based rationale regarding why the controls are not relevant. The key difference is the allowance to justify *not* including security controls with appropriate justification, which is not possible with Tier 1.

Digital medical devices are complex combinations of hardware, firmware, and software. Manufacturers bring together a wide variety of elements to make a single product. When there is an issue with one of these "ingredients," it is difficult for an HDO to know whether the issue impacts their purchased/supported devices. Much like the listing of ingredients in manufactured food, the SBOM advocated for by the HHS HCIC report provides transparency and awareness for the HDO. The SBOM must describe its components, including open source software, as well as any known risks associated with those components to enable HDOs to more quickly determine if they are impacted [14].

In 2014 a vulnerability nicknamed "Heartbleed" was identified in the implementation by OpenSSL (which is an open source software library of encryption tools) implementation of transport layer security (TLS) in client and server implementations [15]. While there was widespread understanding that the OpenSSL implementation of TLS was used on many web servers, it was not nearly as well known that OpenSSL's implementation of TLS was included in many medical devices. Without an SBOM included in the documentation for medical devices, it can be difficult for HDOs, clinicians, and patients to identify, track, and address vulnerabilities.

In 2015 DTS launched a project called DTSec: The DTS Standard for Connected Diabetes Devices Security. Its objective is to protect patients who use wireless diabetes devices from hacking and other types of cybersecurity incidents [16]. Devices such as those for diabetes can communicate wirelessly with each other, the Cloud, and with patient smartphones. Increasingly, vulnerabilities put these devices at risk for cyberattacks, leading to potential breaches of the CIA Triad. DTSec contains security and assessment requirements for wireless products such as CGMs, wireless insulin pumps, blood glucose monitors, smart insulin pens, and closed-loop systems.

Following development and release of the DTSec standard, DTS developed its second cybersecurity standard: the DTS Mobile Platform Controlling a Diabetes Device Security and Safety Standard (DTMoSt). Like DTSec, this guidance is for clinicians, patients, payers, industry, and regulators. DTMoSt, which expanded upon the principles of DTSec, applies these principles to the use of mobile phones to control actions of implantable and wearable diabetes devices. The goal of DTMoSt is to provide assurance that off-the-shelf consumer mobile phones can safely control diabetes devices. DTMoSt supplies extended packages called advanced basic and extended moderate, which together replace the single assurance package provided by DTSec [17]. This standard is not just important for the cybersecurity of digital diabetes monitoring and treatment devices, these principles of sensible cybersecurity can also apply to other types of monitoring and treatment devices intended for other diseases, as well as for other high criticality devices outside of healthcare.

The Cybersecurity Information Sharing Act of 2015, established by the US Congress, required the formation of the HCIC Task Force to identify challenges and opportunities faced by the health-care industry in protecting and securing itself against cybersecurity incidents [18]. The HCIC was formed in 2016 and was comprised of individuals representing several parts of the health-care ecosystem, including health delivery organizations, technology/security vendors, health information technology vendors, medical device manufacturers, and multiple federal agencies, including Centers for Medicare and Medicaid Services (CMS), FDA, HHS, Department of Homeland Security, Department of Defense, Veterans Administration, and the Public Health Service. The task force's report to Congress included a set of recommendations and action items that focused attention on critical gap areas to address six high-level imperatives. One imperative, in particular, addressed the importance of increasing the security and resilience of medical devices and health IT.

In early 2019 the Healthcare and Public Health Sector Coordinating Council (HSCC), an industry-driven public-private partnership of health-care professionals and companies issued the voluntary Medical Device and Health IT Joint Security Plan (JSP). The JSP is a total product lifecycle reference guide to help vendors and providers develop, deploy, and support cyber-secure technology solutions in healthcare, and responds to a set of recommendations issued by the HHS HCIC Task Force in 2017 [18,19].

The JSP recommendations are designed to be globally applicable and to help organizations regardless of size, stage, or maturity address key cybersecurity challenges and enhance their product cybersecurity posture. Specifically, the JSP provides a framework that aims to help organizations implement a continuous improvement program for developing, deploying, and supporting cyber-secure technology in healthcare. Design controls and requirements, risk management, testing, and postmarket management are not inherent to any specific software development methodology. They can be aligned with the methodology used by individual organizations. Adoption and integration into existing practices should improve product security and quality resulting in more resilient and safer patient care overall [19].

How to safeguard security in a health-care environment

The JSP outlines the framework for the vendor and makes recommendations to the HDO in order to determine whether the framework has been consistently applied by the vendor. There are many security best practices to consider when performing vendor due diligence on health IT systems, medical devices, and applications prior to rollout in the enterprise or utilization by a patient. Securely implementing medical devices and systems is critical. Many organizations still believe that that they are not a target for a cyberattack. However, attacks are often opportunistic and not specifically targeted.

Both NIST and OWASP [20] provide guidance on secure deployment of network-connected medical devices. In addition, OWASP provides guidance on Medical Device Purchasing Assessment Criteria [21] to determine the types of questions that should be asked as part of an HDO's due diligence process prior to device and system purchase.

Questions addressed by the OWASP guidance and criteria include information on network controls, software development lifecycle process and methods, and device controls. Additional guidance provided includes information on perimeter and network defenses, including firewalls, intrusion detection/prevention systems (IDS/IPS), proxy servers and web filters, network segmentation, log monitoring, and vulnerability scanning. Device security control guidance is included on changing default credentials, account lockout, secure transport, baseline and backup of device configurations, data encryption, restricted access to management interfaces, and software update mechanisms. Furthermore, interface and central station security addressing operating system (OS) hardening, encrypted transport, and message security is addressed. Finally, security testing and incident response guidance is included [20].

The NIST Special Publication 1800-8: Securing wireless infusion pumps in HDOs applies "security controls to the pump's ecosystem to create a defense-in-depth solution for protecting infusion pumps and their surrounding systems against various risk factors" [22]. Specifically, this document presents guidelines to secure the wireless pump environment, including information on network segmentation, program and file whitelisting, code-signing, hardening of OSs, and using certificates for encryption and authorization. While this document is intended for infusion pumps, the guidance can be applied to other network-connected medical devices throughout IoMT environments.

Closing

Health-care providers, rightfully, have one main focus in mind: the care of the patient. Evidence dictates that the more complete the information providers possess to make clinical decisions, then the better the outcomes [23]. To achieve this focus, information and data need to be available, correct, and confidential. These concepts represent the CIA Triad's three elements. Sharing of this information between HDOs is at the center of the United States "Meaningful Use" program. While all three are important, when the device is connected to or reporting essential patient information, integrity and availability remain paramount. Data confidentiality must be addressed, but not at the cost of data integrity and availability.

Historically, the network was the domain of the chief information officer (CIO) and the CIO alone. As networks increased in complexity and the value of health-care data became evident, the CISO took responsibility for network and data protection. The CISO differs from the chief security officer who is responsible for the overall risk mitigation and compliance with regulatory guidance (i.e., HIPAA). Often the CISO battles the clinical community to maintain the confidentiality and the integrity of the data while attempting to make the data available only to those that need the data, when they need it. The CISO typically attempts to achieve this by strictly limiting accessibility to the network and ultimately, the EHR. The clinical community often insists that they must have unfettered access to all pertinent data to make the best-informed clinical decisions.

This chapter has presented the need to present diabetes data to the CDS to optimize patient outcomes. Furthermore, resources have been provided for HDO leadership to maximize cybersecurity knowledge required to be an informed partner with manufacturers and vendors of these devices and systems. Organizations can take an active role in the protection of their information infrastructure by requiring manufacturers and vendors to provide an SBOM and ensuring that they align with the recommendations of the JSP and the HCIC Task Force, among others, to solve health-care cybersecurity shortcomings and mitigate gaps in cybersecurity posture, vendors, manufacturers, HDOs, health-care professionals, lawmakers, and regulators must all work together.

References

[1] McCulloch, D.K., 2019. UpToDate. [Online]. Available from: <https://www.uptodate.com/contents/glycemic-control-and-vascular-complications-in-type-2-diabetes-mellitus/> [cited 12.04.19.].

[2] Bailey T, Grunberger G, Bode B, Handelsman Y, Hirsch I, Jovanovic, et al. 2016. American Association of Clinical Endocrinologists and American College of Endocrinology outpatient glucose monitoring consensus statement. Endocr Pract 2016;22:231−61.

[3] Shah, V.N., Garg, S.K., 2015. BioMed Central. [Online]. Available from: <https://clindia-betesendo.biomedcentral.com/articles/10.1186/s40842-015-0016-2> [cited 12.04.19.].

[4] Cortez, A., Hsii, P., Mitchell, E., Riehl, V., Smith, P., 2018. HealthIT.gov. [Online]. Available from: <https://www.healthit.gov/sites/default/files/onc_pghd_final_white_paper.pdf>[cited 12.04.19.].

[5] Health and Human Services, 2013. Federal Regiser. [Online]. Available from: <https://www.federalregister.gov/documents/2013/01/25/2013-01073/modifications-to-the-hipaa-privacy-security-enforcement-and-breach-notification-rules-under-the#h-95> [cited 12.04.19.].

[6] Hernandez S, editor. Official (ISC)2 Guide To The HCISPP CBK. first ed. Boca Raton, FL: CRC Press; 2015.

[7] Beardsley, T., 2016. Rapid7 Blog. [Online]. Available from: <https://blog.rapid7.com/2016/10/04/r7-2016-07-multiple-vulnerabilities-in-animas-onetouch-ping-insulin-pump/> [cited 10.04.19.].

[8] U.S. Food and Drug Administration. Medtronic Recalls Remote Controllers for MiniMed Insulin Pumps for Potential Cybersecurity Risks. Published November 18, 2019. Available at: https://www.fda.gov/medical-devices/medical-device-recalls/medtronic-recalls-remote-controllers-minimed-insulin-pumps-potential-cybersecurity-risks. Accessed March 19, 2020.

[9] Department of Homeland Security (DHS), 2015. [Online]. Available from: <https://www.dhs.gov/sites/default/files/publications/ISC-PPD-21-Implementation-White-Paper-2015-508.pdf> [cited 01.04.19.].

[10] Cenerts for Disease Control and Prevention, 2017. CDC.gov. [Online]. Available from: <https://www.cdc.gov/ehrmeaningfuluse/introduction.html> [cited 14.06.19.].

[11] OWASP, 2016. [Online]. Available from: <https://www.owasp.org/index.php/Security_by_Design_Principles> [cited 11.05.19.].

[12] U.S. Food & Drug Administration, 2016. FDA.gov. [Online]. Available from: <https://www.fda.gov/media/95862/download> [cited 11.05.19.].

[13] U.S. Food and Drug Administration, 2014. FDA.gov. [Online]. Available from: <https://www.fda.gov/media/86174/download> [cited 11.05.19.].

[14] Health Care Industry Cybersecurity Task Force, 2017. Public Health Emergency. [Online]. Available from: <https://www.phe.gov/Preparedness/planning/CyberTF/Documents/report2017.pdf> [cited 10.04.19.].

[15] US-Cert. US-Cert.Gov, 2014. [Online]. Available from: <https://www.us-cert.gov/ncas/alerts/TA14-098A> [cited 10.04.19.].

[16] Diabetes Technology Society, 2016. Diabetes Technology. [Online]. Available from: <https://www.diabetestechnology.org/dtsec-standard-final.pdf> [cited 10.04.19.].

[17] Diabetes Technology Society, 2018. Diabetes Technology. [Online]. Available from: <https://www.diabetestechnology.org/dtmost/DTMoSt%20Guidance.pdf> [cited 10.04.19.].

[18] Healthcare and Public Health Sector, 2017. Healthcare and Public Health Sector. [Online]. Available from: <https://www.phe.gov/Preparedness/planning/CyberTF/Documents/report2017.pdf> [cited 10.04.19.].

[19] OWASP, 2018. Open Web Application Security Project. [Online]. Available from: <https://www.owasp.org/images/9/95/OWASP_Secure_Medical_Devices_Deployment_Standard_7.18.18.pdf> [cited 10.04.19.].

[20] OWASP, 2017. Open Web Application Security Project. [Online]. Available from: <https://www.owasp.org/images/7/73/MedicalDevicePurchasing.pdf> [cited 10.04.19.].

[21] NIST, 2018. NIST Virtual Library. [Online]. Available from: <https://nvlpubs.nist.gov/nistpubs/SpecialPublications/NIST.SP.1800-8.pdf> [cited 20.04.19.].

[22] American Diabetes Association. 6. Glycemic targets: standards of medical care in diabetes—2018. Am Diabetes Assoc Diabetes Care 2018;41(Suppl. 1):55—64.

[23] International Electrotechnical Commission (IEC), 2015. Medical Device Software—Software Life Cycle Process.

Index

Note: Page numbers followed by "*f*" and "*t*" refer to figures and tables, respectively.

Printed in the United States
By Bookmasters